# Innovative Approaches for Difficult-to-Treat Populations

# Innovative Approaches for Difficult-to-Treat Populations

Edited by

**Scott W. Henggeler, Ph.D.**
**Alberto B. Santos, M.D.**

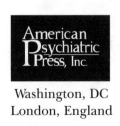

American Psychiatric Press, Inc.

Washington, DC
London, England

**Note:** The authors have worked to ensure that all information in this book concerning drug dosages, schedules, and routes of administration is accurate as of the time of publication and consistent with standards set by the U.S. Food and Drug Administration and the general medical community. As medical research and practice advance, however, therapeutic standards may change. For this reason and because human and mechanical errors sometimes occur, we recommend that readers follow the advice of a physician who is directly involved in their care or the care of a member of their family.

Copyright © 1997 American Psychiatric Press, Inc.
ALL RIGHTS RESERVED
Manufactured in the United States of America on acid-free paper
00  99  98  97      4  3  2  1

American Psychiatric Press, Inc.
1400 K Street, N.W., Washington, DC    20005

**Library of Congress Cataloging-in-Publication Data**

Innovative approaches for difficult-to-treat populations / edited by
   Scott W. Henggeler, Alberto B. Santos.
       p.   cm.
   Includes bibliographical references and index.
   ISBN 0-88048-680-5
   1. Mentally ill—Services for—United States.   Mental health
policy—United States.   I. Henggeler, Scott W., 1950–     .
II. Santos, Alberto B., 1951–     .
   [DNLM: 1. Mental Disorders—therapy.   2. Psychotherapy—trends.
3. Mental Health Services—organization & administration.   WM 420
I584 1997]
RC480.53.I56   1997
362.2′0973—dc20
DNLM/DLC
for Library of Congress                                            96-4744
                                                                        CIP


**British Library Cataloguing in Publication Data**
A CIP record is available from the British Library.

To Jay and Charlie, the T-Ball Kings

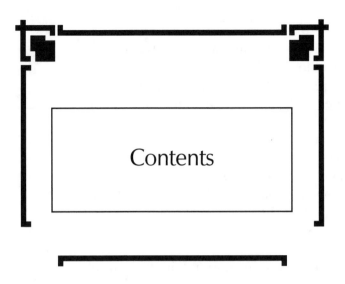

# Contents

## Part I
## Services for Children, Adolescents, and
## Their Families

# Part II
## Approaches for Severely Ill
## Adult Populations

**Part III**
**Policy Issues**

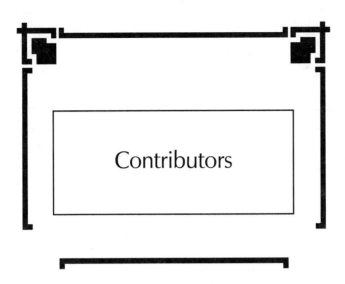

Contributors

George W. Arana, M.D.
Associate Dean for Graduate Medical Education, Medical University of South Carolina, Charleston, South Carolina

Robert J. Battjes, D.S.W.
Deputy Director, Division of Clinical Research, National Institute on Drug Abuse, Rockville, Maryland

Joseph J. Bevilacqua, Ph.D.
State Initiative Director, Bazelon Center for Mental Health Law, Washington, DC

Jack D. Blaine, M.D.
Branch Chief, Treatment Research Branch, Division of Clinical Research, National Institute on Drug Abuse, Rockville, Maryland

Michael Bogrov, M.D.
Assistant Professor, Department of Mental Hygiene and Psychiatry, Johns Hopkins University, Baltimore, Maryland

Roger A. Boothroyd, Ph.D.
Research Scientist, Bureau of Evaluation and Services Research, New York State Office of Mental Health, Albany, New York

J. Donald Bray, M.D.
Visiting Scholar, South Carolina Department of Mental Health, Columbia, South Carolina; Oregon Health Sciences University, Salem, Oregon

Michael J. Brondino, Ph.D.
Instructor, Family Services Research Center, Department of Psychiatry and Behavioral Sciences, Medical University of South Carolina, Charleston, South Carolina

Barbara J. Burns, Ph.D.
Professor of Medical Psychology, Department of Psychiatry, Duke University Medical Center, Durham, North Carolina

Deborah Bybee, Ph.D.
Adjunct Professor, Department of Psychology, Michigan State University, East Lansing, Michigan

Judith A. Cook, Ph.D.
Director, National Research and Training Center on Psychiatric Disability, University of Illinois at Chicago, Chicago, Illinois

Phillippe B. Cunningham, Ph.D.
Instructor, Family Services Research Center, Department of Psychiatry and Behavioral Sciences, Medical University of South Carolina, Charleston, South Carolina

Paul A. Deci, M.D.
Assistant Professor, Department of Psychiatry and Behavioral Sciences, Medical University of South Carolina, Charleston, South Carolina

James K. Dias, Ph.D.
Assistant Professor of Biometry, Medical University of South Carolina, Charleston, South Carolina

Robert E. Drake, M.D., Ph.D.
Director, New Hampshire-Dartmouth Psychiatric Research Center, Lebanon, New Hampshire

Albert J. Duchnowski, Ph.D.
Professor and Deputy Director, Research and Training Center for Children's Mental Health, Florida Mental Health Institute, University of South Florida, Tampa, Florida

Mary E. Evans, Ph.D.
Interim Director, Bureau of Evaluation and Services Research, New York State Office of Mental Health, Albany, New York

Diane Farrell, M.S. (Deceased)
Former Director, Thresholds Loren E. Juhl Young Adult Program, Chicago, Illinois

M. Carolyn Gonzales
President, Resource Systems Design, Isle of Palms, South Carolina

Trevor R. Hadley, Ph.D.
Director, Center for Mental Health Policy and Services Research, Department of Psychiatry, University of Pennsylvania, Philadelphia, Pennsylvania

Nancy M. Halewood, R.N.
Director of Rural Services, Charleston/Dorchester Community Mental Health Center, Charleston, South Carolina

James A. Hall, Ph.D.
Associate Professor of Social Work, School of Social Work, University of Iowa, Iowa City, Iowa

Cindy L. Hanson, Ph.D.
Associate Professor, Department of Psychiatry and Behavioral Sciences, Medical University of South Carolina, Charleston, South Carolina

Susan J. Hardesty, M.D.
Assistant Professor, Department of Psychiatry and Behavioral Sciences, Medical University of South Carolina, Charleston, South Carolina

Scott W. Henggeler, Ph.D.
Professor of Psychiatry and Behavioral Sciences and Director of the Family Services Research Center, Department of Psychiatry and Behavioral Sciences, Medical University of South Carolina, Charleston, South Carolina

Kimberly Hoagwood, Ph.D.
Chief, Child and Adolescent Services Research Program, National Institute of Mental Health, Rockville, Maryland

Michael Hogan, Ph.D.
Director, Ohio Department of Mental Health, Columbus, Ohio

Peter S. Jensen, M.D.
Chief, Child and Adolescent Mental Disorders Research Branch, National Institute of Mental Health, Rockville, Maryland

Jessica A. Jonikas, M.A.
Managing Director and Director of Training, National Research and Training Center on Psychiatric Disability, University of Illinois at Chicago, Chicago, Illinois

Betty King, M.A.
Director of Administration and Operations, The Annie E. Casey Foundation, Baltimore, Maryland

Matthew Koziel, B.A.
Case Manager, Thresholds Loren E. Juhl Young Adult Program, Chicago, Illinois

Krista Kutash, Ph.D.
Assistant Professor and Deputy Director, Research and Training Center for Children's Mental Health, Florida Mental Health Institute, University of South Florida, Tampa, Florida

Kerry R. Lachance, M.A., L.M.S.W.
Program Director, On-Site Program, Charleston/Dorchester Community Mental Health Center, Charleston, South Carolina

Philip J. Leaf, Ph.D.
Professor, Department of Mental Hygiene, School of Hygiene and Public Health, Johns Hopkins University, Baltimore, Maryland

Steven Leff, Ph.D.
Senior Vice President, Human Services Research Institute, Cambridge, Massachusetts

Alan I. Leshner, Ph.D.
Director, National Institute on Drug Abuse, Rockville, Maryland

Gail N. Mattix, M.S.W.
Director, Community Support Services, Lexington County Community Mental Health Center, West Columbia, South Carolina

Cecile B. McAninch, Ph.D.
Assistant Professor, Department of Psychology, Washington State University, Pullman, Washington

Nancy M. McCrohan, Ph.D.
Project Manager, Survey Research Division, Institute for Public Policy and Social Research, Michigan State University, East Lansing, Michigan

Elizabeth C. McDonel, Ph.D.
Outcome and Evaluation Specialist, Tri-County Mental Health Center, Carmel, Indiana

William R. McFarlane, M.D.
Chief, Department of Psychiatry, Maine Medical Center, Portland, Maine

Stephen McLeod-Bryant, M.D.
Assistant Professor, Department of Psychiatry and Behavioral Sciences, Medical University of South Carolina, Charleston, South Carolina

Neil Meisler, M.S.W.
Assistant Professor and Administrative Director of the Division of Public Psychiatry, Department of Psychiatry and Behavioral Sciences, Medical University of South Carolina, Charleston, South Carolina

Gary B. Melton, Ph.D.
Director, Institute for Families in Society, University of South Carolina, Columbia, South Carolina

Judith Meyers, Ph.D.
Consulting Services, Geneva, New York, and Greenwich, Connecticut

John A. Morris, M.S.W.
Interim Director of Mental Health, South Carolina Department of Mental Health, Columbia, South Carolina

Carol T. Mowbray, Ph.D.
Associate Professor, School of Social Work, University of Michigan, Ann Arbor, Michigan

Richard L. Munger, Ph.D.
Associate Professor of Psychiatry, Department of Psychiatry, University of Hawaii School of Medicine, Honolulu, Hawaii

Kristine Nelson, D.S.W.
Professor of Social Work, Graduate School of Social Work, Portland State University, Portland, Oregon

Lisa Simon Onken, Ph.D.
Associate Branch Chief, Treatment Research Branch, Division of Clinical Research, National Institute on Drug Abuse, Rockville, Maryland

Fred C. Osher, M.D.
Associate Professor and Director, Division of Community Psychiatry, School of Medicine, University of Maryland—Baltimore, Baltimore, Maryland

Bernice A. Pescosolido, Ph.D.
Associate Professor and Program Director, Department of Sociology, Indiana University, Evansville, Indiana

Susan G. Pickrel, M.P.H., M.D.
Assistant Professor, Family Services Research Center, Department of Psychiatry and Behavioral Sciences, Medical University of South Carolina, Charleston, South Carolina

Thomas B. Plum, M.S.W.
Director, Community Support Program, Michigan Department of Community Mental Health, Lansing, Michigan

Laura J. Rames, M.D.
Assistant Professor, Department of Psychiatry and Behavioral Sciences, Medical University of South Carolina, Charleston, South Carolina

Frances L. Randolph, D.P.H.
Acting Director, Demonstration and Evaluation Program, Homeless Program Section, Division of Demonstration Programs, Center for Mental Health Services, Substance Abuse and Mental Health Services Administration, Rockville, Maryland

Melisa D. Rowland, M.D.
Assistant Professor, Department of Psychiatry and Behavioral Sciences, Medical University of South Carolina, Charleston, South Carolina

Alberto B. Santos, M.D.
Professor, Director of the Division of Public Psychiatry, and Director of the Psychiatry Residency Training Program, Department of Psychiatry and Behavioral Sciences, Medical University of South Carolina, Charleston, South Carolina

Gretchen E. Schafft, Ph.D., M.H.S.
Applied Anthropologist in Residence, American University, Washington, DC

David G. Scherer, Ph.D.
Assistant Professor of Education, College of Education, University of New Mexico, Albuquerque, New Mexico

Sonja K. Schoenwald, Ph.D.
Assistant Professor of Psychiatry and Behavioral Sciences and Associate Director, Family Services Research Center, Department of Psychiatry and Behavioral Sciences, Medical University of South Carolina, Charleston, South Carolina

Jeanette Semke, Ph.D.
Research Assistant Professor, School of Social Work, University of Washington, Seattle, Washington

Mardi L. Solomon, M.A.
Research Consultant, National Research and Training Center on Psychiatric Disability, University of Illinois at Chicago, Chicago, Illinois

Ralph Warren, Jr., Ph.D.
Senior Research Analyst, Human Services Research Institute, Cambridge, Massachusetts

Mary Bruce Webb, Ph.D.
Research Analyst, Administration on Children, Youth, and Families, U.S. Department of Health and Human Services, Washington, DC

J. Mark Westfall, M.D.
Private Practice, Frank Kay Psychiatric Clinic, Baptist Health Center, Birmingham, Alabama

Eric R. Wright, Ph.D.
Assistant Scientist, Institute for Social Research, Indiana University, Bloomington, Indiana

Joseph J. Zealberg, M.D.
Associate Professor and Director of Mobile Crisis/Emergency Psychiatry Program, Department of Psychiatry and Behavioral Sciences, Medical University of South Carolina, Charleston, South Carolina

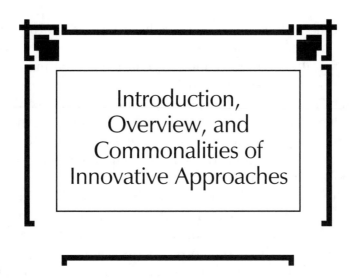

# Introduction, Overview, and Commonalities of Innovative Approaches

**Scott W. Henggeler, Ph.D., and Alberto B. Santos, M.D.**

Current economic trends increasingly call for alternatives to traditional mental health care as both state authorities and private insurers attempt to reduce costs. As the clinical effectiveness and cost-effectiveness of traditional mental health services are examined critically (and often fail the test), opportunities to develop and disseminate innovative models of mental health services are expanding. Yet, regardless of whether services are traditional or innovative, rigorous empirical evaluation is essential to ensure that reform will be meaningful for consumers of mental health services.

The primary purpose of this volume is to suggest directions in the development and dissemination of innovative mental health services, especially for those individuals who consume mental health resources most disproportionately and for whom traditional services have little established effectiveness. Such individuals include youth with serious behavioral and emotional disturbances and adults with severe and persistent mental illness.

Throughout the volume, authors have focused on those treatments and services that have been evaluated empirically. As such, the clinical effectiveness and cost-effectiveness of many of the innovative services featured in this volume have been documented in controlled clinical trials. The effectiveness of others has been supported in quasi-experimental studies and in uncontrolled program evaluations. These empirically tested approaches provide a solid scientific foundation for continued mental health service reform.

Although the innovative approaches reviewed in this volume include diverse treatment methods and although they target varied clinical populations, a qualitative assessment suggests that the approaches share common elements. Commonalities include social-ecological theoretical frameworks; emphases on delivering flexible, comprehensive, pragmatic, and goal-oriented interventions in the persons' natural environments; and increased accountability of service providers. Commonalities are presented more extensively at the conclusion of this chapter, and the implications of such service characteristics for mental health policy are discussed throughout the volume.

Next, brief backgrounds and overviews of the major sections of this volume are presented.

## Mental Health Services for Children, Adolescents, and Their Families

Public sector policy makers, private foundations, and leading academics agree that current systems of mental health care are not meeting the mental health needs of children and adolescents, and may, at tremendous human and financial cost, be doing more harm than good. Some examples are given below.

- The need for services far outweighs availability.
- A grossly disproportionate percentage of mental health dollars is allocated to restrictive and expensive services with no demonstrated effectiveness.

- Communities usually have a limited selection of available programs, which increases the likelihood that children will receive inappropriate services (e.g., overly restrictive services).
- Services often lack cultural competence and blame families rather than supporting them.
- Programs are often categorical, whereas children and families frequently have multiple problems requiring comprehensive services.
- Service systems are highly fragmented, lacking in collaboration and coordination.

Proposed solutions to these problems have tended to target changes in the service systems and in the types of mental health services provided to children and adolescents. Recent attempts at systems-level change have been largely based on the system-of-care principles articulated in 1986 by Stroul and Friedman. Such changes have emphasized reduced use of restrictive services, increased services integration, increased interagency collaboration, reform of mechanisms for financing services, increased use of services that are flexible, comprehensive, and individualized, and increased use of approaches that empower families. In general, demonstration projects such as the Ft. Bragg Demonstration Project and the Ventura County Project and its replications have supported the capacity of the mental health system to change in ways compatible with the system-of-care principles.

On the other hand, it remains to be determined whether reforms in the mental health services provided to children and adolescents will translate to improved psychosocial functioning in youth and families receiving services. Indeed, several research literatures suggest that improving the clinical outcomes for youth with serious emotional disturbance will present a formidable task. Although the child psychotherapies have proven moderately successful in studies conducted in university settings, such success has not transferred to community-based settings. Treatments of serious antisocial behavior have shown minimal long-term effects, and no evidence supports the relative efficacy of any treatment of adolescent substance abuse. Likewise, the effectiveness of innovative services (e.g., family preservation) has often been disappointing when evaluated empirically, and many such services have received little evaluation.

A central purpose of this volume is to address the clinical-effectiveness void in the field of research on mental health services concerning children and adolescents. Specifically, the void pertains to the development and validation of effective interventions for youth presenting serious clinical problems. As such, chapter authors have addressed critical areas of clinical research and have suggested directions that appear most promising.

Richard Munger's persuasive review (Chapter 1) describes the behavioral and emotional problems of youth as being fundamentally multidetermined and ecological in nature, thus requiring interventions that directly address key ecological factors in their natural environments. Mary Evans and Roger Boothroyd (Chapter 2) describe viable family-based alternatives to the restrictive and costly practice of hospitalizing youth who are experiencing a mental health crisis; they also describe plans for evaluating the effectiveness of such alternatives. Krista Kutash, Albert Duchnowski, Judith Meyers, and Betty King (Chapter 3) provide a concise overview of the major federal, state, and private foundation initiatives concerning the reform of mental health services for youth, and provide a cogent rationale for the development of neighborhood-based services.

Sonja Schoenwald, David Scherer, and Michael Brondino (Chapter 4) account for the failure of most existing treatments of serious antisocial behavior, and argue for interventions that directly address the multiple causes of serious antisocial behavior in the youth's natural surroundings. Kristine Nelson (Chapter 5) notes the multidetermined nature of child neglect, and describes family-based intervention approaches that intervene directly with those factors contributing to child maltreatment. Susan Pickrel, James Hall, and Phillippe Cunningham (Chapter 6) argue that emerging approaches to the treatment of adolescent substance abuse should be reconfigured so that less emphasis is placed on individual pathology and more emphasis is placed on systems change. Philip Leaf, Michael Bogrov, and Mary Bruce Webb (Chapter 7) provide an overview of the East Baltimore Mental Health Partnership, which is an exciting federally funded project to reshape and coordinate children's mental health services in a select inner-city community.

Whereas Chapters 1–7 examine important clinical issues in the development of effective mental health services for children and adolescents, Chapter 18 and Chapters 23–25 in the Policy Section of this volume address issues that pertain to the field in its entirety.

Gary Melton (Chapter 18) examines why the types of innovative, cost-effective, and clinically effective services discussed in this volume are rarely adopted by policy makers. Cindy Hanson (Chapter 23) makes a compelling case for the importance of advocating social policies that promote the physical, mental, and social well-being of all individuals. Kimberly Hoagwood, Peter Jensen, and Alan Leshner (Chapter 24) denote the distinctive ethical issues in conducting research on children's mental health, especially applied research that can immediately inform state and local policies. Lisa Onken, Jack Blaine, and Robert Battjes (Chapter 25), focusing on the National Institute on Drug Abuse Behavioral Therapies Development Program, provide an excellent overview of the process needed to translate effective university-based and laboratory-based treatments to real-world community settings.

## Innovative Approaches for Adult Populations

The chapters that address complex adult populations center primarily on initiatives for adults with severe and persistent mental illness (SPMI). The care of this population has historically been, and continues to be, one of society's greatest challenges. Adults with SPMI, a majority of whom suffer from schizophrenic, schizoaffective, or bipolar affective disorders, consume a significant portion of health care costs and other social resources. Aggressive behavior and other disruptive activities of persons with SPMI often result in the involvement of law enforcement and judicial systems. Residual symptoms associated with more stable phases of illness include impoverished cognitive capacities and resultant social and occupational disability. Although recent advances in psychopharmacology hold promise for improved treatment, more effective systems of psychosocial interventions are also needed to facilitate community living.

Since the federal government entered the arena of reform of the public mental health system in the 1960s, there has been a slow but steady transition from centralized care to local care in many states. This volume highlights the work of many individuals who have contributed to the transition to community-based care. For the past decade, case management has been promoted as a means to assist persons with SPMI to live in the community, by linking them to needed human services and monitoring the provision of services to ensure that identified needs are met. However, although such case management functions are important, they often do not address the needs of many persons with SPMI who neither adhere to medication regimens nor attend prescribed psychosocial programs. Even persons with SPMI who comply with treatment often experience chaos on a daily basis because of their susceptibility to ordinary stress, their tendency to distort and misinterpret communication, and so on. These persons often feel hopeless, abuse substances, and experience extreme poverty and/or homelessness. Such factors can make it very difficult for persons with SPMI to interact with complex human service systems, because these persons often require direct assistance with virtually all areas of their life. Case management for persons with SPMI, therefore, must transcend its traditional linking function.

One innovative case management system, which is featured in this volume, has gained considerable popularity among providers and policy makers. Prompted by a recognition of the complexities of treating persons with SPMI and the frustration of the revolving-door phenomenon, a group of mental health professionals (including Mary Ann Test and Len Stein) conceptualized and developed a service delivery system in which a team of clinicians provides patients with flexible, long-term, and intensive care in their natural surroundings. This approach, usually referred to as Training in Community Living (TCL) or Assertive Community Treatment (ACT), allows for the application of pharmacological treatment within an intensive field-based service system; the generalist team of providers is continuously available to monitor and support mentally disabled adults living independently in their communities. In effect, the mental health professionals transposed the work site of a hospital treatment team from the inpatient setting to the community field to address patients' multiple and complex needs in a pragmatic, flexible, and comprehensive manner. Over 35 states currently have such teams in operation. The approach is the only full-service program for persons with SPMI that has been tested in multiple clinical trials. This rich empirical base is now serving as a common scientific foundation for innovations to address special populations and variations in clinical and social problems.

Four of the chapters in this volume (Chapters 9–12) build on the original contributions of Test and Stein and the subsequent worldwide dissemination efforts of Deborah Allness and William Knoedler. Chapter 9 by Neil Meisler describes the early history, clinical principles, and research findings of TCL/ACT. Chapter 10 by Robert Drake and Fred Osher describes the successful integration of substance abuse treatment into the TCL/ACT service system for the care of adults with SPMI who use and abuse substances. Chapter 11 by Bill McFarlane discusses the role of families in the treatment and rehabilitation of adults with SPMI. It features the family psychoeducation intervention and the innovative multiple family psychoeducation context, and presents benefits of the model when integrated into the work of TCL/ACT teams. Finally, the chapter by Kerry Lachance, Paul Deci, Alberto Santos, Nancy Halewood, and Mark Westfall (Chapter 12) describes the adaptation of the TCL/ACT principles for use in rural settings.

In addition, other less rigorously tested approaches to helping individuals with SPMI or acute psychiatric problems maintain community tenure are discussed. Chapter 13 by Paul Deci and Gail Mattix describes a widely disseminated approach to improving community tenure in adults with SPMI: Homeshare, a foster-placement program for adults. Chapters 14 and 15 present innovative approaches to the delivery of acute care services. Joseph Zealberg, Susan Hardesty, Neil Meisler, and Alberto Santos (Chapter 14) describe in detail the operation of a mobile emergency psychiatry service, and Stephen McLeod-Bryant, George Arana, Laura Rames, and Alberto Santos (Chapter 15) illustrate the efficient use of community-based psychiatric hospital beds for acutely ill patients. Chapter 16 by Melisa Rowland, Barbara Burns, Gretchen Schafft, Frances Randolph, and Cecile McAninch provides an overview of state-of-the-art services to elderly populations, including the currently NIMH-funded services demonstration project with this population.

There is little doubt that the ultimate success of community support programs lies in their ability to normalize a patient's daily routine. Arguably, a patient served by the most modern of community support systems is not likely to reach full community integration without gainful employment. The challenge of entering the competitive workforce is especially difficult for patients whose disabilities interfere significantly with their capacity to remain task-oriented, or to discriminate social cues, so often important in competing for employment. Given the importance of employment as an outcome for a service system, we have devoted two chapters to this challenging issue. Judith Cook, Mardi Solomon, Diane Farrell, Matthew Koziel, and Jessica Jonikas (Chapter 8) describe their efforts at helping young adults to achieve community-based employment; Carol Mowbray, Steven Leff, Ralph Warren, Nancy McCrohan, and Deborah Bybee (Chapter 17) discuss innovative methods for promoting the vocational functioning of persons with psychiatric disabilities.

The final section (Chapters 19–22) addresses statewide perspectives on mental health systems for adults. Chapter 19 by Paul Deci, Elizabeth McDonel, Jeanette Semke, Trevor Hadley, Michael Hogan, James Dias, Bernice Pescosolido, and Eric Wright describes several statewide (South Carolina, Indiana, and Washington) efforts at downsizing their centralized, long-term bed census. Chapter 20 by Neil Meisler and Caroline Gonzales and Chapter 21 by Tom Plum describe statewide efforts (Michigan, Delaware, Rhode Island, Wisconsin, and South Carolina) at disseminating and financing innovative mental health services. In Chapter 22, Joseph Bevilacqua, John Morris, and J. Donald Bray describe their strategies for reforming a state mental health care system.

## Commonalities of Innovative Approaches, and Conclusion

The treatment systems discussed in this volume share common elements, which, interestingly, arose through independent lines of investigation with populations of different ages and clinical problems, as explained below.

- The treatment and service approaches assume a social-ecological model of behavior. That is, the approaches maintain that a person's capacity to function in the community is inexorably linked with his or her biological, psychological, and social characteristics and key elements in the environment, such as family, work and school, health care, and neighborhood.
- Interventions are delivered in the patient's natural environment. Such delivery of services addresses the many difficulties associated with care provided in artificial environments (e.g., hospital, residential treatment facility), which have little bearing on the individual's functioning in the real world. Such difficulties include high rates of missed appointments for outpatient services, inaccurate assessment of problems due to limited knowledge about the individual's ecology, and poor generalization of treatment effects from clinic and institutional settings to the community.
- The treatment approaches are pragmatic, with an emphasis on action-oriented and well-specified interventions.

- Clinical outcomes are often monitored continuously to allow rapid feedback regarding the viability of interventions and to assess the possible need to alter or refine treatment plans.
- Therapeutic goals are highly individualized and services are comprehensive and flexible. Essentially, staff are encouraged to do whatever it takes to attain treatment goals that are tailored to the particular strengths and weaknesses of each person and his or her social context.
- Finally, clinicians are held accountable for therapeutic outcomes. Thus, rather than blaming the patient for lack of progress, staff are encouraged to seek creative solutions to intervene successfully with patients.

In addition to the common clinical and services themes of the innovative treatment approaches discussed in this volume, similar barriers exist to the implementation and dissemination of these approaches.

- A major barrier to the acceptance of innovative models of mental health services has been their challenge to the high profit margins of standard institution-based services. Yet, with upcoming health care reform, the pressure to reduce cost will encourage the dissemination of effective home- and community-based services.
- Another barrier has been that these nontraditional community-based services have not been reimbursed through traditional funding sources. However, with the new rehabilitation option under Medicaid, which has not historically paid for in vivo or off-site treatment, initiatives to fund home- and community-based services have developed.
- A third barrier pertains to the fundamental nature of many of these interventions, which challenge the traditions of office-based practitioners who typically specialize in specific approaches (e.g., individual, family, or group therapies) or target specific contributors to maladaptive behavior (e.g., cognitions, family relations, the past). Training programs for mental health professionals will need substantive revision to

provide skilled clinicians in the delivery of such innovative treatment approaches.

In conclusion, and as echoed throughout this volume, authors advocate the development, validation, and dissemination of mental health services that are individualized and comprehensive, and that intervene directly in the individual's environments. In contrast with traditional mental health systems, such services can realistically address the multiple and interrelated difficulties experienced by youth with serious emotional and behavioral problems and adults with SPMI.

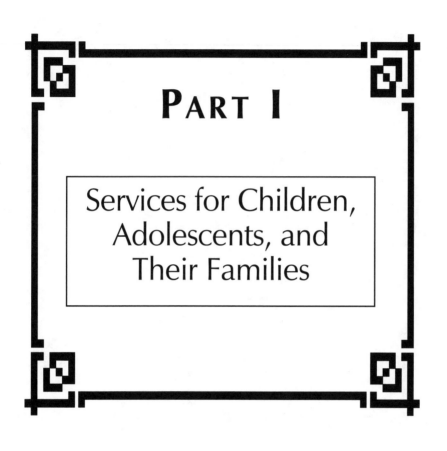

# PART I

## Services for Children, Adolescents, and Their Families

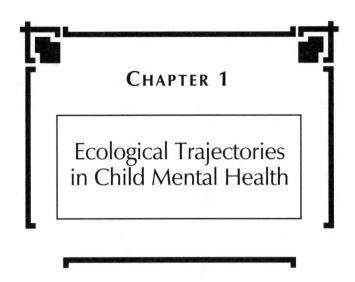

# CHAPTER 1

## Ecological Trajectories in Child Mental Health

**Richard L. Munger, Ph.D.**

In the early 1960s, Americans huddled around television sets to watch the first space flights return to earth. Reporter Walter Cronkite described the tense moments of reentry when the space capsule had to penetrate the earth's atmosphere at the precise trajectory or, if its path veered only slightly, face fiery destruction. The critical path, or trajectory, meant putting the capsule on a course with the proper angle for the crucial dynamics of flight to unfold a corridor of safety.

Just as a space capsule must maneuver through the invisible forces of space, children must navigate their own life spaces or ecosystems. They, too, create their own pathways, some that spin off into positive opportunities, and others that lead to failure and negative outcomes. Finding the proper pathways—that is, trajectories—for children to move through their life spaces might be just as important as finding those trajectories for a space capsule, especially for youths with serious emotional disturbances (SED).

This chapter presents a new strategy for dealing with emotional disturbances in children: the ecological method. The ecological viewpoint challenges the traditional, individualistic, "inner treatment" philosophy in mental health and advocates helping the child with emotional disturbance by making changes in the outer, or ecological, factors that influence behavior. The key in the ecological viewpoint becomes identifying and enabling critical environmental trajectories in the child's life.

The treatment methods ordinarily used in the field of child mental health concentrate on the internal physiological and psychological factors that influence a child's behavior. The principal factors are considered to be the thoughts, feelings, self-concepts, and ego strengths of the child, along with a host of other traits and dispositions. It is usually assumed that when these are treated, the problem will be solved.

It is true that some traditional theories do consider outer factors, from parents and family life to race relations and neighborhood conditions, but this is mainly for the sake of interpretation and diagnosis. Treatment remains highly individualistic. Even those who work with families, and who should, therefore, understand the importance of systems extending beyond the individual, rarely look into environmental factors beyond the child's relatives. The danger in looking only as far as relatives is that the troubled family can easily replace the troubled individual as the focus of attention, with no wider social investigation deemed necessary.

"Ecology" has become a popular word in recent years. Originally its meaning was associated mainly with the natural environment and the threat from pollution. Consider the analogy between this familiar biological concept and ecological intervention in mental health. There are many cases in which corruption of an ecosystem has had a devastating effect on the wildlife within the system. If waters become polluted, fish often die. If smog settles over a forest for a lengthy period, birds can die. It follows logically that a difficult environment can have a deleterious effect on children, who may well flourish in a better, more supportive environment.

The knowledge base of ecological practice is interdisciplinary.

Ecological viewpoints have emerged from such diverse fields as clinical sociology, cultural and social anthropology, environmental psychology, ecological psychology, social work, community psychology, public health, ethology, and biological ecology. The ecological model has antecedents extending back thousands of years, but ecological theory can be summed up in a few words: the environment governs to a large degree the behavior that takes place within it; therefore, changing the environment will often change behavior.

For child clinicians who are willing to change their approaches and add one more theory to those they are already using, the ecological method has much to offer. Child clinicians who learn ecological techniques will find that these techniques are flexible enough to let them master new areas of diagnosis and treatment. The techniques will reveal why a child's environment—whether at home, at school, in the town swimming pool, or anywhere else—is a critical factor in effective treatment. The clinician will see how people the child knows can be drawn into the healing process.

This chapter describes the present status of the ecological therapist in the therapeutic universe. Before beginning, a note of clarification about terminology is in order: the use of the terms *systems* and *ecology* by mental health professionals has resulted in some confusion about differences in their meanings. To "think systems" is to concentrate on relatedness rather than on the basic nature of separate entities (Hartman 1979). For example, much of the literature on family therapy emphasizes systems theory and the significance of interactions, communications, and patterns of relationships. Family therapists, however, tend to focus their efforts exclusively on the family, overlooking both individual personality systems that extend beyond the family and the environmental context of the family life (Mannino and Shore 1984). So, although a systems model is closely connected to ecological approaches in mental health, "thinking systems" and "thinking ecology" are not comparable.

Mannino and Shore (1984) have succinctly characterized the use of the term *ecology*:

The term ecology is broader and includes the concept of system; on the other hand, the concept of system does not necessarily include the concept of ecology. For example, from a system's perspective, one can view the family as a group of individuals interacting within the context of the family. Here, an individual's problem is seen as related to a position of functioning in the family relationship system. An ecological perspective broadens the context to include other relationship systems beyond the family, for example, school, workplace, hospital. Here, an individual's problem may not be restricted to the family context, but may extend to other physical and social contexts within which he or she interacts. Moreover, the ecological perspective forces one to deal with the real problems of social living by emphasizing the environmental context in which one performs roles and creates and interacts with institutions in order to obtain such basic life necessities as food, clothing, medical care, and housing. (p. 75)

## Resistance to Therapeutic Change and Ecology

Ecologists contend that changing the environment is important, sometimes even decisive, in treating clients (Krasner 1980). Therefore, ecological intervention ought to be a major technique to which clinicians can resort when confronting cases not amenable to other techniques. Because the main point in the ecological approach to mental health is to change the environment, rather than the person apart from the environment, professionals can manipulate important variables hitherto ignored, extend their treatment into new areas, and provide assistance to segments of the population never, or only inadequately, served before.

Intervention with children can differ substantially from intervention with adults because the environment is so much more influential on children's behavior. Children are, for the most part, confined within environments that dominate them and over which they have little control. In fact, it has been suggested that the level of ecological intervention needed may be, in part, a function of the level of the child's disturbance. That is, the more troubled the child is and the more pathological the environment is, the greater the need for environmental changes (Schulman 1979).Obviously, the problems of children with SED cannot be properly understood and effectively dealt with if the ecological elements are deemphasized, or worse yet, left out altogether. Henggeler and Borduin (1990), in fact, have argued that the primary reason for historically poor results of treatments with children could be that the interventions used in the studies have almost always addressed only a small portion of the factors that might contribute to a youth's disturbed behavior.

Two groups of children—those from low-income, crisis-prone, multiproblem families and those with a history of removal from the home for institutional treatment—present particular challenges to existing treatment methods. Many of our mental health programs for these children fail. Ecological methods offer hope for preventing many of these failures, as reviewed below.

## Children in Low-Income, Crisis-Prone, Multiproblem Families

Kraft and DeMaio (1982) were among the first to acknowledge that behavioral problems of youths in low-income families could be viewed as disruptions in the social system rather than as isolated personal or family problems. This interpretation, a classic ecological perspective, contends that the maladaptive behavior of youths in such situations is merely a symptom of a much broader-based disorder. The ultimate ecological problem is the family's poor connection with the network of resources provided by the community and society at large. Kraft and DeMaio (1982) note, "To focus on uncovering sensitive, anxiety-laden feelings without providing a payoff increasing the availability of resources could merely inflate expectations, remove a functioning defensive system, and result in even greater anxiety or more drastic coping mechanisms" (p. 133).

The typical family described above is so overwhelmed with problems that the members often cannot benefit from weekly visits to a clinic or an agency. They often lack both a phone to make appointments and a means of transportation to get to the office. For those who do manage to make it to a clinic, the clinical techniques of interview and advice frequently make them feel uncomfortable, sometimes frightened. Moreover, they rarely approach clinicians of their own free will; they are usually forced into treatment by somebody else. This causes them to feel that they are being controlled from the outside, victimized by the process, and threatened by the authorities.

The ineffectiveness of typical approaches to counseling often causes public services to cease referring these families to clinicians or agencies that would expect them to keep office appointments. As a result, whole families become virtually nonexistent to local mental health agencies, although they remain only too well-known to teachers, police officers, judges, and other officials who have to deal with their antisocial behavior. Intervention must improve family life by giving these families environmental supports, letting them see how these supports can diminish their periodic crises, and prompting them to take control of their lives. Outreach programs to families must stress that the solution for any family is to find its place (good fit) within the overall community environment (Clark et al. 1982).

## Children in Institutional Treatment

Children with long histories of multiple placements in institutions have some of the most difficult problems to treat. Institutionalization—removing children from mainstream society and confining them in reform schools, psychiatric hospitals, and residential treatment centers—has been one of the most widely used forms of intervention. This practice is based on the individualistic theory that such children can be led or coerced into modifying their behaviors, that their personalities can be changed more or less permanently, and that they can function adequately upon returning to their old environment or being placed in a new one. To accomplish these tasks, institutions commonly employ psychotherapeutic techniques, educational programs, drugs, or all three.

It is axiomatic, however, that children grow and learn to be human beings through their interactions in families, schools, neighborhoods, and the broader community. The notion that you can remove a child from these settings to an institutional environment for the treatment of an emotional or psychological problem is reminiscent of a predominant practice of a century ago, which was to send mentally ill people to remote hospitals in the countryside as a refuge from the tribulations of daily life. Contrary to this practice, children must be helped in the most normalized environment possible. Therapeutic supports must be put in place around children in their everyday environments so that they can learn to function as they ordinarily would, in homes and classrooms and other environs. There is absolutely no empirical evidence that institutional treatment is effective (Saxe et al. 1988); its perpetuation appears more related to the convenience it provides professionals and the comfort it brings a public offended and frightened by aberrant behavior.

Consignment to an institution should be carefully examined with this in mind, for institutionalization, more than anything, removes the child from relationships and supports conducive to mental health (Swenson 1979). Community-based treatment allows for community involvement and for changes in environmental conditions that have an adverse effect on children's mental health. Lasting changes in children's behavior demand an understanding and manipulation of environmental factors; without ecological intervention, any changes are likely to be only temporary (Bechtel 1984).

To summarize, the environmental dimension of many mental health problems renders them resistant to traditional psychological techniques. The difficulties of children with serious emotional problems in low-income, crisis-prone, multiproblem families and in institutions, reveal quite clearly the nature of the dilemma. The proper approach for the clinician is often the development of concrete, practical, environmental supports. Helping the families of these children improve their environments is essential for effective intervention on their behalf (Mannino and Shore 1984). Table 1–1 contrasts the ecological model with the

**Table 1–1.**  Ecological model contrasted with traditional psychological model

| Factor | Ecological model | Psychological model |
|---|---|---|
| Etiology of mental disorder | Lack of fit with environment | Intrapsychic and familial conflict |
| Location of intervention | Community | Office; institutional setting |
| Level of intervention | Throughout the ecosystem | Individual level; some family level |
| Types of services delivered | Emphasizes consultation with participants in child's environment | Emphasizes therapeutic services within medical model |
| Methods of intervention | Emphasizes indirect services | Emphasizes direct clinical services |
| Strategies of service | Emphasizes strategies aimed at modifying relationship with environment | Emphasizes psychotherapy |
| Kind of planning | Planning focus is closely coordinated with existing services | Unplanned; no overall coordination |
| Who is the change agent? | Collaboration of a full range of community professionals and natural helpers | Traditional mental health professionals |
| Type of planning, locus of decision | Decision making is a joint responsibility of community agents | Mental health professionals maintain control over decision making |

traditional psychological mental health model.

Ecology in mental health is a naturally optimistic idea. By studying environmental factors as causes of behavior, clinical ecologists have opened up new avenues for helping children with serious emotional problems.

# Domains of the Environment

The goals and methods of mental health ecologists can be likened to those of zookeepers, in the sense that the most successful zookeepers build the optimum environments for the animals in their care. Wild animals live and flourish in captivity best when their environments approximate the natural surroundings from which they come. For instance, animals that naturally live on the plains are more healthy and contented when they are let out of their cages and placed in open areas where they can roam at will.

Mental health professionals, it is argued, should be at least as interested in finding the optimum environments for the human beings they are trying to help. What kind of environment is supportive for people? It should allow individuals to accomplish the most critical tasks in their lives; achieve a satisfactory threshold of enjoyable, fulfilling experiences on a regular basis; and avoid undue strain (Lee 1985).

Ironically, although zookeepers are aware of the necessity of making the environment fit the animal, mental health professionals frequently try to make the human being fit the environment. They think that if only they can change the "animal" in suitable ways, everything will be fine. They do not recognize that they are often wasting their time and also are often creating situations that are worse for those involved. For successful mental health intervention, the environment must be viewed as a factor in individual behavior, a factor that can be adjusted and molded to help effect a better person-environment fit.

A critical concept in the ecological viewpoint is that individuals and environments are neither good nor bad. The terms *congruence* and *incongruence* are more useful in referring to how well or how poorly individuals and environments fit. But when one speaks of environmental forces impinging on the individual, what comprises the environment? Generally, the environment is defined by its three components: physical, social, and institutional (Conyne and Clark 1981). Each dimension is briefly discussed below.

## Physical Environment

The physical environment is made up of both natural (geography, weather, animal life, etc.) and manufactured (buildings, streets, telephone poles, etc.) elements—that is, objective things to which people respond as they experience them by way of the five senses (Wohlwill 1981). As an example of how one particular element in the physical environment affects people, it has been shown that parents in crowded homes are more severe than others in punishing their children for misbehavior. Also, there appears to be a correlation between home discipline and school conduct, and specifically between crowded homes and aggression in class or on the playground (Martin 1975).

## Social Environment

This aspect of the total environment is made up of other people or groups of people. The relationships within social environments vary tremendously, from the intimacy between child and parent to the formality of banker and client. For example, the size of a school population is a factor in children's behavior. Smaller schools are preferable to schools with large student populations, as Barker and Gump (1964) demonstrated. Good students do especially well in small schools, but even marginal students profit from such institutions, partly because small schools encourage participation in school life to a greater degree than large schools.

## Institutional Environment

This last subcategory of environment is made up of such things as legal systems, cultural norms, and the rules and regulations of society. Driving on the right-hand side of the street, remaining silent in the library, paying taxes before the government's deadline, practicing agreed-upon civilities in public—all these, and dozens more, fall under the heading of institutional environment. It focuses on the relationship between individuals or groups and nonpersonal controls. People need nonpersonal controls in order to be fully human and socially well adjusted. Personality develops in a healthy way only within an elaborate value system, in which individuals know what to expect of others and what others expect of them, and in which interaction produces stable social life (Glassner and Freedman 1979).

All the environmental elements, or physical, social, and institutional settings, are involved in ecological intervention, so a clinician must consider each when moving from the isolation of the consulting room into the world of the ecosystem. Factors in all of them may have to be modified, directly or indirectly, before an intervention is successful. Any or all of these types of settings can be selected, changed, or created by the interventionist (Price 1979). Setting selection is the process whereby the clinician or the child, or both, look at the child's environment and then select existing settings the child should try in the future because they promise to be helpful. Setting change is a strategy that involves looking into an existing setting to see the extent to which it is beneficial and the extent to which it should be changed to be made more congruent with the child. The settings subject to change may be familial, educational, recreational, or social; indeed, any setting of significance in the child's environment. Setting creation means analyzing an environmental setting, perceiving where the difficulties lie, and establishing a new setting that will function as a positive influence. The new setting will provide the child with resources that were lacking or insufficient in the old setting.

A clinician must identify the variables in the environment that affect the child's conduct. Settings must be defined that will spur the child toward the specific changes desired. Finally, decisions must be made about selecting, changing, and creating settings to address the child's behavior.

## Ecological Assessment and Diagnosis

Gump (1984) reports an experience in the assessment of a young woman outpatient that helped him realize more clearly how the approaches and findings of ecological psychology are relevant to clinical practice. A young woman was assessed by clinicians from a number of different orientations, with each clinician using a particular method: psychiatric interview, Rorschach test, thematic apperception test, and so on. Gump's method was to learn about the woman's behavior over a weekend. He wanted to discover not her personal traits but her activities, which she described to him in detail. Moos (1976) has referred to this assessment of an individual's "ecological niche" as an Environmental Status Exam. When all the evidence of all the assessments was in, Gump realized that the woman's behavior could be explained in a much more satisfactory manner with his form of ecological assessment added to the traditional techniques than with those techniques alone forming the basis of the assessment. Gump puts it well in suggesting that it is not the individual who is "sick" so much as it is his or her lifestyle.

The ecological orientation avoids classic forms of diagnosis. To say that a child is disturbed, or that a child has a disorder, puts the disturbance within the domain of the individual. Saxe et al. (1988) note that traditional diagnoses ignore the essential environmental covariants of children's mental health disorders. What is needed is a way of thinking about and classifying disturbance by locating it within the ecosystem. Hobbs (1975) has proposed such a scheme, which emphasizes the ecological changes that would diminish or eliminate the disturbance. Diagnosis is unambiguous and intuitive. Quite simply, children are not classified according to familiar categories, such as DSM-IV (American Psychiatric Association 1994), but rather according to the services required to obtain some reasonable level of adjustment. Therefore, the child-in-setting, not the individual child, is the unit of classification. Hobbs calls this an ecologically oriented, service-based system for the classification of children, the main element of which is the ecological assessment and enablement plan.

The purpose of the ecological assessment and enablement plan is to organize systematically every step that is necessary to modify the ecosystem so it functions satisfactorily. After identifying what needs to be done, principal ecosystem members meet to delineate, for each step, who will be responsible for getting the task done, who will actually provide the service, if a service is required, by what date the service will be completed or the goal achieved, what, if anything, the service will cost, where the money will come from, what criterion or criteria will be used to determine whether objectives have been met, and what follow-up steps might be required.

# Environmental Intervention

Some of the key theoretical concepts that are brought to bear on clinical ecological intervention are reviewed below.

## Natural Therapy System

Most of the time, children remain in dynamic equilibrium with their surrounding environment and its demands, supported by family, friends, teachers, neighbors, and others. When a child manifests a problem for which professional help is sought, it is assumed that this natural therapy system in the child's life space has reached an impasse (Becvar et al. 1982). When a problem is brought to the community caregiving agency, the child is only a part of a larger network. Sometimes clinicians erroneously assume that they have greater curative skills than exist in the natural therapy system. Such an attitude can work against the possibilities of the natural structures in the child's life, resulting in more stress and turmoil. Ideally, the clinician need not intervene with therapy but need only serve as consultant to the larger natural systems in the child's life in order to overcome the impasse and allow the natural therapy elements to again support the child. Because ecosystems are usually self-restoring, clinicians should avoid doing anything that interferes with this restorative power.

It goes without saying that a mental health professional attempting to help a child must first build a trusting relationship with that child. However, such a relationship can cause more harm than good in the long run. The development of strong bonds between a professional caregiver and a child can disrupt the natural resources in the environment. For example, Fitzgerald and Illback (1993) found that, as a result of intensive in-home services, over time there is less support from informal helpers (e.g., friends, neighbors, extended family), possibly leaving the individual more vulnerable as the intervention program is gradually withdrawn.

Intensive individual therapy naturally creates an intimacy between therapist and child. This intimacy violates the child's ecology and disrupts the child's relationships with natural contextual resources in a careless fashion that is not facilitative of those natural resources. Too often, therapists either consciously or unconsciously substitute themselves for vital linkages in the child's daily world (Combrinck-Graham 1990). In many cases, mental health professionals would do well to relinquish their roles as omnipotent experts upon whom therapeutic success solely depends. Implementing a treatment strategy that acknowledges and involves the natural helping systems in the child's environment is really the logical thing to do. There is no doubt that certain child behavior problems require the expertise and experience that only a child therapist can provide. It is equally true that some people who are integral components of the child's everyday environment have unique knowledge of the child, knowledge that qualifies them to be useful participants in the child's therapy. An effective clinical ecologist serves less as a therapist than as a consultant who orchestrates the relationships among the many domains of a child's life, all of which contribute to solving the child's problems (Combrinck-Graham 1990).

## Interconnectedness

The "web of life" was Charles Darwin's phrase for complex interrelationships among organisms and habitats (environments). Darwin saw the web of life as analogous to a spider's web: touching one strand causes the whole structure to shake. This concept is fundamental to all ecological investigations (Catalano 1979).

An interdependent behavior-environment system means,

quite simply, that everything is connected to everything else; everything is part of the web of life. When any component of the system is altered through some intervention, changes are likely to occur elsewhere in the system. On the positive side, this means that improvement in any part of the system can benefit the entire system. Because all elements of the system affect one another, it is possible to intervene in one area and to see results in another. Consequently, the way to help a child is not necessarily to focus on him or her; it might be more productive to direct efforts to another part of the child's system. On the negative side, this interconnectedness also means that a clinician should not intervene unthinkingly in any environment. To do so could produce an effect similar to the proverbial bull in a china shop, disrupting the child's helpful human relationships and shaking the social support system (Gottlieb 1981).

## Behavior Settings

People are just one component of the larger behavior-setting system, a system of environments that prompt (sometimes require) certain activities and discourage or short-circuit others. A behavior setting is an "arena," a physical arrangement of advantages and obstacles, in which certain activities flourish, others manage only to survive, and still others cannot even get started. As a result of his studies of children's environments, Barker (1968) spoke of behavior settings: "We could predict some aspects of children's behavior more adequately from knowledge of the behavior characteristics of the drugstores, arithmetic classes, and baseball games they inhabited than from knowledge of the behavior tendencies of the particular children" (p. 4).

A behavior setting exerts an environmental press, which is the combined influence of various forces working in a particular setting to shape the behavior of individuals in that setting. Environmental press arises from circumstances confronting and surrounding an individual—circumstances that generate psychosocial momentum tending to guide the individual in a particular direction (Garbarino 1982). Intervention, then, emphasizes linking a youth with an environmental network of behavior settings that facilitate specific behavior changes desired.

Take, for example, Lee's (1985) concept of life-space structures. Lee theorizes that people develop different kinds of life-space patterns, or, as she calls them, "characteristic ways of negotiating time, space, people, and activities in their day-to-day lives" (p. 624). Individuals manipulate these patterns to deal with the environment for the satisfaction of needs and desires. Consider this example demonstrating how, if time cannot be manipulated, the proper use of space, people, and activities can make up for it. Suppose some parents feel that they are not with their children often enough, and they cannot add to the time available. They might then take their work home (space adjustment), or take their children to their workplaces (activity adjustment), or hire somebody in their place to be with the children, who would otherwise be alone (people adjustment).

Benson (1990) has found that as a child's assets in behavior settings increase, high-risk behaviors are likely to decrease. By studying four key environmental assets for sixth-, seventh-, and eighth-graders (positive school climate, family support, involvement in structured youth activities, and involvement in a church or synagogue), Benson made the following observations. Those with no key assets exhibit an average of four at-risk indicators; those with one of the key assets exhibit an average of three at-risk indicators; those with two key assets average only two at-risk indicators; and those with three key assets average 1.4 at-risk indicators. In other words, for almost every asset added, a risk indicator is eliminated. Bogenschneider et al. (1990), too, found that there are protective factors and risk factors in every family system, peer group, school, workplace, and community. They found in addition that increases in protective factors or assets tend to correlate directly with decreases in at-risk indicators.

The core philosophy of ecological intervention in mental health comes down to this: strategies can be targeted primarily toward the environment, as opposed to the individual. Identifying the factor in the environment that promises to work the quickest and provide the most beneficial changes is the first challenge to the ecology-minded clinician. Usually, when the environment is subjected to a "diagnosis," this key factor attracts the attention of the clinician, who can then fashion an intervention based on it (Hartman and Laird 1983).

Therapists seeking to integrate a child's environment into treatment plans will discover an ever-expanding literature base to provide guidance (Munger 1991). Some ecological research has even produced data about scientific correlations between individual problems and environmental factors (cf. Apter 1982; Fine and Carlson 1992; Garbarino 1982; Hobbs 1982; Whittaker and Garbarino 1983).

## Developing Ecological Consciousness

Even though the Children and Adolescent Service System Program (CASSP) model has been a vast improvement over prior child mental health care efforts in communities, it has had an Achilles' heel: the single most frequently cited barrier to CASSP success is the lack of properly trained personnel to implement the programs (Schlenger et al. 1992). Unfortunately, mental health professionals are not trained to address ecosystems; consequently, they typically have trouble viewing the whole child and whole family within a network of coordinated services.

The medical-psychological model, which has been only minimally challenged by the proponents of the CASSP model, often causes a circumscribed approach to mental health therapy, for it deals only with individuals and their internal problems. Anyone using the medical-psychological model is tempted to view a disturbed child as a client who can be cured merely by controlling internal variables with physiological and psychological treatment. The framework of the medical-psychological model and the adherence of the majority of clinicians to this framework actually limit mental health professionals' ability to deliver services using the new models. The medical-psychological model is limited in its explanation and remediation of complex human behaviors. Its methods are so focused on the child's past that professionals using it often fail to formulate successful ways of working with others in the child's present environment. Clinicians must learn to break from psychodynamic psychology, with its premise that past trauma must be addressed before other options are considered (Hobbs 1982).

In contrast to the traditional mental health specialist, the ecological intervener is expected to strengthen the supportive forces in the child's setting and to encourage or to manipulate change in the detrimental forces in the child's settings in order to expedite successful adjustment in the community (Apter 1982). Hence, the training of mental health professionals should emphasize the role of the child's social system in bringing about worthwhile change. Friedman (1993) has recently outlined the kind of academic curriculum needed to produce broadly trained clinicians. His curriculum focuses on training practitioners to understand the entire child as the child participates in family life, neighborhoods, school, and community settings. Furthermore, Friedman believes that the training of mental health professionals should involve working in diverse community settings and should require those who work with children to build a flexible model for the interpretation of children's changing needs throughout childhood.

Personal involvement, including intimate contact with a community, requires dedication. In some cases, as noted earlier, the mental health professional's efforts should not be aimed toward involving the child in the counseling process, but rather toward using or bolstering some other natural therapy system or resource in the environment on the child's behalf (Maluccio 1981). Most mental health professionals are not trained in this kind of indirect consultation and treatment. The ecological intervener must be primed to play whatever role and to perform whatever activity is necessary to confront and alleviate a problem situation. The clinical ecologist wears many hats, providing support and advocacy as well as teaching and coordinating therapy for children and families. Over time, the roles of specialists in emotional and community problems will probably blend together (Mannino and Shore 1984).

The fact remains that many mental health professionals find it difficult to switch to a strategy that contradicts principles to which they have grown accustomed. Individualist psychology has had a very long run of popularity, going back to the time when it was just about the only model available and when its principles were scarcely challenged. Ecological psychology contradicts traditional thinking in mental health and threatens those who cling to the medical-psychological model. The ecological model implies that many established treatment programs would require significant modification with concomitant reductions in status for some individuals (Schmid 1987).

The reliance of the vast majority of mental health professionals on traditional theories will greatly impair their ability to implement the new mental health approaches espoused by the CASSP model. The importance of broadening clinicians' mindsets cannot be overstated. The training and education of mental health professionals in the ecological viewpoint has become a linchpin in the metamorphosis of the present system of child mental health care.

## Summary: Ecological Alternatives

Mental health professionals must extend the same dynamic examination to a child's environment that standard theories have traditionally accorded to individuals. With a broader conceptualization of practice, the environment becomes a strategic component of mental health's potential. But just how willing are mental health professionals to leave their offices and face children's environments, especially in the reality of other community structures, reimbursement issues, and the comfort with business as usual? Since the 1930s, environmental intervention has been considered a subordinate method, a minor intervention that requires less training and ability than "real therapy," a method relegated to the paraprofessional. Intervention into a child's environment is viewed as less prestigious than the present clinical methods.

This must change. Environmental intervention must gain status as a prominent, viable therapeutic method, rather than merely as an incidental effort in comparison with conventional therapies. According to Whittaker and Garbarino (1983), ecological techniques ought to be given equal status with direct, face-to-face, individualistic techniques.

The systematic use of ecological knowledge is crucial in clinical practice, regardless of the disciplinary background or theoretical orientation of the practitioner. Environmental intervention could either make direct psychological intervention unnecessary or supplement it. Furthermore, traditional treatment efforts can be made more permanent by targeting environmental supports such as kin, friends, neighbors, and other informal helpers who can help families sustain and consolidate the gains made in psychotherapy (Whittaker and Tracy 1991). Obviously, mental health clinicians must be prepared to master much broader information and to grasp much more complex interactions than ever before. Hopefully, clinicians will come to appreciate the many complexities of environments and the possibilities they present for successful intervention.

There is good reason to believe that the mental health of children can be fortified and that treatment efforts can meet with a much greater percentage of success if ecology is given its rightful place in intervention. The weaknesses of present mental health programs and the strengths of the ecological viewpoint proposed in this chapter point to the same conclusion: children will be better served by a change in the focus of mental health services.

# References

American Psychiatric Association: Diagnostic and Statistical Manual of Mental Disorders, 4th Edition. Washington, DC, American Psychiatric Association, 1994

Apter S: Troubled Children/Troubled Systems. Elmsford, NY, Pergamon, 1982

Barker R: Ecological Psychology: Concepts and Methods for Studying the Environment of Human Behavior. Palo Alto, CA, Stanford University Press, 1968

Bechtel R: Patient and community, the ecological bond, in Ecological Approaches in Clinical and Community Psychology. Edited by O'Connor WO, Lubin B. New York, Wiley, 1984, pp 216–231

Becvar R, Becvar D, Bender A: Let us first do no harm. Journal of Marital and Family Therapy 8:385–391, 1982

Benson P: The Troubled Journey: A Portrait of 6th–12th Grade Youth. Minneapolis, MN, Lutheran Brotherhood, 1990

Bogenschneider K, Small S, Riley D: An ecological risk-focused approach for addressing youth-at-risk issues. Paper presented at the Youth At Risk Summit of the National Extension Service, Washington, DC, September 1990

Catalano R: Health, Behavior, and the Community: An Ecological Perspective. New York, Pergamon, 1979

Clark T, Zalis T, Sacco F: Outreach Family Therapy. New York, Jason Aronson, 1982

Combrinck-Graham L: Giant Steps: Therapeutic Innovations in Child Mental Health. New York, Basic Books, 1990

Conyne R, Clark R: Environmental Assessment and Design. New York, Praeger, 1981

Fine M, Carlson C: The Handbook of Family School Intervention: A Systems Perspective. Boston, MA, Allyn and Bacon, 1992

Fitzgerald E, Illback R: The measurement and effects of social support to families participating in Kentucky impact. Paper presented at the 6th Annual Research Conference, "System of Care for Children's Mental Health: Building a Research Base," Tampa, FL, March 1993

Friedman R: Preparation of students to work with children and families: is it meeting the need? Administration and Policy in Mental Health 20:297–310, 1993

Garbarino J: Children and Families in the Social Environment. Chicago, IL, Aldine, 1982

Glassner B, Freedman J: Clinical Sociology. New York, Longman, Inc., 1979

Gottlieb B: Social networks and social support in community mental health, in Social Networks and Social Support. Edited by Gottlieb B. Beverly Hills, CA, Sage, 1981, pp 11–39

Gump P: Ecological psychology and clinical mental health, in Ecological Approaches to Clinical and Community Psychology. Edited by O'Connor W, Lubin B. New York, Wiley, 1984, pp 57–71

Hartman L: The extended family as a resource for change: an ecological approach to family centered practice, in Social Work Practice: People and Environments. Edited by Germain C. New York, Columbia University Press, 1979, pp 239–266

Hartman L, Laird J: Family Centered Social Work Practice. New York, The Free Press, 1983

Henggeler S, Borduin C: Family Therapy and Beyond: A Multisystemic Approach to Treating the Behavior Problems of Children and Adolescents. Pacific Grove, CA, Brooks Cole Publishing Company, 1990

Hobbs N: The Futures of Children: Categories, Labels, and Their Consequences. San Francisco, CA, Jossey-Bass, 1975

Hobbs N: The Troubled and Troubling Child. San Francisco, CA, Jossey-Bass, 1982

Kraft S, DeMaio T: An ecological intervention with adolescents in low income families. Am J Orthopsychiatry 52:131–140, 1982

Krasner L: Environmental design in perspective: theoretical model, general principles, and historical context, in Environmental Design and Human Behavior. Edited by Krasner L. New York, Pergamon, 1980, pp 1–35

Lee M: Life space structure: explorations and speculations. Human Relations 38:623–642, 1985

Maluccio A: Competence-oriented social work practice: an ecological approach, in Promoting Competence in Clients: A New/Old Approach to Social Work Practice. Edited by Maluccio A. New York, The Free Press, 1981, pp 1–24

Mannino F, Shore M: An ecological perspective on family intervention, in Ecological Approaches to Clinical and Community Psychology. New York, Wiley, 1984, pp 75–93

Martin B: Parent-child relations, in Review of Child Development Research, Vol 4. Edited by Horowitz F. Chicago, IL, University of Chicago Press, 1975, pp 463–541

Moos R: The Human Context. New York, Wiley, 1976

Munger R: Child Mental Health Practice From the Ecological Perspective. Lanham, MD, University Press of America, 1991

Price R: The social ecology of treatment gain, in Maximizing Treatment Gains: Transfer Enhancement in Psychotherapy. Edited by Goodstein A, Kanfer F. New York, Academic Press, 1979

Saxe L, Cross T, Silverman N: Children's mental health: the gap between what we know and what we do. Am Psychol 43:800–807, 1988

Schlenger W, Etheridge R, Hansen D, et al: Evaluation of state efforts to improve systems of care for children and adolescents with severe emotional disturbances: the CASSP initial cohort study. Journal of Mental Health Administration 19:131–142, 1992

Schmid R: Historical perspectives on the ecological model. The Pointer 31:5–8, 1987

Schulman R: Environmental interventions, in The Basic Handbook of Child Psychiatry. Edited by Noshpitz J. New York, Basic Books, 1979, pp 300–314

Swenson C: Social networks, mutual aid, and the life model of practice, in Social Work Practice: People and Environments. Edited by Germain C. New York, Columbia University Press, 1979, pp 213–238.

Whittaker J, Garbarino J (eds): Social Support Networks: Informal Helping in the Human Services. New York, Aldine, 1983

Whittaker J, Tracy E: Social network intervention in intensive family based preventive services. Prevention in Human Services 9:175–192, 1991

Wohlwill J: The Physical Environment and Behavior: An Annotated Bibliography and Guide to the Literature. New York, Plenum, 1981

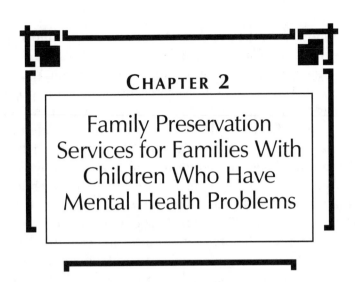

# CHAPTER 2

## Family Preservation Services for Families With Children Who Have Mental Health Problems

**Mary E. Evans, Ph.D., and
Roger A. Boothroyd, Ph.D.**

Every year numerous children and adolescents and their caregivers come to psychiatric emergency settings and other intake sites seeking resolution of behavioral crises and/or help for emotional or behavioral problems. In New York State approximately 56,000 children presented in emergency rooms and crisis settings in 1989 (New York State Office of Mental Health 1992). Although the volume of presenters is difficult to obtain on a national level, there is evidence that children and youth are presenting in increasing numbers (Bristol et al. 1981; Rosenn 1984). Often, presentations at emergency service settings represent a final effort to receive care that is desperately needed and has not been obtained elsewhere in the child service system. Because of the location and general nature of emergency and other crisis settings, children presenting at these settings may be referred, perhaps inappropriately, for a stigmatizing and costly hospitalization.

Compounding the problem of the increasing number of presenters is the fact that the mental health field lacks standardized approaches to the treatment of children in crisis and their families (Rosenn 1984). One relatively recent approach to providing emergency care is to offer intensive services within the context of the family—for example, using approaches modeled on the Homebuilders program (Pecora et al. 1991). The Homebuilders model, originally developed for a child welfare population, has been used in at least 14 states for the treatment of children in psychiatric crisis and their families (H. Bender, personal communication, January 22, 1992). At the time the work discussed in this chapter was initiated, no studies had been published that 1) examined modifications made in the Homebuilders model when applied to a mental health population or 2) assessed the outcomes associated with the intervention when used primarily to resolve mental health crises. The sections that follow review the Homebuilders model and similar intensive in-home service models and examine the research literature related to these interventions as a context for describing Home-Based Crisis Intervention (HBCI) in New York State. One HBCI program in New York State is reviewed in depth as the setting for a research demonstration in crisis care funded by the National Institute of Mental Health and Center for Mental Health Services (Evans 1992).

## Family Preservation Services

Family preservation services go by many names, including in-home services and family-centered or family-based services. The general purposes of these programs are to preserve the integrity of the family, to prevent the unnecessary placement of children in substitute care, to link the family with appropriate community services, and to increase the family's coping skills and community functioning (Stroul and Goldman 1990).

Perhaps the earliest and best known of the family preservation services is the Homebuilders program, which was established in Tacoma, Washington, in 1974. This program has served as a model for the establishment of similar programs across the country. According to Stroul and Goldman (1990), common features of in-home family services include the following:

- The intervention is delivered primarily in the family's home.
- Services are family focused; in other words, the family is the client.
- Services have an ecological perspective, stressing collaboration and coordination with community supports and services.
- Programs are committed to family preservation and reunification unless the child's safety is jeopardized.
- Service delivery hours are comprehensive and flexible to meet the needs of families.
- Services include counseling, skills training, and assisting the family in obtaining needed services, resources, and supports.
- The intensity and duration of services is based upon the program's goals and the family's needs, although most are short-term (1–3 months).
- Staff have small caseloads (2–3 families) thus permitting intensive work with each family.
- Close relationships develop between the home-based worker and the family.
- Programs are committed to empowering families, fostering hope, and assisting families in setting and achieving goals and priorities.

Anecdotal reports and early evaluation efforts of programs designed for child welfare populations have often pointed to positive outcomes, thus fostering the spread of these types of programs nationally. Early studies of family preservation programs tended to show positive outcomes, particularly in rates of out-of-home placement. Later studies with more rigorous designs, however, have shown more mixed results, often with no statistical differences in the proportion of children placed from family preservation and from standard treatment conditions, although children receiving family preservation services may have

been placed at a slower rate. In general, families with more resources and those rated as not having a child at imminent risk
of out-of-home placement have experienced the most positive
outcomes (Berry 1992; Feldman 1991; Henggeler et al. 1992,
1993; Nelson 1991; Pecora et al. 1991; Schwartz et al. 1991; Wells
and Whittington 1993; Yuan and Struckman-Johnson 1991).

Since 1974, at least 30 states have implemented intensive in-
home programs in one or more geographic areas for some target
population. The Omnibus Budget Reconciliation Act of 1993
(H.R. 2264), signed into law in August 1993, is expected to provide a stimulus to states to develop and disseminate home preservation services. Over the next 5 years a billion dollars will be
provided to states for a number of services whose intent is to
strengthen, preserve, support, and/or reunify at-risk children and
their families (Rivera and Kutash 1994). Meanwhile, the field of
mental health continues to lack in-depth descriptions of in-home
programs designed primarily for a child mental health population and lacks studies of the outcomes of such programs. The
following section describes one such in-home program, HBCI,
which is based on the Homebuilders model and has been implemented in New York State. For a comprehensive review of literature on family preservation studies, see Evans (1996).

## The Home-Based Crisis Intervention
## Program in New York State

In 1989 the New York State Office of Mental Health developed
the Home-Based Crisis Intervention Program (HBCI), a family
preservation program based on the Homebuilders model developed in Tacoma, Washington (Kinney et al. 1977). The goal of
this community-based emergency care program in New York
State is to prevent the hospitalization of children and youth by
providing short-term, intensive, in-home emergency services to
a family with a child experiencing a psychiatric crisis. Eight programs are currently operating in five regions of New York State.

Families gain access to the HBCI program through referrals
from either a psychiatric hospital or a general hospital providing

psychiatric emergency services. An HBCI counselor initiates in-home services within 24 hours of referral to the program, and services are typically provided over a 4- to 6-week period. Service delivery is designed to ensure that no child or family is left in a dangerous situation. To maximize family contact, counselors work with only two children and their families at any one time and have flexible working hours, including a 24-hour response capability. The intervention focuses on family strengths and needs, using a multifaceted approach that includes skill building, counseling, and concrete services. Skill building is designed to teach families new problem-solving, behavioral management, and communication strategies, using a cognitive-behavioral treatment approach. The HBCI counselor also establishes linkages for the child and the family with a variety of ongoing support services such as respite care, support groups, intensive case management (ICM), and clinic and day treatment programs. Follow-up contacts with the child and the family are conducted to ensure continued progress.

The target population of children for the HBCI program are 5–17 years of age, are living at home within their biological, foster, or adoptive family, are experiencing a psychiatric crisis that would require hospitalization without immediate intensive intervention, and are willing, along with their parent(s), to receive in-home crisis services.

Children may have had previous or ongoing contact with the juvenile justice system, the Division for Youth, the Department of Social Services, the mental health system, or all four.

### Data Collection Schedule and Instrumentation

Two data collection instruments are completed on all children who receive HBCI services. The Client Description Form (CDF) is completed at intake, and the Program Completion Form (PCF) is completed at discharge. The CDF is used to collect three types of information: 1) basic biographical information about the child, such as the child's age, race, gender, and current living situation, 2) educational information, such as the child's special education classification and current educational placement, and 3) information on the child's psychiatric history, such as diagnosis, symptoms, and behaviors displayed within the past 18 months and prior placements. The PCF is used to collect information on the reason for discharge and any changes in the child's living situation that may have occurred while HBCI services were provided. The CDF and the PCF were developed by the New York State Office of Mental Health to establish a comprehensive database on all children who are clients in seven types of community-based programs. The resulting database conforms to the minimal data standards recommended by NIMH (Leginski et al. 1989). To date, data have been collected on 1,169 children who have received HBCI services. Data are available on children from each of the eight program sites. The greatest number of data are available from HBCI programs located in the Bronx (15%), Erie (17%), and Dutchess (16%) Counties, and the fewest data are available in the HBCI programs located in Queens (7%), Onondaga (10%), Kings (9%), and Suffolk Counties. Findings from these data are summarized in the following paragraphs.

### HBCI Findings

**Classification of children receiving HBCI services.**   To date, more boys than girls have received HBCI services (60% compared with 40%). Over half of the children served are Caucasian (55%), whereas nearly 26% are Hispanic, and 16% African-American. The average age of the children on admission was approximately 11.5 years, and their ages ranged from 3 to 19 years. Nearly all the children who received HBCI (97%) lived at home with either one (55%) or both (33%) biological parents, adoptive parents (1%), or with relatives (8%). Children were most frequently referred to HBCI programs from either hospital emergency rooms (38%), mental health programs (18%), parents (16%), state-operated hospitals (8%), and schools (10%).

**Mental health histories of children receiving HBCI.**   Approximately 37% of the children in HBCI had never received any mental health treatment. Over half of the children (51%) had received mental health treatment in one (39%) or two (12%) different settings, whereas 12% of the children had obtained mental health services in three or more different settings. Approximately 25% of the children in HBCI had experienced one or more out-of-home placements. Most of the children receiving HBCI (82%) had never experienced a psychiatric hospitalization, whereas 11% had one psychiatric hospitalization and 6% of the children had been hospitalized two or more times.

Children exhibited an average of five symptoms or problem behaviors from a list of 26 on the CDF on enrollment to HBCI. Symptoms and behaviors most frequently observed included suicide ideation (57%), depression (59%), anxiety (41%), self-injurious behavior (37%), aggression toward others (38%), destruction of property (35%), physical aggression (49%), and temper tantrums (51%). Four behaviors were used to determine the dangerousness of the children. These included suicide attempts, suicide ideation, other self-injurious behavior, and aggressive behaviors toward others. Almost 80% of children in HBCI exhibited one or more of these dangerous symptoms or behaviors. On average children exhibited 1.5 dangerous symptoms or behaviors, with almost 23% of the children exhibiting three out of four of these symptoms or behaviors.

With respect to functioning, 77% of the children in HBCI were assessed as having impairments related to social relationships, 46% had impairments involving cognitive and communication processes, 44% experienced functional limitations related to self-direction, and 17% experienced impairments involving self-care.

**Average length of stay in the HBCI program.** For the 1,056 children who have been discharged, the average length of stay in HBCI was 36 days (SD = 16 days) and ranged from 1–121 days of service. Approximately 44% of the children served received between 4 and 6 weeks of HBCI services. Approximately 28% of the children were enrolled in the HBCI program less than 4 weeks, whereas a similar percentage (28%) of the children received in excess of 6 weeks of HBCI services.

The average length of stay may be related to how long the program has been in operation. Data from the Bronx HBCI program were examined in more detail because information was available on the 161 children who were enrolled in the program between September 1989, when the program began, and October 1993. The average lengths of stay for children enrolled in the Bronx HBCI program were examined by quarter (i.e., first 4 months, second 4 months, etc.). Figure 2–1 summarizes the average length of stay and a 1-SD confidence interval for each quarter since September 1989. As is shown in this figure, the average lengths of stay during the first four quarters ranged from 34 days to 56 days, whereas the average lengths of stay during the last four quarters ranged from 34 days to 39 days. In general, although the average lengths of stay vary from quarter to quarter, during the past year they were shorter and less variable than during the first four quarters.

The average length of stay for children who were hospitalized while receiving HBCI ($N = 53$) was compared with the average length of stay for children who were not hospitalized ($N = 1003$).

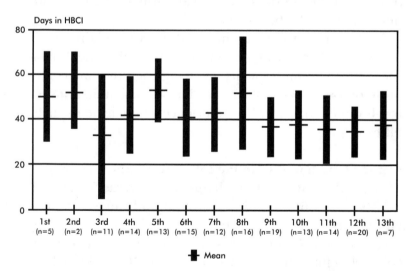

**Figure 2–1.**   Length of stay in Bronx HBCI by quarter.

Although the average length of stay for children who were hospitalized while enrolled in HBCI was 5 days shorter than for children who were not hospitalized ($P < .05$), children who were eventually hospitalized still received about 3 weeks (i.e., 23 days, SD = 14 days) of HBCI services prior to their hospitalization. Children who were not hospitalized received an average of 38 days of HBCI services (SD = 15 days).

**Factors related to the children's length of stay in HBCI.** A regression analysis was conducted to determine what factors were predictive of the length of time children spend in HBCI. Although children who were referred to HBCI from a state-operated hospital and children with cognitive impairments were more likely to have longer lengths of stay in HBCI, these variables accounted for less than 7% of the variance in length of stay. Examination of correlation coefficients indicated that no significant relationships were present between children's lengths of stay and the frequency of prior mental health treatment, number of prior inpatient stays, number of presenting symptoms, or degree of functional impairment. Additionally, length of stay was not significantly associated with demographic variables such as children's age, gender, or racial and ethnic background.

**Percentage of children in the HBCI program who experienced a change in their living situation.** Approximately 18% of the children experienced a change in their living situation during the provision of HBCI. The greatest change occurred among children who were living with relatives when they began receiving HBCI services; nearly one in three children experienced a change in their living situation. For most children a change in their living situation resulted in a more restrictive placement such as moving from living with biological parent(s) to residing with relatives or being placed outside the home. Approximately 5% of the children who received HBCI required hospitalization during the course of treatment.

## A Research Demonstration in the Bronx

Our examination of this in-home intervention left us with several questions and concerns. Chief among these was our concern about the effects of transplanting family-centered interventions from one geographic area to another, because these areas differ significantly in the nature of the cultural groups providing and receiving service. Little has appeared in the professional literature to offer guidance to service providers in identifying the particular needs of ethnic and cultural minorities and in modifying in-home service models to meet these needs. Gray and Nybell (1990) have identified a number of salient issues in African-American family preservation, including the structure and function of the African-American family, African-American cultural values and behaviors, the role of African-American men in the family, the use of physical discipline and Black English, and the resources available in the African-American community. Information of this type needs to be available to assist service providers who are working with other racial and ethnic minorities.

Also, to date, despite the commitment to providing a range of emergency services to children in psychiatric crises, the field has lacked data on the outcomes of commonly used models of care and comparative data on the effectiveness of various models, particularly models of in-family care. Even useful descriptive data are scarce; many of the commonly cited descriptive studies are between 10 and 30 years old. Of particular concern is the lack of data regarding the outcomes experienced by children with different needs and presenting problems; for example, those in crisis who have serious emotional disturbance (SED) and those who do not. Data on the comparative effectiveness of programs are urgently needed for policy development in the area of establishing effective psychiatric emergency services for children and their families.

In response to the lack of comparative information about the outcomes associated with emergency services for children and their families, we developed a proposal to establish and evaluate three in-family psychiatric emergency programs for children and adolescents in the Bronx, New York, an area of high need for such services. Our project, originally funded as a research demonstration by the National Institute of Mental Health and now by the Center for Mental Health Services, established an enhanced HBCI program (HBCI+), which offers staff training in cultural competence and working with violence in families. We also established a crisis case management (CCM) program that has both in-home and out-of-home respite care and a crisis case manager assigned to provide services to children and families on a short-term basis. The salient characteristics of HBCI, HBCI+, and CCM are compared in Table 2–1.

Children presenting to two psychiatric emergency rooms in the Bronx who meet the target population criteria noted earlier are randomly assigned to one of three treatment conditions. The system, child, family, and provider outcomes associated with these programs are being determined when all three programs are operating in the same urban community.

A collaborator of particular importance in this study is the Hispanic Research Center. Working with African-American and Hispanic consultants and community members, the Hispanic Research Center developed a culturally competent HBCI intervention and trained in-home counselors to implement this program. They have also worked with project staff to select culturally relevant instrumentation, and to modify or develop new instruments. The Hispanic Research Center has been responsible for the translation of consent forms and study instruments into Spanish and for pilot testing the study instruments on local African-American and Hispanic community members.

The research component of this project is examining outcomes associated with these three different program models. Child and family characteristics and functioning are being assessed at enrollment, at discharge from service, and at 6 months postdischarge. The study will examine system outcomes (e.g., hospitalization and use of other restrictive settings), child outcomes (e.g., alterations in functioning), and family outcomes (such as self-efficacy in parenting, family adaptability and cohesion, and satisfaction with services). The costs of providing care

**Table 2–1.** A comparison of home-based crisis intervention (HBCI), enhanced home-based crisis intervention (HBCI+), and crisis case management (CCM)

| Program attribute | HBCI | HBCI+ | CCM |
|---|---|---|---|
| Target population | Children and youth living at home who are at risk of an inpatient admission due to psychiatric crisis | Children and youth living at home who are at risk of an inpatient admission due to psychiatric crisis | Children and youth living at home who are at risk of an inpatient admission due to psychiatric crisis |
| Program goals | Resolve immediate crisis, teach skills, improve family relationships, link to needed services | Similar to HBCI with the added goal of providing long-term family support services | Assess needs, provide concrete services, link child and family to needed services |
| Program focus | The child within the context of the family | The child within the context of the family | The child within the context of the family |
| Caseload per worker | Two families in crisis | Two families in crisis | Four families in crisis, four families requiring generic case management services |
| Duration of service | 4–6 weeks | 4–6 weeks | 4–6 weeks |
| Respite | No respite provided | In-home and out-of-home respite available | In-home and out-of-home respite available |

| | | | |
|---|---|---|---|
| Staff training | HBCI training | HBCI training, plus training in cultural competence and working with violence in families and communities | Intensive case management and crisis intervention training |
| Postcrisis family support services | No postcrisis family support services provided | Services available through bilingual, bicultural parent advocate who establishes a parent support group and provides individual parent advocacy | No postcrisis family support services provided |
| Flexible service dollars | Not available | An average of $100 per family available to meet individualized needs | An average of $150 per family available to meet individualized needs |
| In-home visits and supports | Provided within 24 hours of intake and on a regular and frequent basis throughout the crisis period | Provided within 24 hours of intake and on a regular and frequent basis throughout the crisis period | Provided within 24 hours initially, and as needed thereafter |

*(continued)*

**Table 2–1.** A comparison of home-based crisis intervention (HBCI), enhanced home-based crisis intervention (HBCI+), and crisis case management (CCM) *(continued)*

| Program attribute | HBCI | HBCI+ | CCM |
|---|---|---|---|
| Psychiatric services | Psychiatrist available to provide assessment and treatment services within the home | Psychiatrist available to provide assessment and treatment services within the home | Psychiatrist consultation available to crisis case managers and to families for medication review |
| Funding | State resources only | State resources for HBCI components and grant funds for enhancements | State resources for case managers and in-home respite and grant funds for out-of-home respite |

[a]Families receiving generic case management services are not part of this research project.

will be compared with hospitalization costs. The job satisfaction and tenure of the providers (i.e., counselors, case managers, and parent advocates) will also be assessed.

Service delivery began in November 1993 and random assignment of children to the three treatment options will continue for approximately 18 months. During this period of time, between 240 and 260 children and their families will participate in the study. The research involves a positively controlled, randomized study design with repeated measures. A variety of assessments are being conducted at intake, discharge, and at a 6-month follow-up to measure family functioning, child behavior, and parent and child satisfaction. Parents have participated in instrument development and in the design of training components.

Among the research and policy issues the study will address are the following.

- the extent to which intensive, in-home psychiatric crisis services can prevent hospitalization
- the overall effectiveness of each model for families experiencing a child mental health crisis
- the relative importance of program variables such as access to flexible service dollars, respite, and parent support
- differences in effectiveness for children and youth experiencing different types of crises
- risk assessment and decision-making processes in psychiatric emergency settings
- the models' effectiveness for African-American and Hispanic families living in the Bronx
- relative cost-effectiveness of each model as it is implemented compared with hospitalization

## Discussion and Conclusions

Over the course of the last 15 years intensive in-home services have become popular in the child welfare field. More recently such services have been used in at least 14 states for child mental health populations. There have been relatively few systematic evaluations of the outcomes of these programs, and the studies that have been done have not resulted in a consensus regarding program effectiveness. No studies have been published that focus specifically on services provided to children with SED and their families.

There has been little discussion in the literature regarding the program modifications, if any, that should be introduced or that have been introduced into child welfare models when these models are used for child mental health populations. Little has been written specifically about the treatment provided to persons of particular racial and cultural groups who may represent significant numbers of children and families enrolled in family preservation programs. Based on the extant research, it has also been difficult to determine which program components have been associated with successful outcomes; for example, would the same level of success be obtained if counselors did not concentrate on skills building? Faced with issues such as these, and wanting to provide our policy makers with guidance, the Bureau of Evaluation and Services Research at the New York State Office of Mental Health examined our database on children and families who had been served in our family preservation program, HBCI. These data indicated that few of these children, who were identified as being at imminent risk of hospitalization when they were referred to the program, were actually hospitalized during the intervention or shortly following discharge from the intervention. Lacking data, however, on the population from which this sample of children was selected and on a broader range of child and family outcomes, we have designed and implemented a research demonstration to answer many of the unresolved questions that surfaced from our review of the literature and from preliminary data analyses.

Discussions with program staff, service providers, and others about the enhancements that may be needed in the basic Homebuilders model that was the foundation for our HBCI program led us to make some enhancements in the program. These enhancements, such as respite care, flexible service money, use of a parent advocate, cultural competence training, and training in preventing and coping with violence, have been discussed in this chapter. Additionally, because we do not know if an intensive case management model, focused on linkage with existing services rather than providing skills building directly, would be as effective in promoting positive outcomes for children and families, we designed the CCM option. Children and families presenting in psychiatric crisis and who are determined to be at imminent risk of hospitalization are being randomly assigned to one of the three options: HBCI, enhanced HBCI, or CCM.

Although it is still too early in the project to discern even preliminary outcomes, one important lesson has been learned. We have learned that the physical presence of in-home interventions such as HBCI, HBCI+, and CCM does not mean that these services are necessarily available to children and families. For this to occur, clinical staff must accept them as legitimate and viable service options and must be willing to refer children and families. Furthermore, children and families must be willing to accept someone coming to their home and working with them. To the extent that both conditions do not exist, the presence of the interventions does not alter the existing service system. It has been our experience in the Bronx that, although we have increased the capacity of these in-home interventions, referrals have been slow in coming. Referrals are coming from intake sites where staff have had previous experience with these services. However, staff who have not had previous experience with these types of interventions are more reluctant to make referrals. In essence, there is a socialization period that needs to take place.

A primary purpose of this chapter has been to identify some of the issues that exist in interpreting and applying findings from the existing literature on family preservation programs, and to describe our attempts to address some of these issues. Obviously this is a work in progress, but we would like to encourage other researchers, particularly those studying children with emotional and behavioral problems and their families, to engage in systematic study of intensive in-home interventions as these interventions become more widespread for this population.

# References

Berry M: An evaluation of family preservation services: fitting agency services needs. Social Work 37:314–321, 1992

Bristol KM, Giller E Jr, Docherty JP: Trends in emergency psychiatry in the last two decades. Am J Psychiatry 138:623–628, 1981

Evans ME: Outcomes of three children's psychiatric emergency programs. Research demonstration grant funded by the National Institutes of Mental Health (1R18MH48072) and the Center for Mental Health Services (5HD5SM48072), 1992

Evans ME: Family preservation services for children with emotional and behavioral disorders, in Contemporary Society: Childhood and Complex Order. Edited by Pfeffer G. New Delhi, India, Concept Publishers, 1996, pp 287–302

Feldman LH: Evaluating the impact of intensive family preservation services in New Jersey, in Family Preservation Services: Research and Evaluation. Edited by Wells K, Biegel DE. Newbury Park, CA, Sage, 1991, pp 47–71

Gray SS, Nybell LM: Issues in African-American family preservation. Child Welfare 69:513–523, 1990

Henggeler SW, Melton GB, Smith LA: Family preservation using multisystemic therapy: an effective alternative to incarcerating serious juvenile offenders. J Consult Clin Psychol 60:953–961, 1992

Henggeler SW, Melton GB, Smith LA, et al: Family preservation using multisystemic treatment: long-term follow-up to a clinical trial with serious juvenile offenders. Journal of Child and Family Studies 2:283–293, 1993

Kinney J, Madsen B, Flemming T, et al: Home-builders: keeping families together. J Consult Clin Psychol 45:667–673, 1977

Leginski WA, Croze C, Driggers J, et al: Data standards for mental health decision support systems (DHHS Publ No ADM-89-1589). Rockville, MD, U.S. Department of Health and Human Services, 1989

Nelson KE: Populations and outcomes in five family preservation programs, in Family Preservation Services: Research and Evaluation. Edited by Wells K, Biegel DE. Newbury Park, CA, Sage, 1991, pp 72–91

New York State Office of Mental Health: Patient characteristics survey. Bureau of Evaluation and Services Research, 1992

Pecora PJ, Fraser MW, Haapala DA: Client outcomes and issues for program design, in Family Preservation Services: Research and Evaluation. Edited by Wells K, Biegel DE. Newbury Park, CA, Sage Publications, 1991, pp 3–32

Rivera VR, Kutash F: Components of a System of Care: What Does the Research Say? University of South Florida Mental Health Institute, Research and Training Center for Children's Mental Health, Tampa, FL, 1994

Rosenn DW: Psychiatric emergencies in children and adolescents, in Emergency Psychiatry: Concepts, Methods and Practice. Edited by Bassuk EL, Birk AW. New York, Plenum, 1984, pp 303–350

Schwartz IM, AuClaire P, Harris LJ: Family preservation services as an alternative to the out-of-home placement of adolescents: the Hennepin County experience, in Family Preservation Services: Research and Evaluation. Edited by Wells K, Biegel DE. Newbury Park, CA, Sage, 1991, pp 33–46

Stroul BA, Goldman SK: Study of community-based services for children and adolescents who are severely emotionally disturbed. Journal of Mental Health Administration 17:61–77, 1990

Wells K, Whittington D: Child and family functioning after intensive family preservation services. Social Service Review 67:55–83, 1993

Yuan YT, Struckman-Johnson DL: Placement outcomes for neglected children with prior placements in family preservation programs, in Family Preservation Services: Research and Evaluation. Edited by Wells K, Biegel DE. Newbury Park, CA, Sage, 1991, pp 92–118

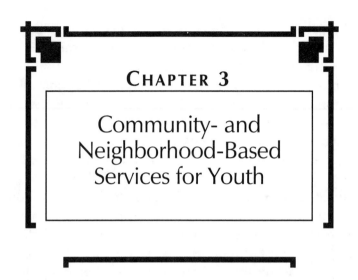

# CHAPTER 3

## Community- and Neighborhood-Based Services for Youth

**Krista Kutash, Ph.D., Albert J. Duchnowski, Ph.D., Judith Meyers, Ph.D., and Betty King, M.A.**

In this chapter we describe a comprehensive, integrated service delivery system for troubled youth that is community and neighborhood based. We describe a proposed system, and we reference empirical support when available. We describe in some detail the newest program in this area, the Mental Health Initiative for Urban Children funded by the Annie E. Casey Foundation, which focuses on inner-city neighborhoods.

## Definition

Little consensus has been achieved in defining emotional or mental disorders in children. This problem has received the attention of advocacy groups as well as researchers. Such groups as the National Alliance for the Mentally Ill (NAMI) have advocated for the use of terms such as *children with neurobiological disorders* (Peschel et al. 1992). NAMI proposes that the system should focus on children who have mental illness that is biological in nature and genetically transmitted. The focus is on conditions such as schizophrenia, depression, and bipolar disorders. This point of view is supported by the extensive neurobiological research program initiated by NIMH, which dubbed the 1990s "the decade of the brain." While researchers wait for the data, some advocates have proposed that antisocial behavior and problems resulting from distressed environmental conditions should not be considered as mental illness and are the responsibility of the child welfare system (Peschel et al. 1992). The causes of mental illness from this perspective are posited to be neurological.

Others have expanded the definition to encompass more children in the target population. The term *emotional or mental disturbance* is usually used in this case and sometimes "behavioral" is added to the list of modifiers. This term has been more characteristic of the approach taken by the Children and Adolescent Service System Program (CASSP) (Lourie and Katz-Leavy 1987). Although emphasizing the need for service for children who are the most seriously impaired, the CASSP definition is broad and does include children who engage in antisocial behavior or who may have emotional problems because of abuse or neglect.

To some degree, the problem of definition has been settled by a request from Congress to the newly created federal Center for Mental Health Services (CMHS). This agency was required to develop standardized definitions and methodologies for states to use in determining prevalence and incidence rates of serious emotional disturbance (SED) in children and adolescents. These rates would assist in planning for services under federal block grant programs, but the expectation is that the definitions will have implications for third-party payments, health care reform, and the broad mental health service delivery system. The following definition was published in the Federal Register on May 20, 1993, and was effective immediately:

> Children with a serious emotional disturbance are persons from birth up to age 18 who currently, or at any time during the past year have had a diagnosable mental, behavioral or emotional disorder of sufficient duration to meet diagnostic criteria specified within DSM-III-R, that resulted in functional impairment

which substantially interferes with or limits the child's role or functioning in family, school or community activities (p. 29425).

Several studies recently have been completed that systematically describe the characteristics of children who have SED and in some cases preliminary causal models are emerging. These studies are the National Longitudinal Study of Special Education Students (Wagner et al. 1991), the Ontario Child Health Study (Offord et al. 1989), the National Child and Adolescent Treatment Study (Silver et al. 1992), and a study by Cullinan et al. (1992).

Although each of these studies was conducted in different parts of the United States and Ontario, Canada, with different methodologies, very striking similarities are found in the results. Children who had SED were overwhelmingly male (approximately 70%). Minority children and low-income families were overrepresented, less than 20% of the children lived in two-parent homes, and an even smaller number lived with both biological parents. About half of the children began to have problems around age 6 and there was a lag of about 2 years before the first service of any type was received. Typically, these youth were 1.5 years behind in math and reading, and average IQ scores were in the low 90s. The graduation rate was less than 40%.

When diagnostic categories were examined, approximately two-thirds of the identified children met the criteria for conduct disorder. Furthermore, over half of these children met criteria for at least one additional diagnosis. Of particular concern is the high prevalence of substance abuse in this population (Greenbaum et al. 1991). These data have been interpreted by some as indicative of strong psychosocial factors creating vulnerability in children for developing emotional disorders. The link between poverty and single-parent homes and emotional and behavioral problems in children is viewed as very strong (Offord et al. 1989).

## Incidence and Prevalence

The difficulty in obtaining reliable and valid incidence and prevalence data has been due in part to the lack of consensus on the definition. Several studies have investigated the prevalence of diagnosable disorders in children and adolescents, in spite of the methodological difficulties that exist. In a review of this research, Brandenberg et al. (1990) concluded that estimates of emotional disturbance range between 14% and 20% of all children.

Using the available data, estimates of 3%–5% frequently are used by states in planning for children identified as having SED and in need of intensive intervention. These figures are higher than those used by NIMH in the 1970s. At that time an estimate of 12% was used as the prevalence of children with a diagnosable disorder (Gould et al. 1980), and 1% was the estimate of the number of children with SED.

## Service Delivery System

This section describes the service delivery system for troubled youth. A model for the design of a service delivery system will be described along with a description of how such a system was implemented in Ventura County, California. Results of the program in Ventura County as well as research from other communities are also presented. Finally, the newest program in this area, the Mental Health Initiative for Urban Children, is described.

Led by CASSP, a new vision of service provision for children and adolescents and their families has emerged (Day and Roberts 1991). This vision emphasizes the need to develop community-based systems of care based on a set of values and principles and the best available research. These systems of care incorporate a range of services, involve several agencies, forge new partnerships between parents and professionals, and provide intensive, individualized, and culturally competent services.

Stroul and Friedman (1986) describe a "system of care" as follows:

> A system of care is a comprehensive spectrum of mental health and other necessary services which are organized into a coordinated network to meet the multiple and changing needs of severely emotionally disturbed children and adolescents (p. iv).

The system-of-care concept represents more than a network of services; it is a philosophy that calls for service systems that are child-centered and family-focused. The services within a system of care are intended to be function-specific rather than agency-specific. Each service area addresses an area of need for children and families, a set of service functions that must be fulfilled in order to provide comprehensive services to meet those needs. All of the functions included in the system-of-care dimensions may be fulfilled by a variety of agencies or practitioners in both the public and private sectors.

The oldest and perhaps best known system of care is located in Ventura County, California. This program, the Children's Demonstration Project, was created in 1984 by the California State Legislature to design a "comprehensive, coordinated children's mental health system that can be replicated in other counties" (Jordan and Hernandez 1990, p. 27). The project successfully implemented a community-based system of care that coordinated four child-serving systems: juvenile justice, education, child welfare, and mental health.

As a result of interagency planning, three categories of programs for children and youth were expanded or developed: family preservation, family reunification, and case management. Family preservation programs include the provision of intensive outpatient services either in a clinic or in the community; enriched classes for youth with SED in the school system; outpatient services for juvenile justice wards; an in-home crisis program; a day treatment program and day care center located in the public schools operated jointly by the mental health system and the school system; therapeutic services for dependents in foster care; and an outreach program to the private sector to obtain needed resources for youth such as clothing and dental care. The family reunification programs are time-limited, local residential alternatives to long-term foster-care group homes or state hospital placements and include a residential facility for juvenile justice wards, which includes on-site mental health day treatment services, a residential program for crisis services, and a group home. In regard to the case management functions, this area monitors and controls residential placements (including state hospital use), sets policy, and resolves disputes between agencies. The committees and teams in this category include a mental health case-management team, a juvenile justice placement screening committee, a protective services placement screening committee, special-education individualized education plan (IEP) teams for residential candidates, and an interagency case-management council, which develops overall policy.

Unlike many communities in which mental health services are independent "stand-alone" programs, all of Ventura County's services and programs are blended into the existing structure and procedures of the child-serving agencies. The only exception is a small outpatient component, which still receives referrals directly from the community and serves as an intake center to capture children at risk for residential placement.

This demonstration program also developed a set of planning principles and procedures to target children who were most in need of services and to identify and develop services to meet the needs of these children. The Ventura Planning Model has five basic components for planning systems of care for children and youth. These components include having a clearly defined target population, a systemwide goal, interagency coalitions, treatment services and standards, and systems monitoring and evaluation. This system is noteworthy not only for being multiagency but also for establishing quantifiable goals and objectives as well as having an ongoing practical system of monitoring and evaluation.

Evaluation data for the Children's Demonstration Project point to reduced rates of admissions to state hospitals, reduced average stay for youth at the state hospital, significantly and consistently lower placement rates in group homes than for the state as a whole, significant gains in school attendance with students present approximately 90% of possible school days, significant gains in school performance, and reduced reincarceration rates for juvenile offenders with reduced total days of incarceration (Goldman 1992).

This model of service delivery currently is being replicated in three counties in California. Accompanying the replication is an independent evaluation effort called the California AB377 Evaluation Project (Rosenblatt and Attkisson 1992), which has a central goal of examining the effects of the creation and maintenance of coordinated community-based services on the rates of admissions to highly restrictive out-of-home placements. The initial results indicate that although the number of per capita group home placements continues to rise steadily in the state of California, the placement rates for group homes in the AB377 counties remain relatively level and constant. This pattern also is found in the expenditures for group home placements, with the AB377 counties having a reduction in expenditures relative to the state as a whole (Rosenblatt et al. 1992).

Another public sector application of the system of care model at the local community level is beginning in Virginia (Macbeth 1993). Each community will develop child planning teams and a local management team, administered by local government, to implement this service delivery system.

One of the latest and most extensive efforts to address the issue of providing a broad range of services is a unique project funded by the Civilian Health and Medical Program of the Uniformed Services (CHAMPUS) program of the Department of Defense and operated by the state of North Carolina and Fayette County in the Ft. Bragg area. Through this program, the 46,000 children and adolescents of military families in the catchment area are eligible to receive whatever types of mental health services are required, rather than being restricted to outpatient care, residential care, and inpatient hospitalization (Behar et al. 1993). The potential benefit of this program is enhanced by a rigorous independent evaluation being conducted by Leonard Bickman and his associates at Vanderbilt University (see Heflinger et al. 1992). Preliminary results of the evaluation document the efficacy of community-based treatment for youth with SED (Bickman 1993).

Private foundations also have played a central role in supporting and developing systems of care for youth. Most notable is the Mental Health Services Program for Youth funded by the

Robert Wood Johnson Foundation (RWJ) and the Mental Health Initiative for Urban Children funded by the Annie E. Casey Foundation.

## Mental Health Services Program for Youth

The Mental Health Services Program for Youth began in 1988 with over $20 million committed by RWJ over 5 years to support the development of community-based systems of care in seven locations. Although each location has its own unique programmatic goals and objectives, all sites share four overarching goals: through effective interagency collaboration, to establish a comprehensive program of care to meet the specific health, mental health, and other needs of children and families; to provide a system of care that results in a decreased likelihood of lifetime dependency upon public service; to provide care in the least restrictive environment; and to modify fiscal policies so that they are more supportive of individualized and home-based care (Beachler 1990; England and Cole 1992).

Each of the seven projects within this initiative is unique. In Kentucky, the RWJ program is called the Interagency Mobilization for Progress in Adolescents' and Children's Treatment (IMPACT Project) and works to provide a full continuum of community-based resources through interagency planning teams. It was funded to operate only in the bluegrass area of the state. However, the state legislature simultaneously provided funding to replicate the program statewide. In Dane County, Wisconsin, the Community Organized to Maintain Parents and Adolescents in Safe, Secure Surroundings (COMPASS Project) has two components: clinical case coordination and crisis services. The program in Multnomah County, Oregon (the Partners Project) has five categorical agencies pooling portions of their budgets to jointly finance flexible services for youth. The Connections project in Cleveland is expanding school-based case management services as one way of meeting the unique needs of inner-city children and their families. The remaining projects are located in North Carolina, San Francisco, and Vermont.

Program evaluation information is being collected by each of the seven projects and is beginning to provide evidence of improved educational status for youth with SED, reduced incarceration and recidivism rates, reduced rates of residential placements, and lower costs in providing services for project participants. The overall initiative is being evaluated by Cross et al. (1993).

## The Mental Health Initiative for Urban Children

Building on the work of Ventura County, CASSP, and RWJ, the Annie E. Casey Foundation designed and funded the Mental Health Initiative for Urban Children in order to apply the insights of these recent reform efforts to a broader range of children and families living in inner-city neighborhoods, where family stresses are compounded by poverty, violence, and drugs, and children are at especially high risk of developing serious mental health problems. The goal of the Mental Health Initiative for Urban Children is to improve outcomes for troubled children, adolescents, and their families through demonstrating new ways of delivering culturally appropriate, family-focused mental health services in high poverty, inner-city neighborhoods and to work with states and cities to improve policies and practices supporting these services. Several states were awarded 1-year planning grants in 1992. Based on the results of the planning year, the states of Florida, Texas, and Virginia were awarded $3 million grants over a 4-year period to implement their plans. The states of Colorado and Massachusetts were funded to continue their planning efforts and will be considered for implementation grants in 1994. Each state selected a city and then neighborhoods for the demonstration. The selected neighborhoods are in Denver, Miami, Boston, Houston, and Richmond. The neighborhoods range in population from 19,000 to 34,000 and include some of the very poorest areas in the United States with child poverty rates over 40%. In three of the neighborhoods the majority of residents are African-American and in the remaining two neighborhoods the majority of the residents are Hispanic.

The Mental Health Initiative for Urban Children seeks to foster, on a neighborhood scale, a community-based system that

- broadens the focus of the work to develop systems of care for the population of individuals who are severely emotionally disturbed to include children and adolescents who are at risk—not just those who have already been identified as having serious mental health problems
- focuses on prevention and early intervention to keep problems from becoming so severe that out-of-home care or out-of-community placements are the only alternatives
- integrates mental health services into existing community settings and activities that offer greater access to needy children and families, and in which the services are less stigmatizing—for example, schools, community health centers, churches, and recreation centers
- emphasizes parent education and involvement

Systems change is to be achieved through restructuring the existing service system at the state, city, and neighborhood levels, increasing the availability of supports and services for children and families in the neighborhood, and increasing neighborhood development activities. Although the focus of this initiative is initially on one neighborhood in each of the participating states, success is based on state and local decision makers reforming policies and practices in conjunction with that neighborhood. The Foundation is seeking ways to reform thinking nationally, based on local efforts, with the work to be replicated in other neighborhoods and communities within each of the states and across other states.

The neighborhood focus envisioned by the Foundation is rooted in the conviction that interventions centered only on children do little to change the factors that give rise to, or increase the incidence of, mental health problems. By building on existing strengths in a neighborhood, and working toward neighborhood ownership and support of a community-based system of care, there is greater likelihood of sustained change over the long term—long after the Foundation's role has ended. A neighborhood focus also provides the opportunity to target efforts on critical aspects of children's lives that are seldom addressed by the large public service systems. Such critical factors, which are key to preventing mental health problems among urban children, include

- opportunities to interact one on one with caring adults in informal learning and recreational settings
- safe, clean facilities for informal and organized sports and recreation
- protection from exposure to violent crimes and victimization by criminal elements in the community
- formal and informal support systems that reinforce positive values and the avoidance of risky behavior, and buffer the impact of negative peer pressure and stressful adult relationships
- caring adults to advocate for youth and to train them in self-advocacy
- opportunities for voluntary community service, which develops leadership skills and teaches young people to value community building
- experiences and information that teach young people the value of work and economic enterprise

The Mental Health Initiative is designed to build on the strengths of residents and traditional community institutions. Churches, social clubs, fraternal organizations, parent groups, business associations, and the like are viewed as important neighborhood resources for support to children and families.

The Foundation looks to the neighborhood sites to create innovative, flexible, and integrated systems that provide the necessary interventions while reducing reliance on the formal service delivery system, and that reflect the characteristics of effective systems. It is expected that the resulting service system will be responsive to the stresses of poverty, crime, violence, racism, family disruption, and other stressors that place children at risk for emotional disturbance. Services are expected to be responsive, accessible, convenient, comprehensive, and culturally appropriate. Services for children identified as having more severe mental health problems are to be family- and community-based, with a reduction in the need for more restrictive placement through hospitalization or incarceration evident over time.

## Components of the Mental Health Initiative

Central to the success of the initiative are the components of restructuring financing patterns, managing information, and developing family advocacy and support systems. A description of each component follows.

### Restructuring Financing Patterns

A basic premise of the Foundation's initiative is that existing public investments can be more effectively used. Currently the greatest portion of public dollars is spent on the fewest children, to pay for institutional and residential treatment center placements for the most seriously disturbed children. The least amount is spent for prevention and family support services. The Foundation envisions a markedly different pattern of resource allocation in an effective multiagency system of care, with a shift in spending from the most expensive placement to front-end services, such as early intervention programs.

The effort to reform funding policies and practices is perceived as closely tied to the development of a plan for a local system of care. Fiscal reform is central to achieving long-term change in the structure and practice of services at the neighborhood level, and will pave the way for future replication in other areas within the state. Financing reforms may include the decategorization of funding, the development of community funding pools that include both public and private sector funds, the development of flexible funding for wrap-around services, the maximization of federal, state, and third-party reimbursement mechanisms, the provision of managed care and capitation mechanisms, and reinvestment of funds from out-of-home placements to community services. Collaboration among state agencies and the legislature in refinancing services will be significant in determining how new dollars, particularly those received as the result of maximizing federal funding, will be reinvested to support the reform of children and family services.

In addition to providing more resources to support early intervention and prevention services in the community, it is anticipated that restructuring finances will result in a reduction of revenue outflow from the neighborhoods. Most of the money currently spent on children in poor urban areas tends to go to agencies and services located in other parts of the city or state and therefore is of no economic benefit to the neighborhood. By redirecting the dollars to community-based services, the money can be used to support jobs for neighborhood residents and to benefit businesses in the community, thus helping to bolster the local economy.

### Managing Information

To develop better interventions and more responsive policies, communities need reliable information about the incidence and trends in indicators relevant to the children and families in the community. A fundamental principle of the Mental Health Initiative is that an integrated data management system is essential to a well-designed and well-functioning service system. Such a system should have the capacity to combine information about children and families across service systems, to be accessed by the various service systems so that families do not have to be subjected to multiple intakes and assessments, and to track the services received by children and families over time. Only with a managed data system will communities succeed in accurately defining their problems, establishing meaningful and measurable goals, and gaining the feedback needed to modify and strengthen their interventions. Each state is expected to design and develop a management information system that will support a family-focused, community-based model of services.

## Developing Family Advocacy and Support

The Foundation places a high value on the involvement of family members in all aspects of this Initiative, from the initial planning through the design of service systems and the evaluation. The Foundation has awarded a grant to the Federation of Families for Children's Mental Health to provide technical assistance to states and communities to develop family support networks in the demonstration communities. The Federation is a national, parent-run organization dedicated to improving research, training, services, and policies that pertain to children with emotional, behavioral, and mental disorders, and to support their families. The Federation is working with the states and communities so that they can assist families in becoming aware of the concept of family-centered services and approaches, enable families to advocate for family-centered services and approaches, enhance the ability of families to provide ongoing support for each other through local support groups, provide information to families to improve their abilities to access resources, and enable families to identify their strengths and decide what support and services will enhance those strengths.

## Evaluation of the Mental Health Initiative

A comprehensive, independent evaluation is being conducted by the Florida Mental Health Institute of the University of South Florida, and with input and participation from each of the sites, will quantitatively and qualitatively describe the Initiative and measure outcomes. The primary focus for the implementation evaluations will be on the specific strategies selected at the sites to achieve their goals, the rationale for the selection of these strategies, and the manner in which these strategies are employed. The role of the neighborhood governance structures also will be closely examined. In examining outcomes, the evaluation will focus on a series of questions about changes in patterns of service delivery, changes in patterns of expenditures, and impact on the children and families living in the project sites.

# Summary

In summary, a model of providing comprehensive services to troubled youth that are community and neighborhood based is emerging in the children's field. The CASSP model, the system of care, is being implemented at sites across the country through the effort of the federal government, state governments, and private foundations. The latest and possibly most unique effort in this area is the Annie E. Casey Foundation's Mental Health Initiative for Urban Children. The intent of this initiative is to promote and protect the emotional well-being and behavioral health of all children and their families, not just to prevent or treat mental illness.

Initial research results are beginning to document the success of providing comprehensive services to children that are community-based and individualized. As noted by Knitzer (1993), there have been gains in the service delivery system for youth; however, these gains are "fragile, and a second generation of reform is needed to ensure their survival and spread" (p. 14).

# References

Beachler M: The Mental Health Services Program for Youth. Journal of Mental Health Administration 17:115–121, 1990

Behar LB, Macbeth G, Holland JM: Distribution and costs of mental health services within a system of care for children and adolescents. Administration and Policy in Mental Health 20:283–295, 1993

Bickman L: Evaluation and research issues surrounding systems of care for children and families. Paper presented at the 6th Annual Research Conference on Children's Mental Health Services, Tampa, FL, March 1993

Brandenburg NA, Friedman RM, Silver SE: The epidemiology of childhood psychiatric disorders: prevalence findings from recent studies. J Am Acad Child Adolesc Psychiatry 29:76–83, 1990

Cross T, Fallon T, Gardner J, et al: Evaluation of the Robert Wood Johnson Foundation Mental Health Services for Youth Program, in the Fifth Annual Conference Proceedings, A System of Care for Children's Mental Health: Expanding the Research Base. Edited by Alagrin A, Friedman RM. Tampa, FL, Research and Training Center for Children's Mental Health, Florida Mental Health Institute, University of South Florida, 1993, pp 177–187

Cullinan D, Epstein MH, Sabornie EJ: Selected characteristics of a national sample of seriously emotionally disturbed adolescents. Behavior Disorders 17:273–280, 1992

Day C, Roberts M: Activities of the child and adolescent service system program for improving mental health services for children and families. Journal of Clinical Child Psychology 20:340–350, 1991

England MJ, Cole RF: Building systems of care for youth with serious mental illness. Hosp Community Psychiatry 43:630–633, 1992

Goldman S: Ventura County, California, in Profiles of Local Systems of Care for Children and Adolescents with Severe Emotional Disturbances. Edited by Stroul B, Goldman S, Lourie I, et al. Washington, DC, Georgetown University Child Development Center, CASSP Technical Assistance Center, 1992, pp 287–338

Gould MS, Wunsch-Hitzig R, Dohrenwend BP: Formulation of hypotheses about the prevalence, treatment, and prognostic significance of psychiatric disorders in the United States, in Mental Illness in the United States. Edited by Dohrenwend B. New York, Praeger, 1980, pp 9–44

Greenbaum PE, Prange ME, Friedman RM, et al: Substance abuse prevalence and comorbidity with other psychiatric disorders among adolescents with severe emotional disturbances. J Am Acad Child Adolesc Psychiatry 30:575–583, 1991

Heflinger CA, Bickman L, Lane T, et al: The Fort Bragg Child and Adolescent Demonstration: implementing and evaluating a continuum of care, in The Fourth Annual Conference Proceedings, A System of Care for Children's Mental Health: Expanding the Research Base. Edited by Alagarin A, Friedman RM. Tampa, FL, Research and Training Center for Children's Mental Health, Florida Mental Health Institute, University of South Florida, 1992, pp 87–96

Jordan DD, Hernandez M: The Ventura Planning Model: a proposal for mental health reform. Journal of Mental Health Administration 17:26–47, 1990

Knitzer J: Children's mental health policy: challenging the future. Journal of Emotional and Behavioral Disorders 1:8–16, 1993

Lourie IS, Katz-Leavy J: Severely emotionally disturbed children and adolescents, in The Chronic Mental Patient, Vol II. Edited by Menninger WW, Hannah GT. Washington, DC, American Psychiatric Press, 1987, pp 159–187

Macbeth G: Collaboration can be elusive: Virginia's experience in developing an interagency system of care. Administration and Policy in Mental Health 20:259–282, 1993

Offord DR, Boyle MH, Racine Y: Ontario Child Health Study: correlates of disorder. J Am Acad Child Adolesc Psychiatry 28:856–860, 1989

Peschel E, Peschel R, Howe C, et al: Neurobiological Disorders in Children and Adolescents. San Francisco, CA, Jossey-Bass, 1992

Rosenblatt A, Attkisson C: Integrating systems of care in California for youth with severe emotional disturbance, I: a descriptive overview of the California AB377 evaluation project. Journal of Child and Family Studies 1:93–113, 1992

Rosenblatt A, Attkisson C, Fernandez A: Integrating systems of care in California for youth with severe emotional disturbance, II: initial group home expenditure and utilization finding from the California AB377 evaluation project. Journal of Child and Family Studies 1:263–286, 1992

Silver SE, Duchnowski AJ, Kutash K, et al: A comparison of children with serious emotional disturbance served in residential and school settings. Journal of Child and Family Studies 1:43–59, 1992

Stroul BA, Friedman R: A System of Care for Severely Emotionally Disturbed Children and Youth. Washington, DC, Georgetown University Child Development Center, CASSP Technical Assistance Center, 1986

Wagner M, D'Amico R, Marder C, et al: What Happens Next? Trends in Postschool Outcomes of Youth with Disabilities: The Second Comprehensive Report from the National Transitional Longitudinal Study of Special Education Students. Menlo Park, CA, SRI International, 1991

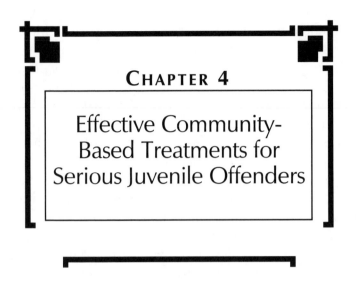

# CHAPTER 4

## Effective Community-Based Treatments for Serious Juvenile Offenders

**Sonja K. Schoenwald, Ph.D., David G. Scherer, Ph.D., and Michael J. Brondino, Ph.D.**

**D**espite decades of social science research and massive expenditures of public sector resources on treatment for juvenile delinquents, serious and violent adolescent offending appears to be on the rise. The Uniform Crime Reports for 1991 (Federal Bureau of Investigation 1992) indicated that juveniles accounted for nearly 29% of the crimes committed in the United States, which was a 7.5% increase over the previous decade. Even more alarming has been the increase in the frequency and savagery of adolescent crime (Kantrowitz 1993; Mulvey et al. 1990). In 1991, juveniles accounted for more than 17% of

Preparation was supported in part by Grant R01DA08029-01 from the National Institute on Drug Abuse (NIDA) to the Medical University of South Carolina and by Grant 5HD5SM48136 from the Center for Mental Health Services, Substance Abuse and Mental Health Services Administration, to the South Carolina Department of Mental Health.

the violent crime arrests that occurred in the United States (Federal Bureau of Investigation 1992).

The majority of the violent and serious crimes perpetrated by juveniles, however, are committed by a small percentage of delinquents (Farrington 1987; Henggeler 1989; Mulvey et al. 1990). They and their families account for disproportionate amounts of the crime in their communities. These chronic and serious offenders are considered to be the "deep end" of the delinquent population (Blaske et al. 1989; Henggeler 1989). The public service systems charged with their care—juvenile justice, child mental health, and child welfare—and the treatments typically delivered by them have failed to address the needs of these youths and their families, and, by extension, their victims and communities. In this chapter we focus on treatment and service-system innovations that have demonstrated clinical and cost effectiveness with this population. Emphasis is placed on treatments that have been subjected to controlled clinical trials. Models of service delivery that appear to hold promise for this population are also described, and issues related to their evaluation are discussed.

Although a heavy intellectual debt is owed to many contributors to the extensive literature on delinquency treatment that preceded current developments, space constraints preclude discussion of their work. Therefore, the reader is referred to reviews and meta-analyses that highlight the major developments in that literature over the last two decades (e.g., Andrews et al. 1990; Basta and Davidson 1988; Gendreau and Ross 1987; Gordon and Arbuthnot 1987; Greenwood and Zimring 1985; Mulvey et al. 1990). Recently completed meta-analyses have clarified critical methodological and treatment characteristics associated with the differential treatment effects reported in the literature (Lipsey 1992). The innovations described in this chapter embody many of these characteristics.

To wit, the results of Lipsey's analysis suggest that multimodal behavioral treatment programs and treatments that led to involvement with prosocial peers reduced recidivism an average of 10% relative to the control-group baseline, although the effect size varied greatly across studies. Traditional counseling and case work, special school classes and tutoring programs, and deterrence-based programs (e.g., shock incarceration, "boot camps") had no, or even negative, effects. Thus, the modalities most often used in community settings (e.g., individual counseling) and those that reflect political strategies to "get tough on crime" (e.g., boot camps) are either ineffective, or have negative treatment effects (Lipsey 1992). Moreover, such strategies are not cost effective. Boot camps, for example, are as or more expensive than other institutional placements (training schools, residential treatment centers, incarceration) and cost much more than even the most intensive probation programs (MacKenzie and Parent 1992).

The failure of these individually oriented approaches to have an impact on serious antisocial behavior is not surprising, given the overwhelming evidence demonstrating that antisocial behavior is multidetermined (Henggeler 1991a), encompassing individual, family, peer, school, and neighborhood factors (Elliott et al. 1985; Patterson and Dishion 1985; Simcha-Fagan and Schwartz 1986). Evidence also suggests that interventions focusing solely on family subsystems (e.g., the adolescent or the parents alone) are less effective with multistressed families (see generally Linblad-Goldberg et al. 1988). Indeed, favorable findings from primary and secondary prevention programs (Olweus 1992; Zigler et al. 1992) have confirmed theorists' suggestions (Hammond and Yung 1993; Henggeler 1989; Kazdin et al. 1992) that effective interventions address multiple systems in which youths are embedded and target the known correlates of serious antisocial behavior (for reviews see Henggeler 1991a; Mulvey et al. 1990).

Lipsey's findings also indicated that larger effect sizes were associated with greater treatment intensity (e.g., duration, number of contacts per week, total contact hours) and integrity (researcher involvement in implementation, monitoring of treatment), as would be expected on the basis of the psychotherapy literature (see Kazdin 1991; Scott and Sechrest 1989; Yeaton and Sechrest 1981). Findings from a recently completed meta-analysis of family-based interventions for youthful offenders (Andrews et al. 1993) highlight the importance of treatment integrity.

Those findings suggest that the efficacy of even well-structured, behaviorally oriented family treatments is attenuated when they are not delivered with high integrity (e.g., specificity of model, training and supervision of therapists, monitoring of treatment process, adequate dosage, and availability of printed manuals).

Reviewers have suggested that the effectiveness of researcher-overseen interventions follows from the close links between theories of causality and treatment (Gordon and Arbuthnot 1987; Lipsey 1988) and from the attention to treatment integrity that characterize such interventions (Andrews et al. 1993). However, even well-specified, well-monitored, theoretically driven treatments (e.g., behavioral parent training, cognitive-behavioral therapy, functional family therapy) that have some impact on antisocial behavior (e.g., Bank et al. 1991; Gordon et al. 1988; Guerra and Slaby 1990; Kazdin et al. 1992) may not sustain long-term effects. There are two major reasons why this might be the case. One is that the treatment theory is too narrowly focused (Henggeler 1991a; Kazdin et al. 1992; Scott and Sechrest 1989). The second is that treatments are not tested with the more seriously troubled youths typically treated in community clinical settings (Weisz and Weiss 1989; Weisz et al. 1992).

The lack of evidence for longer-term effects has led some to conclude that "seriously delinquent youths can be maintained in their communities only as long as their social environment is carefully designed to provide them with structured support and supervision" (Chamberlain 1990, p 33). This observation anticipates the lessons learned from the clinical trials of innovative treatments described in this chapter: in order to be effective over time, interventions must enhance the capacities of multiple aspects of the social environment to provide needed structure, support, and supervision on an ongoing basis.

## Treatment Innovations

### Multisystemic Treatment (MST)

Evidence from clinical trials of multisystemic therapy (MST; Henggeler and Borduin 1990) support this contention. MST has demonstrated both short- and long-term efficacy in controlled clinical trials with confirmed serious, chronic, and violent offenders (Borduin et al. 1995; Henggeler et al. 1986, 1992, 1993). MST is an intensive, time-limited treatment approach predicated on family systems and socio-ecological (Bronfenbrenner 1979) models of behavior, and is informed by findings from causal modeling studies that explicate the multidetermined nature of delinquency in general (Elliott et al. 1985; Patterson and Dishion 1985; Simcha-Fagan and Schwartz 1986). Thus, interventions target the family, peer, school, and neighborhood in which the youth is embedded, as well as the relations between these systems (Henggeler 1991b; Henggeler and Borduin 1990).

Consistent with the family preservation model of service delivery (for a review, see Nelson and Landsman 1992), MST is intensive, pragmatic, and delivered in home and community settings to increase cooperation and to enhance generalization (Henggeler and Borduin 1995). Families are viewed as valuable treatment resources, even when they are characterized by serious and multiple needs. Thus, MST interventions are designed to empower parents and youths to address the developmental, academic, social, and situational challenges that arise throughout adolescence. Problems and treatment goals are specified conjointly by family members and the therapist. Within the context of support and skill building, the therapist places developmentally appropriate demands on the adolescent and family for responsible behavior. Family interventions address the disciplinary, communications, and affective problems shown to characterize families of delinquents (e.g., high rates of conflict, low levels of affection, and inadequate parental monitoring). Peer intervention strategies are designed to enable parents and youths to minimize the youth's antisocial peer contact and maximize affiliation with prosocial peers and activities. School interventions are designed to coordinate the efforts of school personnel and parents to improve an adolescent's behavioral and academic performance.

A variety of therapeutic modalities are used to reach these goals, including strategic family therapy (Haley 1976), structural family therapy (Minuchin 1974), behavioral parent training (Patterson 1979), cognitive behavioral and social skills training (Kendall and Braswell 1985), and effective community consultation techniques. Treatment sessions focus on facilitating attainment of goals that were defined conjointly by family members and the therapist. Emphasis is placed on efficient use of treatment sessions, each typically lasting 30–75 minutes, concluding with the assignment of explicit tasks related to identified goals. Sessions are held as often as every day in the early phases of treatment and as infrequently as once a week later in treatment.

Findings from controlled clinical trials comparing family preservation using MST with the usual services provided for juvenile offenders indicate that MST is more effective with respect to ultimate outcomes such as official and self-reported offenses (Henggeler et al. 1986, 1992) and drug use (Henggeler et al. 1991) and with respect to instrumental outcomes, such as family warmth, cohesion, association with delinquent peers, and aggressive behavior with peers (Borduin et al. 1995; Henggeler et al. 1986) that are believed to facilitate the attainment of such outcomes. Moreover, these gains are sustained over time, as evidenced by the favorable results of MST obtained in 2-year (Henggeler et al. 1993) and 4-year (Borduin et al. 1995) follow-up studies.

## Adventure Programming With Families

Like MST, adventure programming with families, a variant of wilderness therapy (Kelly and Baer 1978; Stewart 1978), changes the contexts in which families operate. In contrast with MST, however, adventure programming accomplishes this by temporarily removing the family from those contexts. This approach has recently demonstrated small treatment effects (Bandoroff and Scherer 1994; Clapp and Rudolph 1990). Wilderness therapies feature experiential learning (e.g., Skipper 1974; Zwart 1988), high arousal (Kelly and Baer 1968), and physical and emotional stresses thought to challenge the maladaptive social behaviors of problem youths (Kelly and Baer 1971; Zwart 1988) and their families in a context that emphasizes the necessity of working cooperatively within a society, and that provides around-the-clock opportunities to develop trust, effective communication, and problem-solving skills.

The bulk of the research on wilderness therapy suggests that such programs change attitudes and self-perceptions more readily than behaviors (Burton 1981; Gaar 1981; Stewart 1978). Because the variant that involved families demonstrated small treatment effects, however, it warrants further investigation. Clinical trials are needed to determine whether changes are maintained when the family returns to the community, and whether they are effective with serious offenders and their multiply stressed families.

## Therapeutic Foster Care

Although the two treatments described thus far focus on the offender's natural environment, the fact remains that many youths are ordered to institutional and residential placements for treatment. Indeed, Melton and Spaulding (in press) have noted that the complexity of serious adolescent antisocial behavior has often led to overintervention in the form of restrictive, costly, and ineffective out-of-home placements. Primary among these is institutionalization. A promising alternative to the long-standing practice of institutionalization being evaluated in clinical trials is therapeutic foster care. Therapeutic foster care programs have developed rapidly in recent years (Burns and Friedman 1990). A variety of models have been implemented with juvenile delinquents. In the group home model, several delinquents reside with professionally trained foster parents, and both the foster parents and the other delinquents are believed to facilitate treatment. In the foster family model, individual youths are placed with foster families in which the parents are seen as critical change agents. The advantages of the latter model include the nonrestrictiveness of placement, opportunities for family learning, increased exposure to prosocial peers, lower costs, and the ability of a single program to treat youths with diverse needs (Chamberlain 1990).

Although several models of therapeutic foster care exist (for a review, see Hawkins et al. 1985), experimental evaluations of their efficacy are rare. Recently, however, Patricia Chamberlain at the Oregon Social Learning Center has undertaken an experimental study (youths are randomly assigned to conditions) of the effectiveness of treatment foster care (TFC) and community-based group care (CBGC) with felonious juvenile offenders. The two types of foster care are being evaluated with respect to the quantity and quality of three parenting variables previously correlated with aggressive and antisocial behavior and their remediation (Bank et al. 1991). These are the quality and quantity of adolescent supervision and monitoring, the consistency with which caretakers use well-suited discipline, and the use of strategies to encourage, reinforce, or teach prosocial skills to adolescents.

Preliminary data (Chamberlain 1993) suggest that youths in the TFC condition experience more adult monitoring, supervision, and discipline relative to youths in the CBGC condition. Immediate and follow-up data will be available with respect to official and self-reported delinquency (ultimate outcomes) and with respect to the parent variables (e.g., monitoring, consistent and appropriate discipline, and induction into prosocial activity) thought to mediate delinquency.

One question raised by these promising findings is whether the training and support offered foster parents in this program would also benefit the biological parents of serious offenders. To this end, the results of a post-hoc comparison of treatment foster care and usual services conducted by Chamberlain (1990) may be instructive. In that study of 16 serious offenders, family therapy was also provided to 10 biological families, although it is not clear that these parents received the same systematic training and treatment program offered to the foster parents. Youths whose parents received family therapy did not fare better with respect to further incarceration than youths whose parents did not receive family therapy. Methodological problems with this study, however (i.e., post-hoc comparison, small sample size, and unclear specification of treatment offered biological families), may account for this finding. Thus, it is not known whether parents of juvenile offenders would benefit from the training and treatment provided to foster parents. Indeed, little appears to be known about the characteristics of, and services that would benefit, the biological parents of children in therapeutic foster placements in general (Thomlison 1993).

## Service System Innovations

In the 14 years since Jane Knitzer's landmark report on the nation's failure to serve the mental health and educational needs of youth (Knitzer 1982), reforms designed to increase the accessibility, array, cost-effectiveness, and coordination of services have been undertaken in all three public systems—child welfare, mental health, and juvenile justice—that serve youths and their families (see Burns and Friedman 1990). As a result, three models of community-based service delivery—family preservation, individualized care, and intensive case management—have been implemented with juvenile offenders in several states, resulting in substantial cost savings relative to institutional and residential programs (City of New York, Department of Juvenile Justice 1992; Jordan and Hernandez 1990). Moreover, placement in restrictive settings has been postponed for youths receiving services via the family preservation (Nelson and Landsman 1992; Wells and Biegel 1991) and individualized-care models of service delivery (Burchard and Clarke 1990). Because rigorous evaluations of these innovations have only recently begun, evidence regarding their impact on serious antisocial behavior is not available for most of them. In the absence of such evidence, placement rate data have historically been considered indirect evidence for the efficacy of these community-based programs.

### Family Preservation

Studies comparing placement rates have been conducted with samples that combine child welfare, mental health, and juvenile offender (but not serious offender) populations (AuClaire and Schwartz 1986; Haapala and Kinney 1988; Schwartz et al. 1991).

Findings suggest that family preservation services were associated with shorter-term placements and fewer days in placement, but not with number of placements. One study that used random assignment of families to family preservation versus standard community services (Feldman 1991) found better placement results for family preservation at 3, 6, and 9 months after treatment, but by 12 months, treatment effects had dissipated. Again, however, the sample was heterogeneous, and juvenile delinquents were combined with the out-of-control cases that made up 59% of the sample.

A variety of family preservation programs have been used specifically with juvenile offenders in several states. In reviewing these programs, Nelson and Landsman (1992) have identified program and family characteristics associated with the subsequent placement, but comparisons of recidivism and placement rates of the youths receiving family preservation services relative to those receiving usual services are not available. Since that review was published, the City and State of New York have instituted the Family Ties program for juvenile offenders (City of New York, Department of Juvenile Justice 1992). The program is based on the Homebuilders model of family preservation (Haapala and Kinney 1979). This model is a short-term (4- to 6-week), crisis-oriented program, which has been widely used with families facing imminent removal of a child due to neglect or abuse, but its efficacy has not yet been evaluated in controlled clinical trials. Data on placement and rearrest up to 1 year after treatment suggest that the impact of Family Ties is greatest in the first 3–6 months after service. Again, however, conclusions about its clinical effectiveness cannot be drawn in the absence of data from a comparison group. Cost savings data were unequivocal, however: the City and State of New York each saved $35,000 for each placement averted by enrollment in Family Ties.

## Individualized Care

An often-cited demonstration of individualized care is the Alaska Youth Initiative. After 2 years of individualized care, almost all youths, including juvenile offenders who had previously been housed in residential treatment programs outside of the state of Alaska, were in less restrictive programs within the state (Burchard and Clarke 1990). The Ventura Planning Model is also consistent with the model of individualized care, in which a single team or subsystem tailors a full array of mental health services to the needs of a particular child and family and coordinates educational and community services to the same end. Data available in 1990 indicated that 85% of those treated by intensive in-home services remained at home at least 6 months. Although a significant reduction in recidivism was obtained (episodes down 22%), the number of days incarcerated increased when youths were rearrested, as judges apparently meted out longer sentences for recidivists (Jordan and Hernandez 1990).

## Intensive Case Management

Intensive case management is the cornerstone of the Willie M. program developed in North Carolina in response to a class action suit on behalf of seriously emotionally, neurologically, or mentally handicapped youth who are violent or assaultive. Each Willie M. youth is assigned a trained case manager who works with a clinical and educational treatment team to determine that youth's needs and arrange for an array of services to target those needs (Weisz et al. 1990). Weisz and his colleagues devised a methodology for indirectly testing the effectiveness of this program; short-term and long-term participants were compared with respect to time to rearrest. The indirect test was necessary because the legislative mandate for Willie M. services precludes the availability of an appropriate comparison group (as all members of such a group would be mandated to receive Willie M. services). Results did not provide strong evidence that receipt of Willie M. services significantly reduces the risk of later arrest among violent and assaultive youth. In discussing these results, the authors noted that one possible explanation for their findings is that, although individualized case management is reasonable in theory, its effectiveness depends on the extent to which a case manager has an array of effective services from which to choose. This observation anticipates a potential pitfall in service system reform, namely, that providing increased access and variety will be perceived as a proxy for efficacy (Henggeler et al. 1994). It seems logical to conclude that the value of increased services is only as great as the efficacy of the services provided.

## Conclusions

Although recently completed meta-analyses suggest that some types of treatment (e.g., well-structured, behaviorally focused, researcher-overseen) have some effect on some delinquents, reviewers of delinquency treatments (Andrews et al. 1992; Hoge et al. 1993) and of the child and adolescent psychotherapy research (Weisz et al. 1992), have concluded that even those elements of effective service identified in research literatures are seldom well-represented in routine practice. A combination of theoretical, methodological, and service system factors have hampered the development and dissemination of clinically effective treatment programs for serious juvenile offenders. Some factors discussed in this chapter include limitations in treatment focus and specification, problems with evaluation methods, and differences between the youths served in research and "real world" settings.

The treatment approaches described in this chapter have successfully addressed many of these limitations. Moreover, in most cases (Adventure Programming with Families notwithstanding), treatment occurs within the context of community-based models that have demonstrated cost-effectiveness. The favorable clinical and cost-effectiveness findings reviewed in this chapter are testimony to the benefits of integrating the strengths of good treatment research with the principles and goals underlying mental health services reform. That is, interventions that are empirically based, directed toward multiple contexts, tested with "deep end" offenders, and rigorously evaluated should inform service system efforts to develop appropriate, accessible, comprehensive, and coordinated child- and family-focused services. Similarly, the needs of these offenders and their families, and of the service systems charged with their care, should inform researchers' efforts to develop community-based interventions that have lasting effects.

# References

Andrews DA, Zinger I, Hoge RD, et al: Does correctional treatment work? A clinically relevant and psychologically informed meta-analysis. Criminology 28:369–404, 1990

Andrews DA, Leschied AW, Hoge RD: Review of the profile, classification and treatment literature with young offenders: a social-psychological approach. Toronto, Canada, Ministry of Community and Social Services, 1992

Andrews DA, Gordon DA, Hill J, et al: Program integrity, methodology, and treatment characteristics: a meta-analysis of effects of family intervention with young offenders. Paper presented at the annual meeting of the American Society of Criminology, Phoenix, AZ, October 1993

AuClaire P, Schwartz IM: An evaluation of the effectiveness of intensive home-based services as an alternative to placement for adolescents and their families. Minneapolis, Hubert H. Humphrey Institute of Public Affairs, University of Minnesota, 1986

Bandoroff S, Scherer DG: Wilderness Family Therapy: an innovative treatment approach for problem youth. Journal of Child and Family Studies 3:175–191, 1994

Bank L, Marlowe JH, Reid JB, et al: A comparative evaluation of parent-training interventions for families of chronic delinquents. J Abnorm Child Psychol 19:15–33, 1991

Basta JM, Davidson WS: Treatment of juvenile offenders: study outcomes since 1980. Behavioral Sciences and the Law 6:355–384, 1988

Blaske DM, Borduin CM, Henggeler SW, et al: Individual, family, and peer characteristics of adolescent sex offenders and assaultive offenders. Developmental Psychology 25:846–855, 1989

Borduin CM, Mann BJ, Cone L, et al: Multisystemic treatment of serious juvenile offenders: long-term prevention of criminality and violence. J Consult Clin Psychol 63:569–578, 1995

Bronfenbrenner U: The Ecology of Human Development: Experiences by Nature and Design. Cambridge, MA, Harvard University Press, 1979

Burchard JD, Clarke RT: The role of individualized care in a service delivery system for children and adolescents with severely maladjusted behavior. Journal of Mental Health Administration 17:48–60, 1990

Burns BJ, Friedman R: Examining the research base for child mental health services and policy. Journal of Mental Health Administration 17:87–97, 1990

Burton L: A critical analysis and review of research on Outward Bound and related programs (doctoral dissertation, Rutgers University). Dissertation Abstracts International 42:1581B, 1981

Chamberlain P: Comparative evaluation of specialized foster care for seriously delinquent youth: a first step. Community Alternatives: International Journal of Family Care 2:21–36, 1990

Chamberlain P: Mediators of male delinquency: preliminary findings from a clinical trial. Paper presented at the annual meeting of the Foster Family Based Treatment Association, Chicago, IL, August 1993

City of New York, Department of Juvenile Justice: Family Ties: The First Eighteen Months. New York, City of New York, Department of Juvenile Justice, 1992

Clapp C, Rudolph S: The Family Challenge Program, in Proceedings Journal of the 18th Annual AEE Conference. Edited by Flor R. Boulder, CO, Association for Experiential Education, 1990, pp 87–89

Elliott DS, Huizinga D, Ageton SS: Explaining Delinquency and Drug Use. Beverly Hills, CA, Sage, 1985

Farrington DP: Early precursors of frequent offending, in From Children to Citizens, Vol. 3: Families, Schools, and Delinquency Prevention. Edited by Wilson JQ, Loury GC. New York, Springer-Verlag, 1987, pp 27–50

Federal Bureau of Investigation, U.S. Department of Justice: Uniform Crime Reports. Washington, DC, Federal Bureau of Investigation, U.S. Department of Justice, 1992

Feldman LH: Evaluating the impact of intensive family preservation services in New Jersey, in Family Preservation Services Research and Evaluation. Edited by Wells K, Biegel DE. Newbury Park, CA, Sage, 1991, pp 47–71

Gaar L: Interpersonal interaction in youth offenders during a therapeutic wilderness experience: a social learning perspective. Unpublished doctoral dissertation, Emory University, Atlanta, GA [Dissertation Abstracts International 42:2055B, 1981]

Gendreau P, Ross RR: Revivication of rehabilitation: evidence from the 1980s. Justice Quarterly 4:348–407, 1987

Gordon DA, Arbuthnot J: Individual, group, and family interventions, in Handbook of Juvenile Delinquency. Edited by Quay HC. New York, Wiley, 1987

Gordon DA, Arbuthnot J, Gustafson KE, et al: Home-based behavioral-systems family therapy with disadvantaged juvenile delinquents. The American Journal of Family Therapy 16:243–255, 1988

Greenwood RW, Zimring FE: One More Chance: The Pursuit of Promising Strategies for Chronic Criminal Offenders. Santa Monica, CA, Rand Corporation, 1985

Guerra NG, Slaby RG: Cognitive mediators of aggression in adolescent offenders, 2: intervention. Developmental Psychology 26:269–277, 1990

Haapala D, Kinney J: Homebuilders approach to the training of in-home therapists, in Home-based Services for Children and Families. Edited by Maybanks S, Bryce M. Springfield, IL, Charles C. Thomas, 1979, pp 248–259

Haapala D, Kinney J: Avoiding out-of-home placement of high-risk status offenders through the use of intensive home-based family preservation services. Criminal Justice and Behavior 15:334–348, 1988

Haley J: Problem Solving Therapy. San Francisco, CA, Jossey-Bass, 1976

Hammond WR, Yung B: Psychology's role in the public health response to assaultive violence among young African-American men. Am Psychol 48:142–154, 1993

Hawkins RP, Meadowcroft P, Trout BA, et al: Foster family based treatment. Journal of Clinical Child Psychology 14:220–228, 1985

Henggeler SW: Delinquency in Adolescence. Newbury Park, CA, Sage, 1989

Henggeler SW: Multidimensional causal models of delinquent behavior and their implications for treatment, in Context and Development. Edited by Cohen R, Siegel AW. Hillsdale, NJ, Lawrence Erlbaum Associates, 1991a, pp 211–231

Henggeler SW: Treating Conduct Problems in Children and Adolescents: An Overview of the Multisystemic Approach with Guidelines for Intervention Design and Implementation. Columbia, SC, South Carolina Department of Mental Health, 1991b

Henggeler SW, Borduin CM: Family Therapy and Beyond: A Multisystemic Approach to Treating the Behavior Problems of Children and Adolescents. Pacific Grove, CA, Brooks/Cole, 1990

Henggeler SW, Borduin CM: Multisystemic treatment of serious juvenile offenders and their families, in Family and Home-Based Services. Edited by Schwartz IM. Lincoln, University of Nebraska Press, 1995, 113–130

Henggeler SW, Rodick JD, Borduin CM, et al: Multisystemic treatment of juvenile offenders: effects on adolescent behavior and family interaction. Developmental Psychology 22:132–141, 1986

Henggeler SW, Borduin CM, Melton GB, et al: Effects of multisystemic therapy on drug use and abuse in serious juvenile offenders: a progress report from two outcome studies. Family Dynamics of Addiction Quarterly 1:40–51, 1991

Henggeler SW, Melton GB, Smith LA: Family preservation using multisystemic therapy: an effective alternative to incarcerating serious juvenile offenders. J Consult Clin Psychol 60:953–961, 1992

Henggeler SW, Melton GB, Smith LA, et al: Family preservation using multisystemic treatment: long-term follow-up to a clinical trial with serious juvenile offenders. Journal of Child and Family Studies 2:283–293, 1993

Henggeler SW, Schoenwald SK, Pickrel SG, et al: The contribution of treatment outcome research to the reform of children's mental health services: multisystemic therapy as an example. Journal of Mental Health Administration 21:229–240, 1994

Hoge RD, Leschied AW, Andrews DA: The repeat offender project: a survey of programs for young offenders. An unpublished report to the Ontario Ministry of Community and Social Services, 1993

Jordan DD, Hernandez M: The Ventura Planning Model: a proposal for mental health reform. Journal of Mental Health Administration 17:26–47, 1990

Kantrowitz B: Teen violence—wild in the streets. Newsweek 122:40–46, 1993

Kazdin AE: Effectiveness of psychotherapy with children and adolescents. J Consult Clin Psychol 59:785–798, 1991

Kazdin AE, Siegel TC, Bass D: Cognitive problem-solving skills training and parent management training in the treatment of antisocial behavior in children. J Consult Clin Psychol 60:733–747, 1992

Kelly F, Baer D: Outward Bound: an alternative to institutionalization for adolescent delinquent boys. New York, Fandel Press, 1968

Kelly F, Baer D: Physical challenge as treatment for delinquency. Crime and Delinquency 17:433–445, 1971

Kendall PC, Braswell L: Cognitive-Behavioral Therapy for Impulsive Children. New York, Guilford, 1985

Knitzer J: Unclaimed Children: The Failure of Public Responsibility to Children and Adolescents in Need of Mental Health Services. Washington, DC, Children's Defense Fund, 1982

Linblad-Goldberg M, Dukes JL, Lasley JH: Stress in Black, low-income, single-parent families: normative and dysfunctional families. Am J Orthopsychiatry 58:104–120, 1988

Lipsey MW: Juvenile delinquency intervention, in Lessons From Selected Program and Policy Areas: New Directions for Program Evaluation. Edited by Bloom HS, Cordray DS, Light RJ. San Francisco, CA, Jossey-Bass, 1988, pp 63–84

Lipsey MW: The effects of treatment on juvenile delinquents: results from meta-analysis. Paper presented at the NIMH Meeting for Research to Prevent Youth Violence, Bethesda, MD, November 1992

MacKenzie DL, Parent DG: Boot camp prisons for young offenders, in Smart Sentencing: The Emergence of Intermediate Sanctions. Edited by Byrne JM, Lurigio AJ, Petersilia J. Newbury Park, CA, Sage, 1992, pp 103–119

Melton GB, Spaulding WJ: No Place To Go: Civil Commitment of Minors. Lincoln, University of Nebraska Press, in press

Minuchin S: Families and Family Therapy. Cambridge, MA, Harvard University Press, 1974

Mulvey EP, Arthur MA, Reppucci ND: Review of programs for the prevention and treatment of delinquency. Washington, DC, Office of Technology Assessment, U.S. Government Printing Office, 1990

Nelson KE, Landsman MJ: Alternative Models of Family Preservation: Family Based Services in Context. Springfield, IL, Charles Thomas, 1992

Olweus D: Bullying among schoolchildren: intervention and prevention, in Aggression and Violence Throughout the Life Span. Edited by Peters R DeV, McMahon RJ, Quinsey VL. Newbury Park, CA, Sage, 1992, pp 100–125

Patterson GR: Living With Children. Champaign, IL, Research Press, 1979

Patterson GR, Dishion TJ: Contributions of families and peers to delinquency. Criminology 23: 63–79, 1985

Schwartz IM, AuClaire P, Harris LJ: Family preservation services as an alternative to the out-of-home placement of adolescents: the Hennepin County experience, in Family Preservation Services Research and Evaluation. Edited by Wells K, Biegel DE. Newbury Park, CA, Sage, 1991, pp 33–47

Scott AG, Sechrest LB: Strength of theory and theory of strength. Evaluation and Program Planning 12:329–366, 1989

Simcha-Fagan O, Schwartz JE: Neighborhood and delinquency: an assessment of contextual effects. Criminology 24:667–703, 1986

Skipper K: A comprehensive evaluation of a therapeutic camping intervention for emotionally disturbed boys. Unpublished doctoral dissertation, University of Texas at Austin [Dissertation Abstracts International 35:2814A, 1974]

Stewart M: Effects of the Connecticut Wilderness School on selected personality characteristics and attitudes of troubled youth. Unpublished doctoral dissertation, University of Utah, Salt Lake City [Dissertation Abstracts International 39:3834A, 1978]

Thomlison B: Child, family, and service characteristics associated with placement outcome in treatment foster family care programs. Paper presented at the annual meeting of the Foster Family Based Treatment Association, Chicago, IL, August 1993

Weisz JA, Weiss B: Assessing the effects of clinic-based psychotherapy with children and adolescents. J Consult Clin Psychol 57:741–746, 1989

Weisz JA, Walter BR, Weiss B, et al: Arrests among emotionally disturbed violent and assaultive individuals following minimal versus lengthy intervention through North Carolina's Willie M Program. J Consult Clin Psychol 58:720–728, 1990

Weisz JA, Weiss B, Donenberg GR: The lab versus the clinic. Am Psychol 47:1578–1585, 1992

Wells K, Biegel DE: Family Preservation Services Research and Evaluation. Newbury Park, CA, Sage, 1991

Yeaton WH, Sechrest L: Critical dimensions in the choice and maintenance of successful treatments: strength, integrity, and effectiveness. J Consult Clin Psychol 49:156–167, 1981

Zigler E, Taussig C, Black K: Early childhood intervention: a promising preventative for juvenile delinquency. Am Psychol 47:997–1006, 1992

Zwart T: The effects of a wilderness/adventure program on the self concept, locus of control orientation, and interpersonal behavior of delinquent adolescents (doctoral dissertation, Western Michigan University). Dissertation Abstracts International 49:1709A, 1988

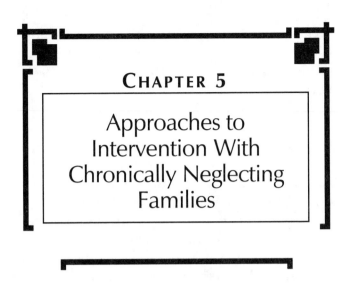

# CHAPTER 5

## Approaches to Intervention With Chronically Neglecting Families

**Kristine Nelson, D.S.W.**

Chronically neglecting families—who are often afflicted by multiple problems, including mental illness in adults and behavior disorders in children—are among the most difficult of families to engage in helping relationships. Ever since the St. Paul project discovered that a small proportion of families consumed a major share of the available resources (Buell 1952), families with multiple problems have been of concern to providers of human services. However, even the most comprehensive treatment programs, designed to reach out and engage families resistant to service involvement, have a lower level of success with child neglect (Berry 1992; Nelson and Landsman 1992; Yuan and Struckman-Johnson 1991).

The finding that family-based services are less effective with families referred to child welfare agencies for neglect than with those referred for physical abuse, sexual abuse, or parent-child conflict has spurred efforts to identify characteristics that differentiate chronically neglecting families from other types of maltreating families and to develop more effective treatment modalities that take these differences into account (DiLeonardi and Johnson 1993; Landsman et al. 1992; Mugridge 1991; Nelson et al. 1993).

# Characteristics

Several characteristics appear to differentiate families with serious and continuing problems that result in child neglect from those involved in other types of maltreatment. Extreme poverty, large families, inadequate housing, unemployment, lower levels of formal education, lack of parenting skills, health and mental health problems, placement, and developmental delay in both children and adults have all been found to be associated with serious neglect (Nelson and Landsman 1992; Nelson et al. 1993).

The most distinctive characteristics of chronically neglecting families—extreme poverty, larger families, multiple problems, and problems in parenting—were identified in one of the first and most comprehensive studies of neglect (Wolock and Horowitz 1979). Poverty and its correlates, low educational levels and high unemployment, have also been documented as characteristic of neglect by other researchers (Giovannoni and Billingsley 1970; Martin and Walters 1982; Nelson et al. 1993; Ory and Earp 1980; Polansky et al. 1972; Zuravin 1988a). In addition, large families with older children and inadequate housing are at higher risk of both neglect and placement in foster care (Giovannoni and Billingsley 1970, Martin and Walters 1982; Nelson and Landsman 1992; Nelson et al. 1993a, 1993b; Ory and Earp 1980; Polansky et al. 1981, 1985a; Zuravin 1988a; Zuravin and Greif 1989).

At the individual level, a lack of parenting knowledge and skills and psychological problems in various forms, including depression and character disorders, have long been associated with neglect (Friedrich et al. 1985; Giovannoni and Billingsley 1970; Herrenkohl et al. 1983; Jones and McNeely 1980; Nelson et al. 1993b; Polansky et al. 1981; Twentyman and Plotkin 1982; Wolock and Horowitz 1979; Zuravin 1988b). Although difficult to measure accurately, substance abuse has also been found to be associated with neglect in several studies (MacMurray 1979; Wolock and Horowitz 1979; Zuravin and Greif 1989).

Earlier findings on social isolation and neglect have not, however, been supported in recent studies (Nelson et al. 1993a, 1993b; Wodarski et al. 1990b) perhaps due to measurement and sampling differences among the studies (Giovannoni and Billingsley 1970; Jones and McNeely 1980; Nelson and Landsman 1992; Polansky et al. 1981, 1985a, 1985b; Wolock and Horowitz 1979; Zuravin and Greif 1989).

## Effects on Children

The impact of neglect on children, reflected in developmental delay in preschool children, low levels of academic achievement, and higher placement rates, is increasingly being documented by research (Nelson et al. 1993a; Paget et al. 1993; Starr and Wolfe 1991). Findings of developmental delay in neglected preschool children (Hoffman-Plotkin and Twentyman 1984; Polansky et al. 1981) have been expanded longitudinally (Erickson et al. 1989) and into the school years (Wodarski et al. 1990a) where neglected children have been found to lag significantly behind their peers in academic achievement (Reyome 1989; Wodarski et al. 1990a). Prior placement has been found in studies of placement prevention programs to be a strong predictor of repeated placement (Fraser et al. 1991; Nelson and Landsman 1992; Yuan and Struckman-Johnson 1991), and repeated placement has been found to exacerbate the effects of neglect on child mental health and behavior (Wodarski et al. 1990b).

# Intervention

Despite the replication of findings about neglect, little progress has been made in treating families with multiple problems. Efforts to identify and to clearly define subtypes of neglect, essential to developing more effective interventions and more sensitive research, are in the early stages of development (Zuravin 1991).

In addition, little is known about ethnically and culturally based variations in neglect. Nonetheless, recent studies and demonstration projects have provided some insight into the treatment of serious neglect.

The multiplicity of problems in chronically neglecting families suggests that a comprehensive, in-home, longer-term service is needed that includes the provision of concrete and paraprofessional services to increase household and parenting skills and informal sources of support (Daro 1988; Gaudin 1988; Howing et al. 1989). Group interventions and family therapy have also been shown to be effective in developing skills, increasing social support, and improving extended family relationships (Cohn and Daro 1987; Daro 1988; Howing et al. 1989).

Researchers caution against relying solely on a narrow educational approach (Daro 1988; Howing et al. 1989). One study tested the efficacy of parent education alone against a multifaceted approach to improving parenting and family relationships (Brunk et al. 1987). Forty-three abusing and neglecting families were randomly assigned to two treatment groups. Both groups received 90-minute weekly therapy sessions for 8 weeks. Parent training took place in clinic-based groups. Multisystemic therapy was provided both in the families' homes and in the clinic. Although both interventions were effective in reducing stress, psychiatric symptomatology, and identified problems, parent training groups were more effective in reducing identified problems and multisystemic therapy was more effective in restructuring parent-child relationships and in changing key behaviors in both parents and children.

A second study examined the effectiveness of social network interventions (Gaudin et al. 1990–1991). Over a 2-year period, 52 neglecting families were randomly assigned to the Social Network Intervention Project and 36 to the usual casework and case management services provided by protective services workers. Families received services—including intensive casework, case management, advocacy, and interventions to strengthen informal network linkages—for 2–23 months (median 10 months). At 6 and 12 months, experimental families had improved significantly more than control families on three measures of parenting adequacy and on the size and supportiveness of their social networks. Families who received at least 9 months of service improved the most. Despite these positive results, workers estimated that almost two-thirds of the families would relapse under stress-producing conditions.

## Motivation

Before any treatment modality can be effective, families must successfully be engaged in services (Dale and Davies 1985; Green et al. 1981; Orenchuk-Tomiuk et al. 1990; Weitzman 1985). Partly a predisposition of the client and partly a product of the success of the worker in engaging the family, motivation and cooperation are key to success in family-based services as well as in other types of therapy.

Motivating neglecting caregivers is a particularly challenging task that is more likely to succeed when comprehensive family-based services, including parent education, transportation, counseling, and paraprofessional services, are provided to families served primarily in their own homes (Ayoub and Jacewitz 1982; Colon 1980; Hartley et al. 1989; Kagan and Schlosberg 1989; Kaplan 1986).

Empowerment-oriented practices, which are fundamental to family-based services, such as encouraging families to set their own goals as well as acknowledging their strengths and instilling hope for positive change, are also supported by psychological research on motivation (Gold 1990; Gutierrez 1990).

However, the provision of comprehensive home-based services, by itself, is insufficient to ensure success. One analysis of 66 families receiving family-based placement prevention services found that, although caregiver attendance at sessions is the most important factor in avoiding placement in cases of child neglect, only 60% of these families were successfully engaged in services (Nelson and Hunter 1993). Of most interest were the 41% of caregivers who increased in motivation over the course of service, according to case readers' ratings of the Child Well-Being Scales

(Magura and Moses 1986). In these scales, motivation is defined as concern about children's needs, confidence that problems can be overcome, and competence in problem solving.

The findings of this study suggested that families who are reluctant to become involved in services are most likely to be engaged by working with them to increase social support and to address school-aged children's behavior problems. A mixture of counseling and concrete services are needed, but merely teaching parenting skills or accompanying the caregiver to other services do not seem to be effective in increasing hopefulness and feelings of capability. Fairly intensive intervention in the first 3 months of service, averaging 7.3 (SD 2.7) home visits a month, followed by another 6 months of maintenance contacts, seemed to be the most effective pattern in increasing family competence while nurturing self-sufficiency (Nelson and Hunter 1993).

## Innovative Demonstration Projects

Several recent demonstration projects have attempted to operationalize the findings of prior research in the treatment of chronically neglecting families.

### The Family Support Center

Drawing on research findings about neglect (summarized by Hartley 1987) and chronic neglect (Nelson et al. 1993b), Mugridge (1991) designed a year-long home-based treatment program for chronically neglecting families. Participating families had at least three referrals for neglect in the prior year, including at least one that resulted in protective supervision. Of the first 12 families in the program, over 75% scored at high risk of child maltreatment on the Adult, Adolescent Parenting Inventory (AAPI) (Bavolek 1984) due to their attitudes toward physical punishment, their inappropriate expectations of children, and reversal of parent-child roles. In addition, 75% had inadequate housekeeping, budgeting, time management, and nutritional knowledge and skills. Over 80% reported incidents of severe, recurring diaper rash and over 60% of the children were behind in their inoculations and had never been to a dentist (Mugridge 1991).

The Family Support Center's model of intervention included skill building, in-home role modeling, parenting classes, and a monthly support group, as well as environmental interventions to improve housing, increase employment, and build social networks. A key element of the intervention was Bavolek's Nurturing Program (Bavolek and Comstock 1983), which teaches parenting skills appropriate for children from birth to 5 years while increasing the self-esteem and self-concept of parents (Mugridge 1991).

A 1-year follow-up of the first 12 families to complete the program found substantial improvement in expectations, empathy, attitudes to physical punishment, and role reversal. In addition, despite an average of 6 founded complaints of neglect per year prior to intervention, there were no new complaints up to 2 years following the program. The elements thought to contribute to the program's success were clear expectations, constant feedback and praise, the encouragement of involvement and hope, decreasing social isolation, and increasing parenting skills. For staff, essential elements were clear expectations, having only 1 chronically neglecting case at a time, 24-hour availability over a 1-year period of time, intensive contact of at least two 2-hour contacts a week, and a sense of accomplishment and recognition (Mugridge 1991).

## Chronic Neglect Consortium Projects

In 1989 the National Center on Child Abuse and Neglect funded six projects to demonstrate different approaches to treating chronic neglect. Although the six projects were located in different parts of the country, provided various kinds of service under different auspices, and served differing populations, they were drawn together in a consortium for the purpose of providing a common evaluation (DiLeonardi and Johnson 1993). Definitions of neglect and recruitment of families for the projects varied, but all projects used a multidisciplinary approach and included services delivered by paraprofessionals. In addition, several included peer support or therapy groups.

As a whole the projects served a primarily Caucasian population, although half the projects included significant numbers of Latino, African-American, or Native-American families as well. All the families were poor and the caregivers averaged less than a high school education. Nearly three-fourths were single parents, although this varied by site. Compared with population statistics for their areas, project families had more children (an average of three), less education, and lower incomes than the average for their communities. Three-quarters had prior referrals for neglect, almost half had had at least one child placed due to neglect, and over three-quarters were assessed as not motivated to change their behavior. In addition, 57% reported a history of drug or alcohol abuse by a caregiver. Over half were rated at high risk of continuing to neglect their children on a risk assessment scale (Baird 1988) developed for the State of Alaska (DiLeonardi and Johnson 1993).

Success was measured by improvement in Childhood Level of Living Scores (CLL) (Polansky et al. 1978), which initially were in the neglectful range for all the projects. Of the three most successful projects, two were operated by private child welfare agencies and one was sponsored by a family service agency. All were in the Midwest. One project worked primarily through groups to provide support and improve parenting; a second provided treatment day care for children, along with parenting, General Education Degree (GED), and job training classes for parents; and the third followed the Nurturing Program model (DiLeonardi and Johnson 1993).

Of the three less successful projects, according to change on the CLL, one was under the auspices of a public child protective services agency, one was in a family service agency, and one was conducted by a community-based agency with an educational focus. All three served diverse populations, including Latino and Native-American families, or families in which neglect was combined with physical or sexual abuse. The lack of change on the CLL may have been due in part to these population differences (DiLeonardi and Johnson 1993).

In most of the sites, positive change on the CLL was related to length of treatment, which averaged 18 months. Although responding families were very positive about the projects and the changes they had been able to make in their lives (separating from an abusive partner, completing a GED), project staff were more pessimistic, citing as barriers to success a lack of motivation on the part of the families or a lack of service resources. In a majority of the cases, staff thought that the chance of a reoccurrence of neglect in the family was at least moderately high (DiLeonardi and Johnson 1993).

## The Self-Sufficiency Project

One of the projects took an empowerment approach, leaving the design of services to the participating families (Landsman et al. 1992). The families, referred by public agency protective service and family workers, scored at high risk of both continued neglect and physical abuse on the Alaska scales (Baird 1988). Over 70% had prior referrals for physical abuse as well as for neglect. Over 75% acknowledged a history of substance abuse and almost all the caregivers reported having been neglected as children. Ninety percent scored at high risk of continued neglect.

The core service of the Self-Sufficiency Project was a series of support and treatment groups for parents and children of differing ages. Transportation was arranged if needed—including transportation of children in placement—and a dinner, which followed the group meetings, was provided by local restaurants. The 4-hour weekly sessions ended with multiple-family group meetings. Families also received support and parent education from a paraprofessional staff member, family therapy, and substance abuse treatment as needed. Families attended an average of 12 group meetings and received an average of 4 hours a month of parent aide services (hours of individual family therapy were not available; Landsman et al. 1992).

Several standardized measures were employed at the outset, with the result that on the Index of Self-Esteem and the Generalized Contentment Scale half the primary caregivers scored in the problem range for self-esteem and 65% scored in the problem range for depression (Hudson 1982). By the end of service there were significant improvements on both of these scales, as well as on the role-reversal subscale of the AAPI (improvement on the empathy subscale approached significance). Only 4 of the 31 families who participated in the project had further confirmed reports of neglect, three of which led to placement. Additional reports of maltreatment included three of sexual abuse and one of physical abuse, none of which resulted in the placement of a child (Landsman et al. 1992).

Families who showed little improvement in the project were those with substance abuse problems, those involved in negative social relationships, and those with subsequent reports of sexual abuse. In addition, families scoring at high risk of continued abuse did less well, indicating that the project, as intended, was of most benefit to families at high risk of continued neglect who were not involved in physical or sexual abuse. Finally, families who entered a group after it had started and those who had to wait for a group to form had lower levels of success (Landsman et al. 1992).

Validating the empowerment approach, families in the first study cohort, who designed the program, were seen by staff as the most successfully engaged. However, families in all three cohorts who stayed with the project longer (an average of 12 months) showed the most change. The final evaluation credited successes to peer support in groups facilitated by skilled therapists. These groups enabled caregivers to work through issues such as neglect in their own childhood, increase their self-esteem, reduce depression, and free energy for their children's needs. Indeed, one of the key recommendations to the evaluators from the parents was the need for more services for children (Landsman et al. 1992).

## Conclusions and Recommendations

These findings indicate that the personal problems of caregivers, including low levels of motivation, which contribute to family instability, lack of support, and neglect (Polansky et al. 1992; Webster-Stratton 1989) may be successfully addressed through a combination of group and individual interventions. However, the individual and family problems that lead to neglect occur in a social context of extreme deprivation. Failure to address the poverty and lack of support with which many of these families contend limits the effectiveness of intervention at the family level. Other programs and policies needed to increase family stability and reduce neglect include substance abuse treatment programs especially designed for low-income mothers with children, greater access to family planning services, and stable employment with remuneration adequate to keep a family out of poverty. Increasing the educational achievement of mothers from deprived backgrounds would help to raise their aspirations and increase self-sufficiency as well.

Finally, parental stress would be reduced and family stability enhanced by programs and policies to improve the quality of housing and neighborhoods of poor families. The availability of adequate housing for large families is particularly important in reducing foster care placement. It is, of course, critical in the design of treatment and prevention programs to attend to cultural variations in child rearing and to recognize the contribution that extended kin and ethnic communities can make in supporting vulnerable families (Cross 1986; Fischler 1985; Gray and Cosgrove 1985; Long 1986; Nelson et al. 1993a; Saunders et al. 1993).

Further research, especially longitudinal study, is needed on differences in etiology and treatment of neglect in ethnic subgroups and on the role of fathers in neglecting families. Studies with more adequate measures of mental illness and intellectual functioning are also needed to further delineate their contribution to neglect. Research on programs to increase empathy for children and understanding of their needs among caregivers from troubled families seems especially important, as does research on the prevention of the child abuse, sexual abuse, neglect, and placements that contribute to the inadequate parenting of the next generation in vulnerable families. Finally, research is needed to identify subtypes of neglect and culturally appropriate instruments to assess neglect and to measure improvement in the many factors that contribute to chronic child neglect.

# References

Ayoub C, Jacewitz MM: Families at risk of poor parenting: a descriptive study of sixty at risk families in a model prevention program. Child Abuse Negl 6:413–422, 1982

Baird C: Development of risk assessment indices for the Alaska Department of Health and Social Services, in Validation Research in CPS Risk Assessment: Three Studies. Edited by Tatara T. Washington, DC, American Public Welfare Association, 1988, pp 85–121

Bavolek S: Handbook for the Adult-Adolescent Parenting Inventory. Schaumburg, IL, Family Development Associates Inc, 1984

Bavolek S, Comstock CM: The Nurturing Program for Parents and Children. Schaumburg, IL, Family Development Associates Inc, 1983

Berry M: An evaluation of family preservation services: fitting agency services to family needs. Social Work 37:314–321, 1992

Brunk M, Henggeler SW, Whelan JB: Comparison of multisystemic therapy and parent training in the brief treatment of child abuse and neglect. J Consult Clin Psychol 55:171–178, 1987

Buell B: Community Planning for Human Services. New York, Columbia University Press, 1952

Cohn AH, Daro D: Is treatment too late: what ten years of evaluative research tell us. Child Abuse Negl 11:433–442, 1987

Colon F: The family life cycle of the multiproblem poor family, in The Family Life Cycle: A Framework for Family Therapy. Edited by Carter E, McGoldrick M. New York, Gardner Press, 1980, pp 343–377

Cross T: Drawing on cultural traditions in Indian child welfare practice. Social Casework 67:283–289, 1986

Dale P, Davies M: A model of intervention in child-abusing families: a wider systems view. Child Abuse Negl 9:449–455, 1985

Daro D: Confronting Child Abuse. New York, Free Press, 1988

DiLeonardi JW, Johnson P: Evaluation of the Chronic Neglect Consortium. Chicago, IL, Children's Home and Aid Society, 1993

Erickson MF, Egeland B, Pianta R: The effects of maltreatment on the development of young children, in Child Maltreatment: Theory and Research on the Causes and Consequences of Child Abuse and Neglect. Edited by Cicchetti D, Carlson V. New York, Cambridge University Press, 1989, pp 647–684

Fischler R: Child abuse and neglect in American Indian communities. Child Abuse Negl 9:95–106, 1985

Fraser MW, Pecora PJ, Haapala DA: Families in Crisis: The Impact of Family Preservation Services. New York, Aldine, 1991

Friedrich WN, Tyler JD, Clark JA: Personality and psychophysiological variables in abusive, neglectful, and low-income control mothers. J Nerv Ment Dis 173:449–460, 1985

Gaudin JM: Treatment of families who neglect their children, in Mental Illness, Delinquency, Addictions, and Neglect: Families in Transition. Edited by Nunnally EW, Chilman CS, Cox FM. Beverly Hills, CA, Sage, 1988

Gaudin JM, Wodarski JS, Arkinson MK, et al: Remedying child neglect: effectiveness of social network interventions. Journal of Applied Social Sciences 15:97–123, 1990-1991

Giovannoni JM, Billingsley A: Child neglect among the poor: a study of parental adequacy in families of three ethnic groups. Child Welfare 49:196–204, 1970

Gold N: Motivation: the crucial but unexplored component of social work practice. Social Work 35:49–56, 1990

Gray E, Cosgrove J: Ethnocentric perception of childrearing practices in protective services. Child Abuse Negl 9:389–396, 1985

Green AH, Power E, Steinbook B, et al: Factors associated with successful and unsuccessful intervention with child abusive families. Child Abuse Negl 5:45–52, 1981

Gutierrez LM: Working with women of color: an empowerment perspective. Social Work 35:149–153, 1990

Hartley R: A Program Blueprint for Neglectful Families. Salem, OR, Children's Services Division, 1987

Hartley R, Showell W, White J: Outcomes of Oregon's family treatment programs: a descriptive study of 1752 families. Paper presented at the Intensive Family Preservation Services Research Conference, Cleveland, OH, September 1989

Herrenkohl RC, Herrenkohl EC, Egolf BP: Circumstances surrounding the occurrence of child maltreatment. J Consult Clin Psychol 51:424–431, 1983

Hoffman-Plotkin D, Twentyman C: A multimodal assessment of cognitive and behavioral deficits in abused and neglected preschoolers. Child Dev 55:794–802, 1984

Howing PT, Wodarski JS, Gaudin JM, et al: Effective interventions to ameliorate the incidence of child maltreatment: the empirical base. Social Work 34:330–338, 1989

Hudson W: The Clinical Measurement Package. Homewood, IL, Dorsey Press, 1982

Jones J, McNeely R: Mothers who neglect and those who do not: a comparative study. Social Casework 61:559–567, 1980

Kagan R, Schlosberg S: Families in Perpetual Crisis. New York, WW Norton, 1989

Kaplan L: Working with Multiproblem Families. Lexington, MA, Lexington Books, 1986

Landsman MJ, Nelson K, Allen M, et al: Family Based Treatment for Chronically Neglecting Families: The Self-Sufficiency Project. Iowa City, IA, National Resource Center on Family Based Services, 1992

Long K: Cultural considerations in the assessment and treatment of interfamilial abuse. Am J Orthopsychiatry 56:131–136, 1986

MacMurray V: The effect and nature of alcohol abuse in cases of child abuse. Victimology: An International Journal 4:29–45, 1979

Magura S, Moses BS: Outcome Measures for Child Welfare Services: Theory and Applications. Washington, DC, Child Welfare League of America, Inc, 1986

Martin MJ, Walters J: Familial correlates of selected types of child abuse and neglect. Journal of Marriage and the Family 44:267–276, 1982

Mugridge GB: Reducing Chronic Neglect. Paper presented at the Ninth National Conference on Child Abuse and Neglect, Denver, CO, September 1991

Nelson K, Hunter R: Empowering families through home-based services. Paper presented at Education and Research for Empowerment Practice: A Working Conference, Seattle, WA, October 1993

Nelson K, Landsman M: Alternative Models of Family Preservation: Family Based Services in Context. Springfield, IL, Charles C Thomas, 1992

Nelson K, Landsman M, Cross T, et al: Family Functioning of Neglectful Families. Iowa City, IA, National Resource Center on Family Based Services, 1993a

Nelson KE, Saunders EJ, Landsman MJ: Chronic child neglect in perspective. Social Work 38:661–671, 1993b

Orenchuk-Tomiuk N, Matthey G, Pigler-Christensen C: The resolution model: a comprehensive treatment framework in sexual abuse. Child Welfare 69:417–431, 1990

Ory M, Earp J: Child maltreatment: an analysis of familial and institutional predictors. Journal of Family Issues 1:339–356, 1980

Paget KD, Philp JD, Abramczyk LW: Recent developments in child neglect, in Advances in Clinical Child Psychology, Vol 15. Edited by Ollendick TH, Prinz RJ. New York, Plenum, 1993, pp 121–174

Polansky NA, Borgman RD, DeSaix C: Roots of Futility. San Francisco, CA, Jossey-Bass, 1972

Polansky NA, Chalmers MA, Buttenweiser E, et al: Assessing adequacy of child caring: an urban scale. Child Welfare 57:439–449, 1978

Polansky NA, Chalmers MA, Buttenweiser E, et al: Damaged Parents: An Anatomy of Neglect. Chicago, IL, University of Chicago Press, 1981

Polansky NA, Ammons PW, Gaudin JM: Loneliness and isolation in child neglect. Social Casework 66:38–47, 1985a

Polansky NA, Gaudin JM, Ammons PW, et al: The psychological ecology of the neglectful mother. Child Abuse Negl 9:265–275, 1985b

Polansky NA, Gaudin JM, Kilpatrick AC: Family radicals. Children and Youth Services Review 14:19–26, 1992

Reyome ND: A comparison of the school performance of sexually abused, neglected, and non-maltreated children. Paper presented at the Eighth National Conference on Child Abuse and Neglect, Salt Lake City, UT, September 1989

Saunders EJ, Nelson K, Landsman MJ: Racial inequality and child neglect: findings in a metropolitan area. Child Welfare 72:341–354, 1993

Starr RH, Wolfe DA: The Effects of Child Abuse and Neglect. New York, Guilford, 1991

Twentyman C, Plotkin R: Unrealistic expectations of parents who maltreat their children: an educational deficit that pertains to child development. J Clin Psychol 38:497–503, 1982

Webster-Stratton C: The relationship of marital support, conflict, and divorce to parent perceptions, behaviors, and childhood conduct problems. Journal of Marriage and the Family 51:417–430, 1989

Weitzman J: Engaging the severely dysfunctional family in treatment: basic considerations. Fam Process 24:473–485, 1985

Wodarski JS, Kurtz PD, Gaudin JM, et al: Maltreatment and the school-aged child: major academic, socioemotional and adaptive outcomes. Social Work 35:506–513, 1990a

Wodarski JS, Kurtz PD, Gaudin JM, et al: Maltreatment and the School-Aged Child: Developmental Outcomes and System Issues. Athens, GA, School of Social Work, The University of Georgia, 1990b

Wolock I, Horowitz B: Child maltreatment and material deprivation among AFDC-recipient families. Social Service Review 53:175–194, 1979

Yuan YT, Struckman-Johnson DL: Placement outcomes for neglected children with prior placements in family preservation programs, in Family Preservation Services: Research and Evaluation. Edited by Wells K, Biegel DA. Newbury Park, CA, Sage, 1991, pp 92–118

Zuravin SJ: Child maltreatment and teenage first births: a relationship mediated by chronic sociodemographic stress. Am J Orthopsychiatry 58:91–103, 1988a

Zuravin SJ: Child abuse, child neglect, and maternal depression: is there a connection? in Child Neglect Monograph: Proceedings from a Symposium. Washington, DC, U.S. Department of Health and Human Services, National Center on Child Abuse and Neglect, 1988b, pp 20–43

Zuravin SJ: Research definitions of child physical abuse and neglect, in The Effects of Child Abuse and Neglect. Edited by Starr RH, Wolfe DA. New York, Guilford, 1991, pp 100–128

Zuravin SJ, Greif GL: Normative and child-maltreating AFDC mothers. Social Casework 70:76–84, 1989

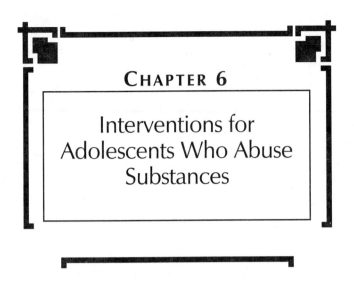

# CHAPTER 6

## Interventions for Adolescents Who Abuse Substances

**Susan G. Pickrel, M.P.H., M.D., James A. Hall, Ph.D., and Phillippe B. Cunningham, Ph.D.**

Adolescent substance abuse represents one of the major health concerns facing our nation (Blau et al. 1988; Matarazzo 1982; Paulson et al. 1990; U.S. Congress, Office of Technology Assessment 1991). Although the overall rate of illicit substance use among American youth has shown an appreciable decline during the 1980s, their rate of use remains the highest among similarly aged youth in the industrialized world (Johnston et al. 1993). For many adolescents, substance use does not become so problematic that their use is labeled drug or alcohol abuse or dependence (Kaminer and Bukstein 1989). The issue of problem definition and who to treat, either with actual clinical treatment or with a prevention intervention, con-

Preparation of this chapter was supported by Grant R01DA08029 from the National Institute on Drug Abuse (NIDA) to the Medical University of South Carolina.

fuses the prevention and treatment picture. This, along with a lack of a common definition of positive treatment outcome, makes an understanding of the success of programs that treat adolescent substance abuse very difficult. In this chapter we delineate the prevalence and consequences of adolescent substance abuse, examine the scope and content of current treatment options, and present research on treatment and prevention of adolescent substance abuse. These topics serve as a springboard for exploring the need for innovative approaches in this area and for the exposition of existing promising new approaches to this difficult problem.

That substance use has reached epidemic proportions among youth in our society is borne out by studies such as the one conducted by the National Institute on Drug Abuse (1992), a nationwide survey of 8th, 10th, and 12th graders, and of college students. This survey found that among 8th graders, 69% had tried alcohol and 27% had been drunk, 45% had tried cigarettes, 34% had used smokeless tobacco, 11% had tried marijuana, 11% had used stimulants, 3.2% had used LSD, 1.6% had tried crack—a particularly dangerous form of cocaine— 2.4% had used other cocaine products, and 1.4% had used heroin. Among older adolescents, 28% of high school seniors reported having 5 or more drinks in the 2 weeks preceding the study, 8.4% of high school seniors had at some time smoked marijuana daily for at least a month, and 2.5% of high school seniors had tried crack.

These numbers are disturbing but fail to provide a complete picture of the drug epidemic among our nation's youth. The survey conducted by the National Institute on Drug Abuse (1992) and other national drug surveys that canvas adolescent school samples measure frequencies in a select, high-functioning group and fail to account for school dropouts (representing 15%–20% of this age cohort), who are more prone to substance abuse than their peers who attend school (Allen et al. 1990; Brown et al. 1990; Johnston et al. 1993). It is clear that substance use is prevalent among both problem and nonproblem American youth.

# Consequences

The short- and long-term consequences of adolescent substance use—physiological, psychological, and social—are considerable. The acute health consequences of alcohol have been well documented (Kandel et al. 1986; Newcomb and Bentler 1988; U.S. Congress, Office of Technology Assessment 1991). These include death in alcohol-related vehicular accidents (3,000 15- to 19-year-olds in 1988), fatal pedestrian and bicycle accidents (35% associated with alcohol use), and adolescent drownings (40% associated with alcohol use) (Howland and Hingson 1988; U.S. Congress, Office of Technology Assessment 1991).

The potential long-term consequences of adolescent substance abuse for later life include criminality and deviant behavior as well as problems with sexual behavior, educational pursuits, livelihood pursuits, mental health, and social integration (Newcomb and Bentler 1988). Longitudinal studies of adolescent substance abusers have found that substance abuse is associated with a number of negative psychosocial outcomes, including divorce and lower educational level (Kandel et al. 1986; Newcomb and Bentler 1988; Robins et al. 1970; Yamaguchi and Kandel 1985). Additionally, the association between drug use and delinquency seems to be well established (Kandel et al. 1986; Newcomb and Bentler 1988).

# Treatment

Adolescent substance abuse as a biopsychosocial problem has been difficult to treat due to a variety of factors. These include the reinforcing nature of drug taking behavior, the developmental fit of drug experimentation with the adolescent individuation process, and the inconsistent societal messages to adolescents about drug use (Catalano et al. 1991; Ungerleider and Siegel 1990). Additionally, services for treating adolescent substance abuse are often poorly defined operationally and are fashioned as stepchildren of adult treatment approaches and systems, with unknown amounts of attention, if any, paid to specializing services to accommodate age, family, socioeconomic, and cultural factors (U.S. Congress, Office of Technology Assessment 1991).

Service systems for treating adolescents with substance abuse are either not present in communities or are often fragmented and overwhelmed. Behar (cited in Friedman 1992) notes that there has been less developmental work on models of systems of care for adolescents with substance abuse problems than for youth with serious emotional problems. Like systems of care for adolescents who are seriously emotionally disturbed, systems of care for adolescents who abuse substances need to be integrated into the national agenda for children's and youths' mental health care adopted from Stroul and Friedman's (1986) landmark document. Treatment programs that fit this agenda address an adolescent's physical, emotional, social, and educational needs with an individualized treatment plan implemented in the least restrictive environment, with coordinated, therapeutic case management, which involves the family as full participants in the planning and delivery of services and is responsive to cultural differences (Stroul and Friedman 1986). The available data about numbers and kinds of treatment services for adolescents indicate that current treatment falls far short of the Stroul and Friedman principles. This gap in treatment is one indication of the need for innovative services.

What is known about treatment services for adolescents who abuse substances comes from several data sources. These include the National Drug and Alcohol Treatment Unit Survey (NDATUS), a 10/30/87 cross-sectional census of public and private treatment programs; the Chemical Abuse Treatment Outcome Research (CATOR) network, a network providing outcome data for private treatment programs; and the Treatment Outcome Prospective Study (TOPS), a prospective study of drug (not alcohol) abuse treatment (U.S. Congress, Office of Technology Assessment 1991). These sources include substance abuse clients of all ages, and data for adolescents are not always broken out. The NDATUS had 22% nonresponders, and reported figures are extrapolated to corrected estimates of numbers of adolescents in treatment. In this survey, 76,000 adolescents under age 18 were in treatment in public and private programs on 10/30/87. From this number, it is estimated that 272,000 adolescents in this broad age group were treated during 1987. Of these, an estimated 157,000 were in drug treatment, and 115,000 were in alcohol treatment. The number of adolescents in drug treatment represented 15% of all ages in drug treatment, and those in alcohol treatment represented only 6% of all ages in alcohol treatment (U.S. Congress, Office of Technology Assessment 1991).

It is interesting to note that, although alcohol is the most frequently abused substance among adolescents, there are more adolescents in drug treatment than in alcohol treatment, and adolescents are proportionately less represented in the alcohol treatment population. Understanding the limitations of the reported data, this may be a by-product of the existence of fewer age-specific alcohol treatment programs. Fifty percent of drug treatment programs for adolescents are age-specific, whereas only 15% of adolescent alcohol treatment programs are age-specific (U.S. Congress, Office of Technology Assessment 1991). Large numbers of our youth are being treated in substance-abuse treatment programs. What are these programs and what treatments do they implement with what outcomes?

Traditional treatment programs for adolescent substance abuse include self-help programs, outpatient treatment, residential programs (including therapeutic communities and halfway houses), inpatient programs, and other types of programs (including drop-in centers) (Kusnetz 1985; U.S. Congress, Office of Technology Assessment 1991). Inpatient and residential treatments are the most expensive and most restrictive, followed by outpatient therapy and self-help programs. Within all of these programs, various treatment techniques are used, including individual counseling, individual psychotherapy, various group approaches, self-support groups (based on the "anonymous" self-help model), family therapy, recreation therapy, and employment counseling. Unfortunately, in many of these programs a "shotgun" approach is used for each adolescent treated, with all treatments (of unknown efficacy) applied in each case without individualizing them to the adolescent's and the family's needs (Kaminer and Bukstein 1989).

## Self-Help Programs

Self-help programs include all of the "Anonymous" 12-step programs, which are often used as an alternative or adjunct to professional treatment for substance abuse (Sunshine and Wright 1988). Alcoholics Anonymous (AA) and Narcotics Anonymous (NA) collect their own data on membership and resist rigorous outside research studies. Their surveys show that in 1986, 47,000 of the 1 million AA members and 18,000 NA members were under 20 years old (U.S. Congress, Office of Technology Assessment 1991). The AA/NA approach has the appeal of structure (i.e., 12 steps) and the support of a "higher power." However, even AA's own outcome surveys do not include data for adolescent members. The 12-step approach is integrated into most formal adolescent treatment programs; yet there are no outcome data to document its efficacy in adolescent substance-abuse treatment.

## Outpatient Treatment

Outpatient treatment for adolescents who abuse substances includes both office-based counseling and more intensive day treatment. The latter is patterned after inpatient treatment but is less restrictive because the adolescent attends only during the day and returns home at night (U.S. Congress, Office of Technology Assessment 1991). In a private facility, day treatment costs an average of $3,000 per month (Sunshine and Wright 1988).

## Residential Programs

Residential treatment programs remove adolescents from their usual environment and provide 24-hour supervision with competent adults and recovering peers. These programs range from halfway houses to therapeutic communities to boot camps (U.S. Congress, Office of Technology Assessment 1991). One advantage of this approach is that removal from the usual environment limits access to substances and provides a positive milieu for working on problems related to substance abuse (Needle et al. 1988). However, the literature on delinquent behavior shows that the extent of involvement with delinquent peers is a powerful and direct predictor of delinquent behavior (Elliot et al. 1985; Hanson et al. 1984). Isolation in a group with other substance-abusing peers may support and consolidate further antisocial patterns rather than effect long-term changes in substance use. Additionally, removal from the environment may produce short-term sobriety, but does not address the environmental factors that encouraged or failed to prevent substance abuse in the first place. Cost for residential treatment is less than hospital-based care, but is still considerable, especially in light of there being no evidence for or against its efficacy in adolescent substance abuse (Catalano et al. 1991; Sunshine and Wright 1988).

## Inpatient Programs

Inpatient programs provide the most restrictive treatment environment and occur in psychiatric hospitals, general hospitals, and independent addiction facilities (National Academy of Sciences 1990). The NDATUS numbers indicate that over one-half of inpatient adolescent treatment for alcohol abuse in 1987 occurred in primary adult inpatient settings, with only a few states funding inpatient treatment programs specifically designed for adolescents (U.S. Congress, Office of Technology Assessment 1991). Adolescents are treated in inpatient units for longer lengths of stay than their adult counterparts under the assumption that adolescents need an even longer period away from their previous environment to achieve sobriety (Sunshine and Wright 1988). This increases the cost of an already expensive intervention. The cost of an average stay in a private inpatient treatment program may average $10,000. Public programs cost about half this amount, which still makes their cost considerable (Sunshine and Wright 1988). Treatment numbers also indicate a dichotomy, with 70% of adolescents placed in restrictive alcohol treatment going to inpatient treatment programs and the majority of those placed in restrictive drug treatment going to residential treatment programs (U.S. Congress, Office of Technology Assessment 1991).

## Other Types of Programs

Drop-in centers for adolescents who abuse substances provide peer-group social opportunities in a drug-free environment, some drug and alcohol counseling, and in some instances school-support activities and career counseling. These centers provide low-intensity community-based services that allow adolescents to work on their substance abuse problem within their community environment. However, as in residential treatment programs, adolescents in these programs socialize with other substance-abusing peers, which may support and consolidate antisocial patterns rather than effect long-term changes in substance use.

## Conclusion

In their review of adolescent substance abuse treatment, the U.S. Congress, Office of Technology Assessment (1991) concluded that treatment modalities are seldom provided in age-specific settings, often occur in highly restrictive settings, involve high attrition rates from treatment, are not differentiated as a function of the adolescent's presenting problem, and do not pay attention to social and cultural issues. These problems parallel Stroul and Friedman's (1986) identified treatment issues of individualized treatment planning, treatment in the least restrictive environment, and cultural sensitivity. Additionally, rigorous outcome research is not available for most existent treatments (Catalano et al. 1991; U.S. Congress, Office of Technology Assessment 1991). Treatment innovations to address both these therapeutic and evaluation issues are critically needed.

# Research

## Prevention

Although the focus of this chapter is on innovative treatment programs, many prevention programs for adolescent substance abuse have been described in the empirical and clinical literature. The purpose of mentioning these programs is to identify possible linkages with treatment innovations and to emphasize the much greater extent of prevention research when compared with existing treatment research. A great deal of money has been invested in providing and sometimes evaluating prevention programs for adolescent substance abuse. Most have targeted early teens in schools, usually in grades 6–9. Skills training in various forms has been used as either the main approach or as a part of the overall program in several prevention interventions. Given the lack of rigorous evaluation designs and the complexity of most programs, no one program, approach, or intervention technique has been shown to be consistently effective.

However, in identifying the complexity of substance abuse and targeting more than just the individual adolescent, prevention studies point the way to innovations in prevention that are salient for treatment innovations. Kumpfer and Turner (1991) propose a "social ecology" model that advocates improving the school and family climates as well as improving the adolescent's skills and self-esteem. Forman and Linney (1988) also recommend that prevention interventions target "personal, social, and ecological variables" due to the complexity of the problem. Additionally, in an extensive review of the curriculum-based programs published from 1980 to 1990, Hansen (1992) analyzed the format and results of 45 programs and recommended that "comprehensive and social influence" programs are the most successful in preventing substance abuse.

As noted in the prevention literature, there is considerable evidence that substance abuse in adolescents is a complex problem, involving multiple systems. It has also been postulated that drug involvement in adolescence is significantly correlated with a number of other problem behaviors such as delinquency and precocious sexual behavior. This constellation has been identified as a "syndrome of problem behaviors" (Donovan and Jessor 1985; Jessor and Jessor 1977; Jessor et al. 1986). In support of this, Barnes and Welte (1986) found that alcohol abuse was strongly associated with illicit drug use, the negative social consequences of illicit drug use, and general school misconduct. Evidence has also accumulated suggesting that the correlates and risk factors associated with adolescent substance abuse are the same as those of juvenile delinquency (Henggeler 1992). Elliot et al. (1985) found that adolescent substance abuse and delinquency were directly predicted from prior antisocial behavior, association with drug-using peers, and familial and school difficulties.

## Treatment

Given this understanding of the correlates of adolescent substance abuse, what is known about the efficacy of current treatment modalities? There are problematic methodological issues in the treatment evaluation literature that make conclusions about treatment efficacy difficult. Most studies lack reliable measures of abuse, dependency, and therapeutic success. In other words, success rates are reported only for those completing therapy, whereas attrition ranges from 50% to 90%. Outcome research is limited and poorly designed, with poorly defined variables and little attention to controls and factors associated with effectiveness (U.S. Congress, Office of Technology Assessment 1991). Catalano et. al. (1991) came to a number of conclusions.

1. Research evaluating treatment effectiveness is only at a beginning stage.
2. Treatment should be evaluated using rigorous designs (i.e., including control and comparison groups, defining treatment programs in detail, and measuring as many treatment factors as possible).
3. Researchers should use standard definitions of outcome variables.
4. More research should be conducted on promising approaches to preventing relapse.

Treatment reviews have focused on subjective descriptions of characteristics of successful treatment programs (Friedman and

Glickman 1986), and program effectiveness as defined by prevention of relapse (Catalano et al. 1991). In their review, Catalano et al. (1991) concluded that no one treatment approach was significantly better than any other. Similarly, in comparing inpatient versus outpatient treatments, the U.S. Congress, Office of Technology Assessment (1991) review found no conclusive evidence that either setting was more effective in decreasing adolescent substance abuse. This review additionally found that the services that were most clearly associated with positive outcomes for the adolescents in treatment were educational and recreational services, social skills training, and family therapy components seen as adjunctive to the actual substance abuse treatment.

## Innovations

What innovations are needed in adolescent substance abuse treatment? From the evidence that substance abuse in adolescents is associated with other problem behaviors and family dysfunction, and that positive outcomes for adolescents in treatment are related to school, peer, and family interventions, it appears that treatments that directly address these variables are needed. Additionally, treatment programs that avoid removing adolescents from their immediate environment and that address treatment issues within the context of adolescents' local community would allow testing of the assumption that increasingly restrictive environments are needed to help adolescents achieve short- and long-term sobriety. Programs that individualize treatment around the unique set of problems of adolescents and their families, that are culturally sensitive, and that incorporate parents into treatment planning and implementation are needed. Additionally, innovative interventions must be rigorously evaluated with attention to outcome definition and measurement against control groups.

Two innovative programs that address these issues are Positive Adolescent Life Skills (Project PALS), a unique skills training program now being tested with pregnant and nonpregnant teens, and Multisystemic Therapy (MST), an empirically developed community-based treatment implemented successfully with serious juvenile offenders and currently being tested in a population of delinquent adolescents who abuse substances.

## Social Skills Training

Project PALS, one of the Perinatal 20 programs funded in 1989 and 1990 by the National Institute on Drug Abuse (NIDA), is a research demonstration project that targets drug-using pregnant women and women at risk for drug use during pregnancy. The purpose of the project is to evaluate the effectiveness of two treatment approaches with drug-using and at-risk pregnant and nonpregnant adolescents. The primary treatment approach is PALS training and focuses on cognitive-behavioral or social skills and network skills. The secondary treatment approach is case management, originally developed to maintain adolescent compliance with activities and medical appointments. It includes assisting adolescents in their local environment in overcoming barriers to treatment. The overall goal of Project PALS is to eliminate or significantly reduce drug use and criminal activity in adolescents who abuse substances or who are at risk for abusing substances. The treatment approaches are being rigorously evaluated using a two-factor randomized research design. Project PALS is now in its third year of treatment evaluation. The project serves a culturally diverse population with 37% African-American, 13% Caucasian, and 44% Hispanic (Mexican-American). The project includes several innovations in social skills training, including networking skills, some community-based case management interventions, and a rigorous evaluation component using random assignment and standardized instruments.

## Multisystemic Therapy

MST was developed to intervene with adolescents who are chronic juvenile offenders and who have significant problems involving multiple systems. Henggeler and Borduin (1990) describe MST in detail. MST is based largely on family-systems theory conceptualizations of behavior and behavior change (Haley 1976; Minuchin 1974). Systems theory emphasizes the reciprocity of interpersonal relations and posits that child behavior problems typically reflect dysfunctional family relations.

Although MST has much in common with traditional family therapies, MST also includes substantive differences that are pertinent to the discussion of adolescent substance abuse treatment. The most important of these differences is that, consistent with Bronfenbrenner's (1979) theory of social ecology, the multisystemic approach views individuals as being nested within a complex of interconnected systems that encompass individual (e.g., biological and cognitive), family, and extrafamilial (peer and school) factors. Behavior problems can be maintained by dysfunctional transactions within and/or between any one or combination of these systems. MST, then, is not limited to interventions within the family, but encourages treatment of dysfunction in other systems as needed. In further contrast with most family therapy approaches, MST emphasizes the consideration of child development variables and often incorporates interventions that are not necessarily systemic (e.g., behavioral parent training). With regard to adolescent substance abuse, MST naturally includes the environmental systems variables that may contribute to or fail to prevent adolescent substance use. MST also allows for biological contributors to be identified and psychopharmacological treatment to be integrated with psychosocial treatments.

A crucial aspect of MST is its emphasis on promoting behavioral change in the youth's natural environment. Treatment takes place in the family's home, although meetings in community locations (e.g., school, recreation center, project office) are often needed. Parent involvement is crucial, with all family members identifying problems targeted for change, and participating in developing and implementing solutions. Additionally, therapists are from ethnic backgrounds that correspond to the ethnic makeup of the community and attend to issues of cultural sensitivity.

MST is now being evaluated in Charleston, South Carolina, in a NIDA-funded project with juvenile delinquents who abuse substances. As with Project PALS, the study is ongoing and results will be available in several years. This rigorous, randomized, controlled outcome study involves random assignment of substance-abusing juvenile delinquents to either an MST treatment or usual services control group. Treatment occurs over 3–4 months, with pre-, post-, and 6- and 12-month follow-up assessments using standardized instruments. Following completion of the treatment phase, MST-treated adolescents are randomized into either monitoring or no-monitoring groups. The long-term effects of monitoring with short-term booster treatment as needed will be assessed in these latter groups.

This evaluation of MST in the treatment of adolescents who abuse substances is innovative in several respects. Delivering treatment within the adolescent's natural environment both provides the least restrictive treatment setting and facilitates the development of an individualized treatment plan. This treatment plan directly involves adolescents, parents, and other family members, and has ecological validity. By facilitating parent and adolescent interventions in the involved extrafamilial systems, therapists directly address family, peer, school, and community variables that are associated with the adolescent's substance abuse. Additionally, since MST involves 24-hour therapist availability, the intensity of services can be tailored to the specific family situation, with increased intensity around crisis times as needed. Also, by going to the family's environment, therapists operationalize their commitment to helping adolescents and their families overcome their denial and resistance to substance abuse treatment. An especially effective repertoire of strategies has been developed to overcome low adolescent and parental cooperation with behavior change efforts (Henggeler and Borduin, in press; Robins and Foster 1989). As therapists join with families in a persistent commitment to solutions, the problem of attrition from treatment is reduced substantially. Finally, a rigorous outcome research design, with attention to the multiple variables associated with adolescent substance abuse and the long-term effects of a monitoring and booster therapy intervention, provides an avenue for assessment of this innovative approach.

# Conclusion

Clearly, innovations are needed in our attempts to understand and treat substance abuse in adolescent populations. Several directions of innovation seem to be indicated by previous research and clinical experience. In addition to developing systems of care for substance-abusing adolescents that conform to Stroul and Friedman's (1986) recommendations, treatment providers and treatment researchers need to work more closely together to define and evaluate treatment approaches. The problem of adolescent substance abuse should be reconfigured so that less emphasis is placed on individual pathology and more emphasis is placed on systems change (i.e., family, school, juvenile justice, and community). Both outcome and process research should be included in treatment effectiveness studies so that both effectiveness and change mechanisms can be identified. More research on risk and resiliency factors is needed to advance prevention efforts. Finally, treatment programs and procedures that have been shown to be ineffective, or even harmful, should be identified and discarded. This is a tall order, but certainly worthy of our attention in this area, which has such serious consequences for adolescents and society.

# References

Allen JP, Leadbeater BJ, Aber JL: The relationship of adolescents' expectations and values to delinquency, hard drug use, and unprotected sexual intercourse. Development and Psychopathology 2:85–98, 1990

Barnes GM, Welte JW: Adolescent alcohol abuse: subgroup differences and relationships to other problem behaviors. Journal of Adolescent Research 1:79–94, 1986

Blau GM, Gillespie JF, Felner RD, et al: Predisposition to drug use in rural adolescents: preliminary relationships and methodological considerations. Journal of Drug Education 18:13–22, 1988

Bronfenbrenner U: The Ecology of Human Development: Experiments by Nature and Design. Cambridge, MA, Harvard University Press, 1979

Brown SA, Mott MA, Myers MG: Adolescent alcohol and drug treatment outcome, in Drug and Alcohol Abuse Prevention. Edited by Watson RR. New York, The Humana Press, 1990, pp 373–403

Catalano RF, Hawkins JD, Wells EA, et al: Evaluation of the effectiveness of adolescent drug abuse treatment, assignment of risks for relapse, and promising approaches for relapse prevention. Int J Addict 25:1085–1140, 1991

Donovan JE, Jessor R: Structure of problem behavior in adolescence and young adulthood. J Consult Clin Psychol 33:890–904, 1985

Elliot DS, Huizinga D, Ageton SS: Explaining Delinquency and Drug Use. Beverly Hills, CA, Sage, 1985

Forman SG, Linney JA: School-based prevention of adolescent substance abuse: programs, implementation and future directions. School Psychology Review 17:550–558, 1988

Friedman AS, Glickman NW: Program characteristics for successful treatment of adolescent drug abuse. J Nerv Ment Dis 174:669–679, 1986

Friedman RM: Mental health and substance abuse services for adolescents: clinical and service system issues. Administration and Policy in Mental Health 19:159–178, 1992

Haley J: Problem Solving Theory. San Francisco, CA, Jossey-Bass, 1976

Hansen WB: School-based substance abuse prevention: a review of the state of the art in curriculum, 1980–1990. Health Education Research 7:403–430, 1992

Hanson CL, Henggeler SW, Haefele WF, et al: Demographic, individual, and family relationship correlates of serious and repeated crime among adolescents and their siblings. J Consult Clin Psychol 52:528–538, 1984

Henggeler SW: Multisystemic treatment of serious juvenile offenders: implications for the treatment of substance abusing youths. Paper presented at the National Institute of Drug Abuse Technical Review: Behavioral Treatments for Drug Abuse and Dependence, Bethesda, MD, September 1992

Henggeler SW, Borduin C: Family Therapy and Beyond. Pacific Grove, CA, 1990

Henggeler SW, Borduin CM: Multisystemic treatment of serious juvenile offenders and their families, in Home-based Services for Troubled Children. Edited by Schwartz IM, AuClaire P. Lincoln, University of Nebraska Press, 1995

Howland J, Hingson R: Alcohol as a risk factor for drownings: a review of the literature. Accident Analysis and Prevention 20:19–71, 1988

Jessor R, Jessor SL: Problem Behavior and Psychosocial Development: A Longitudinal Study of Youth. New York, Academic Press, 1977

Jessor R, Donovan JE, Costa F: Psychosocial correlates of marijuana use in adolescence and young adulthood: the past as prologue. Alcohol, Drugs, and Driving 2:31–49, 1986

Johnston LD, O'Malley PM, Bachman JG: National Survey Results on Drug Use From the Monitoring the Future Study, 1975–1992, Volume 1: Secondary School Students, National Institute of Drug Abuse (Publication No. 93-3597). Rockville, MD, Department of Health and Human Services, 1993

Kaminer YM, Bukstein O: Adolescent chemical use and dependence: current issues in epidemiology, treatment, and prevention. Acta Psychiatr Scand 79:415–424, 1989

Kandel DB, Davies M, Karus D, et al: The consequences in young adulthood of adolescent drug involvement: an overview. Arch Gen Psychiatry 43:746–754, 1986

Kumpfer KL, Turner CW: The social ecology model of adolescent substance abuse: implications for prevention. Int J Addict 25:435–463, 1991

Kusnetz S: Services for adolescent substance abuse, in Teen Drug Use. Edited by Beschner GM, Friedman AS. Lexington, MA, Lexington Books, 1985, pp 123–162

Matarazzo JD: Behavioral health's challenge to academic, scientific, and professional psychology. Am Psychol 37:1–14, 1982

Minuchin S: Families and Family Therapy. Cambridge, MA, Harvard University Press, 1974

National Academy of Sciences, Institute of Medicine, Division of Health Care Services, Committee for the Substance Abuse Coverage Study: Treating Drug Problems. Washington, DC, National Academy Press, 1990

National Institute on Drug Abuse: National household survey on drug abuse: population estimates 1991 (DHHS Publ No ADM-92-1887). Rockville, MD, U.S. Government Printing Office, 1992

Needle R, Lavee Y, Su S, et al: Familial, interpersonal, intrapersonal correlates of drug use among adolescents: a longitudinal comparison of adolescents in treatment, drug-using adolescents not in treatment, and non-drug using adolescents. Int J Addict 23:1211–1240, 1988

Newcomb MD, Bentler PM: Consequences of Adolescent Drug Use: Impact on the Lives of Young Adults. Newbury Park, CA, Sage, 1988

Paulson MJ, Coombs R, Richardson MA: School performance, academic aspirations, and drug use among children and adolescents. Journal of Drug Education 20:289–303, 1990

Robins AL, Foster SL: Negotiating Parent Adolescent Conflict: A Behavioral-Family System Approach. New York, Guilford, 1989

Robins LN, Darvish HS, Murphy GE: The long-term outcome for adolescent drug users: a follow-up study of 76 users and 146 nonusers, in The Psychopathology of Adolescence. Edited by Zubin J, Freedman AM. New York, Grune & Stratton, 1970, pp 159–178

Stroul BA, Friedman RM: A System of Care for Severely Emotionally Disturbed Children and Youth. Washington, DC, CASSP Technical Assistance Center, 1986

Sunshine L, Wright J: The 100 Best Treatment Centers for Alcohol and Drug Abuse. New York, Avon, 1988

Ungerleider JT, Siegel NJ: The drug abusing adolescent: clinical issues. Psychiatr Clin North Am 13:435–442, 1990

U.S. Congress, Office of Technology Assessment: Adolescent health, Volume II: Background and effectiveness of selected prevention and treatment services (Publ No OTA-H-466). Washington, DC, U.S. Government Printing Office, 1991

Yamaguchi K, Kandel DB: On the resolution of role incompatibility: a life event history analysis of family roles and marijuana use. American Journal of Sociology 90:1284–1325, 1985

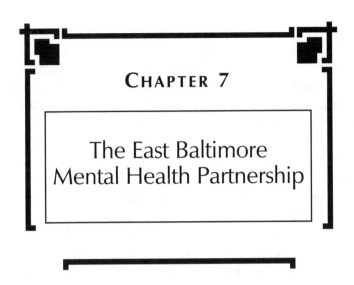

# CHAPTER 7

## The East Baltimore Mental Health Partnership

**Philip J. Leaf, Ph.D., Michael Bogrov, M.D.,
and Mary Bruce Webb, Ph.D.**

Limited service alternatives exist in most communities for children and adolescents with serious emotional disturbances (SED) (Duchnowski and Friedman 1990; Knitzer 1982). During the past decade, a consensus has developed concerning the array of services that should be included in a system of service for these children (e.g., England and Cole 1992; Friedman et al. 1989; Stroul and Friedman 1986; Zirul et al. 1989). Although federal (e.g., Child and Adolescent Service System Program [CASSP]) and foundation (e.g., Robert Wood Johnson, Annie E. Casey) initiatives have stimulated community-based and family-focused services in many localities, few published reports exist describing these efforts. In this chapter, we describe one ongoing effort, the East Baltimore Mental Health Partnership (EBMHP), a joint state, city, and community effort begun in October 1993 with funds provided by the Center for Mental Health Services (CMHS) of the Substance Abuse and Mental

Health Services Administration. Among the model service demonstration programs funded by the CMHS during the first funding cycle, the East Baltimore Mental Health Partnership is unique because its service area is limited to an inner-city community where the majority of children are African-Americans living in households with incomes below the federal poverty level.

The East Baltimore Mental Health Partnership has been developed to establish a comprehensive, multiagency system of care for children with SED living in an inner-city environment. As with most mental health initiatives, funds are targeted to improve and expand traditional mental health services, to improve access to existing services, and to develop services not currently available for children in the target population. In addition to the remediation of clinical problems, considerable effort is devoted to improving the environments in which children spend the majority of their time: the family (both biological and foster) and the school.

A priority for this project is to increase the capacity of caregivers to promote the health and well-being of their children. Parents from the local community will be included in policy decisions related to the needs of the children with SED. The EBMHP involves these and other caregivers along with community agencies and community leaders in activities aimed at reducing the stigma of mental illness; providing children with access to the same educational, recreational, and social opportunities as their peers; and reducing the stresses and strains that exacerbate psychiatric problems and that contribute to the disabilities associated with these disorders.

## Organizing a System of Services

The EBMHP builds on changes at the national as well as at the state and local level that have moved children's mental health services toward a coordinated community- and family-based system of care. Without these earlier activities and policy initiatives, the EBMHP would not have been possible. At the state level, a subcabinet consisting of the Secretaries of the Departments of Education, Social Services, and Juvenile Services has been established and charged with the development, coordination, and integration of children's services in the state. Governor William Donald Schaefer also established the Governor's Office for Children, Youth and Families to facilitate the promotion of statewide policies.

One of the major undertakings of the Governor's Office has been a Systems Reform Initiative (SRI), initially developed with the assistance of funding from the Annie E. Casey Foundation. In Baltimore, the SRI has focused on the provision of wraparound services to families whose children are at risk for out-of-home placement or who are currently in out-of-state placements. These activities have been important in stimulating interagency, family-focused, community-based treatment alternatives.

The State Mental Hygiene Administration has also created a strong foundation for the EBMHP through several initiatives that give local jurisdictions more control over the planning and implementation of mental health services. These efforts by the State Mental Hygiene Administration include the creation of core service agencies, with primary responsibility for the development and administration of mental health within each county and the city of Baltimore. At the time of the development of the EBMHP, the core service agency in Baltimore—Baltimore Mental Health Systems, Inc. (BMHS), a not-for-profit corporation—had operated adult services in the community for a number of years, and had a record of providing innovative, coordinated services for the adult population. BMHS did not, however, assume the oversight responsibility for children's mental health services until July 1993.

Currently, BMHS administers services through a system of lead agencies, which are the major providers of mental health services in each of seven geographic catchment areas in Baltimore. The lead agency for the East Baltimore Catchment Area is the Johns Hopkins Hospital, which has operated the Children's

Mental Health Center (CMHC) for a number of years. It is within this catchment area that the EBMHP operates.

Another initiative on which the EBMHP has been built is the Consortium for Child and Adolescent Mental Health Services. The Consortium was organized in the spring of 1991 by the Departments of Mental Hygiene and Psychiatry at the Johns Hopkins University, the State Mental Hygiene Administration, and the City Health Department to develop a better understanding of factors affecting the detection, referral, and treatment of children with SED. This group has grown to over 100 service providers, policy makers, academic researchers, advocates, and family members who meet to discuss issues of relevance to the provision of services to children with SED and their families. The discussions held by participants in this consortium over a 2-year period were the foundation for the proposal that resulted in obtaining the federal funds for the EBMHP.

The committee that developed the proposal for the EBMHP consisted of senior staff from the Baltimore City Departments of Health, Social Services, and Police; the Baltimore City Public Schools; the Mayor's Office of Children and Youth; the State Department of Juvenile Services; the Baltimore City Family Preservation Initiative; Baltimore Mental Health Systems, Inc.; Clergy United for the Renewal of East Baltimore; The Johns Hopkins Hospital; Liberty Medical Center; the Johns Hopkins Schools of Public Health and Medicine; and representatives from local family and advocacy groups. What is unique in the program is the strong collaboration with and leadership supplied by school personnel, staff from other social and human services agencies, parents and child advocates, and leaders from the local churches.

## Characteristics of Target Population for EBMHP

The EBMHP was created to consolidate and expand services for children and adolescents living in East Baltimore (the catchment area consisting of 23 census tracts surrounding the Johns Hopkins Hospital) who have SED and who are served by or are in need of services from multiple public agencies, including schools. In 1990, the population of the East Baltimore Catchment Area was 70,067 living in 21,713 households; 19,587 of these residents were age 17 or younger. African-Americans constitute the largest racial and ethnic group in the catchment area. Over half the children live in households with incomes below the poverty level, making the East Baltimore community one of the poorest in the nation.

Although all agencies in Baltimore consider children with SED to be an underserved population, data are not available concerning the number of SED youth served by multiple agencies. We have been able to determine that in 1992, 2,612 children citywide received an out-of-home placement, not including hospitalization on a psychiatric unit. Reviews of available data indicate that the overwhelming majority of these children had a diagnosable psychiatric disorder. At the end of 1992, 17,769 children in Baltimore were receiving special education services, with 1,172 receiving services because of an SED. We estimate that there are approximately 177 children from the catchment area receiving special education services for an SED. Many of these children are served by special schools outside the catchment area.

In 1992, the Johns Hopkins Children's Mental Health Center conducted intakes on 315 children. A review of active cases found that over 80% were being served by another public agency, and all of the children had at least one psychiatric disorder. Although systematic assessments of functioning were not available for these children, most had encountered severe problems in school, at home, or both.

The target population for the EBMHP consists of children and adolescents living in the East Baltimore catchment area for the Johns Hopkins Children's Mental Health Center with the following characteristics:

1. *Age.*   Children under 18 years for initial service contact up through age 21 for clients receiving services prior to age 18 (transition to adult services).

2. *Diagnosis.*    DSM-III-R disorder (with the exception of DSM-III-R V-Codes, substance use disorders, and developmental disorders unless they co-occur with another diagnosable SED).

3. *Disability.*    Substantial inability to perform in family, school, community, or all three. Criteria for determining functional impairment included in the latest draft of the state's 5-year plan (1995–1999) include "inability to learn which is not explained by intellectual, sensory, or health factors; inability to build or maintain satisfactory interpersonal relationships with peers, teachers, and/or parents; inappropriate relationships with peers, teachers, and/or parents; inappropriate types of behavior or emotional tone under normal conditions; and tendency to develop marked physical symptoms, pain, or fears associated with personal or school problems."

4. *Services.*    Currently being served by two or more community agencies or in need of services from two or more community agencies.

5. *Duration.*    Present for 1 year or expected to last more than 1 year.

A child's eligibility for this project is determined by a multiagency case-management team. Because services for children with severe developmental disabilities are coordinated by a separate agency, these children are excluded from the target population. We also exclude youth serving criminal sentences of 2 years or longer.

## Priorities for the Project

The Partnership emphasizes the support and empowerment of families and other caregivers. Although children with SED and their caregivers require access to effective professional services, the foundation of any system of services for children with SED must be the parent, the family, and others who care for the child. The availability of professionals and others capable of working effectively with families and in settings outside the traditional mental health and residential treatment settings is critical if we are to expand and improve systems of services for children who have SED.

Priorities for the East Baltimore Partnership include the following:

1. The empowerment of consumers (parents, other caregivers, and the child when age-appropriate) to become true partners in the development and implementation of services, and the inclusion of the parent in the development of procedures for client identification, treatment, and program evaluation.
2. Development of a coordinated, comprehensive system of services for children with SED and for families, in which services are provided in the least restrictive setting possible.
3. Development of an integrated program of case management for children being served by multiple agencies.
4. Enhancement of the cultural competence of service providers and the cultural appropriateness of programs.
5. Strengthening mechanisms for the early detection of children with SED and the reduction of disability accompanying these disorders.
6. Integration of services for adults and children in order to develop a transition program for children with SED who are growing out of child-oriented services, and to develop a program for children with SED who are living with an adult with a serious emotional disorder.
7. Modification of funding streams as health care policy and funding opportunities change.
8. Integration of service delivery and training efforts so that adequate personnel will be available for the implementation of model services elsewhere in Baltimore and Maryland, and so that personnel working in health, social service, educational, and juvenile services are capable of collaborating with caregivers in the development and implementation of services.

The East Baltimore Project uses a three-pronged approach to improving the quality of life experienced by children in the target population: increasing the capacity of parents and caregivers to participate in the planning and implementation of services, improving the services infrastructure, and working with community agencies and leaders to ensure maximum participation of children with SED in community activities.

## Increasing Parent/Caregiver Involvement at the Individual and Systems Levels

Efforts to develop systems of services for children with SED must begin with a focus on the child and the child's family. No community has adequate resources for the replacement of the care and coordination activities of parents and other family members. Even if money were not an obstacle, there are not enough trained professionals available to manage and coordinate the care required by all children with SED. Communities must find ways of supporting and increasing the capacity of parents and family members to care for children with serious emotional and behavioral problems, and to provide these supports as early as possible. Communities also must find ways to assist existing agencies and organizations (e.g., schools, social services, health care providers, and the religious community) in their efforts to support and include parents of children with SED.

Efforts to continue to increase the involvement of parents involves a multifaceted strategy. First, we work to involve parents in the planning of programs for their children, and in monitoring and modifying the course of the Partnership. Second, we work to expand the capacity of existing parent support groups. Third, the Partnership provides funds to facilitate participation of parents and their children in the full range of activities that exist in the community.

To encourage parents' participation in the planning of programs, funds have been built into the project for the hiring of parents to serve on the project's executive committee and to participate in other activities aimed at developing and monitoring new programs. Parents employed by the project are included on the committees developing and implementing individual service plans (ISPs), and in coordinating the implementation of these plans.

Although Baltimore contains several organizations that support parents who have children with SED, few of the parents of children in our target population have participated in these programs. In fact, one difficulty in developing the EBMHP was that most parents participating in the planning process lived outside of East Baltimore. One goal of the Partnership is the development of parent support groups for parents living in East Baltimore that are similar to those active in other areas of the state. We also are exploring other mechanisms for parent support activities that may fall outside the traditional support-group structures.

It is important that parents and their children be able to participate in the full range of activities existing in the community. Parents are engaged as consultants and facilitators in efforts to develop an array of activities that support and empower parents to take an active role in the development and implementation of programs for their children. With parental input, programs are being developed to meet the special needs of children in our target population, most of whom are African-Americans living in households with limited incomes and in a community with few services available to them.

## Improving the Services Infrastructure

The goal of the Partnership is to provide services in the least restrictive environment possible, and to ensure that services are child-centered and family-focused, community-based, and culturally sensitive. The array of services coordinated or developed by the EBMHP include case management services, diagnostic and evaluation services, outpatient services, school-based services, therapeutic nursery services, outreach and community-based services, emergency services, intensive home-based services, intensive day-treatment services, respite-care services, therapeutic foster-care services, and assistance in transition to adult services.

## Case Management Services

The EBMHP has established a Multiagency Case Management and Coordination Committee (MACCC) to develop and implement the procedures for the creation of ISPs, and to meet with parents and children to coordinate services and case management activities. Case management teams include staff from the agencies providing services to the child along with case management, outreach staff, and parents employed by the EBMHP. The MACCC serves as the single point of entry and exit for the East Baltimore Mental Health Partnership. Because some children enter services as the result of a crisis, this office works closely with the crisis response team, emergency room personnel, and the family preservation alternatives that have been implemented for the target population.

Four levels of case management are available:

1. For children at imminent risk for out-of-home placement, staff from the existing Family Preservation Initiative operated under the auspices of the Systems Reform Initiative will assume intensive case-management functions. These programs employ staff serving two or three families at one time, with interventions lasting less than 12 weeks.
2. For children who are not at imminent risk for out-of-home placement, but who nonetheless require intensive services, case-manager-to-client ratios of approximately 1:10 will be provided. These clients may be, for example, children returning from the hospital or who are being followed up after a crisis.
3. The next level of case management intensity provides case-manager-to-client ratios of approximately 1:20. This is for children whose needs are less intense than those above, but who still require frequent contact and strong family support

to stabilize the situation for the child and family.

4. Some children can be ensured necessary services with a less active form of case management, which we refer to as case coordination. These are children whose ISP is well underway and who are making satisfactory progress. In these cases, each child will be assigned a primary case coordinator from one of the agencies providing services to the child.

For all children, it is our goal that the parent, legal guardian, or full-time caregiver become as effective as the professional staff for the implementation and monitoring of the ISPs. We recognize that some parents will not be able to assume the role of case manager at the start of the program or have the capacity to act in the role for periods of time because of personal situations or crises. We expect our professional staff to act as advocates in those situations while helping the parents to assume as much of this role as possible.

## Diagnostic and Evaluation Services

Clinical evaluations conducted prior to the establishment of the EBMHP generally focused on the perspective of the assessing agency, with little concern for the coordination of services of other providers. Further, there is often a waiting period of several weeks before a mental health evaluation is begun, forcing most schools and social service agencies to develop and implement plans in the absence of guidance from mental health professionals.

In the EBMHP, the emphasis and rationale of the assessment or evaluation is the development of an ISP to be implemented by the child, parent, and multiple agencies. As a result, staff conducting the evaluation, the parent or caregiver, and the child will be involved in identifying the issues to be addressed by the evaluation, and results must be made available in a timely fashion to all agencies providing services. Evaluation includes a multifaceted assessment, including psychological and educational assessments, speech and language assessments, physical examinations, identification of the strengths and needs of the family, and determination of the child's strengths and level of functioning within school, family, and community settings.

One goal of the EBMHP is to ensure more rapid assessments, because agencies and families need timely feedback from mental health specialists before they take actions. An evaluation unit has been developed at the Johns Hopkins Children's Mental Health Center and staffed with the goal of providing a written evaluation within 72 hours of a request. The evaluation procedures used by inpatient and outpatient programs have been standardized so that children do not require a new evaluation immediately upon discharge from an inpatient unit. Full-time coordinators have been placed in the Departments of Juvenile Services, Social Services, and the Baltimore City schools to facilitate the dissemination of information and coordination of services.

## Outpatient Services

Additional clinicians were hired through the CMHC to provide clinical services in conjunction with other community services targeted for children in or being diverted from the juvenile service system and in the foster care system. Clinical services are also provided to children who are in transition from the Family Preservation Project. Each of these agencies recognizes the need to strengthen relationships with the mental health service system, and all have agreed to participate in the development of the multiagency case-management system.

## School-Based Services

Because of their natural ties to the communities in which they are located, schools play pivotal roles in the provision of services through the EBMHP. Locating services within schools provides an opportunity to have a greater impact on environmental factors that may influence the course of SED among children within the target population. The presence of mental health services within the schools allows us to institute primary and secondary prevention activities for children who are at risk but who are not part of the target population.

The EBMHP is building on an innovative program initiated in 1991 by the Baltimore public schools and the city Health Department, which created funding mechanisms to place mental health clinicians in 20 schools in the city, including 5 within the East Baltimore catchment area. A range of activities are provided at school sites in the catchment area, including school-based mental health workers, after-school and summer programs, school-based case coordination, training and coordination, transition from hospitalization and out-of-home placements, and a school-based evaluation unit for children with SED.

### School-Based Mental Health Workers

During the first year of operation, the EBMHP was designed to have a full-time clinician in each of six schools in the catchment area. In the second year, the number of schools with full-time mental health clinicians was to increase to 12, with all 18 schools located in the catchment area having full-time mental health clinicians by the third year of the project. Clinicians in these schools work closely with other personnel in the schools and with case managers and outreach workers to ensure that the program provides coordinated and comprehensive services.

### After-School and Summer Programs

After-school and summer programs are conducted by the school-based clinicians, case managers, outreach workers, neighborhood liaisons, and recreational therapists. These personnel work with other agencies to develop additional clinical and support services for children in the target population and their family members. These are coordinated with existing efforts within the schools during the summer and will increase the opportunities of children in the target population to participate in recreational, educational, and social activities with other children.

### School-Based Case Coordination

The school system has established school support teams (SSTs). These teams bring together school psychologists, social workers, master teachers, counselors, and administrators to provide services to students in need before they reach the point of being referred for special education. The school-based mental health worker joins these teams, and the SSTs are used to coordinate services for children in the target population, to facilitate changes in school environment, to link school personnel and children with resources available outside of the school, and to coordinate linkages with other components of the Partnership.

### Training and Coordination

The project has implemented a program that combines school and classroom management techniques with the provision of mental health services. This program seeks to coordinate both the therapeutic and educational aspects of the school, and to facilitate learning by children with SED in local schools and regular classrooms to the greatest extent possible. The Partnership sponsors training of teachers and other staff to facilitate the implementation of these schoolwide programs. Additional funding has been secured from the State Department of Education to support the participation of teachers and other school personnel in the planning process and to provide ongoing technical support.

### Transition From Hospitalization and Out-of-Home Placements

For children in the target population who are hospitalized, centralized staff will be available through this project to represent the school system in the coordination of discharge planning. This may include contacting the appropriate personnel at the local school, participating with the hospital team to create the discharge plan, coordinating school services for the ISP, and monitoring to ensure that appropriate school follow-up services are received.

### School-Based Evaluation Unit for Children With SED

Baltimore schools have planned a centralized diagnostic and prescriptive unit to serve children in the school system who are at risk for hospitalization or placement in residential treatment centers, or who are being released from those facilities. The goals for this unit are the prevention of restrictive placements and maintenance of children within their local schools; and the facilitation of the reintegration of previously hospitalized children back into their local schools. This facility will be able to capitalize on existing personnel with considerable expertise in planning for and working with children with SED and their families in order to perform comprehensive assessments, design a treatment plan, and work with the local school personnel and the child's family in implementing the plan when the child returns to his or her community school. Funds from the Partnership will support the mental health services component of the unit.

## Therapeutic Nursery Services

The identification of and delivery of services to preschool-age children in the target population presents special problems because these children may have very limited contact with individuals trained to recognize psychiatric disorders in young children. As one of our major mechanisms for serving the preschool population and their families, we are adding a therapeutic nursery component to the Head Start centers in the catchment area and to the community development center, which serves children ages birth–3 years and their families. These centers are particularly appropriate to this purpose because Head Start has a family focus and also has a mandate to provide mental health services to children. This program will provide direct therapeutic services to children and their families as well as consultation to teachers surrounding specific children, and will address child development and classroom management issues in general.

## Outreach and Community-Based Services

Partnership funds support outreach workers and neighborhood liaisons who are recruited from the catchment area. These individuals are involved in case management and case coordination, as well as the provision of outpatient services and support to children and families within their own communities. Services are provided in the schools, in the homes, and in conjunction with local clergy and local service agencies. These staff constitute a community mental health center without walls, having access to all resources of the Partnership and affiliated agencies but not limited by anything other than the interests and needs of the child in developing and implementing the treatment plan.

## Emergency Services

Currently, many of the children who receive psychiatric hospitalizations enter through the emergency room. The Johns Hopkins Hospital has already hired personnel to work in the emergency room so that staff are available to develop plans for alternatives to hospitalization when appropriate. The Partnership will implement programs in conjunction with the Department of Social Services, the Department of Juvenile Services, and the Baltimore schools to defer unnecessary hospitalizations before they enter the emergency room. These efforts include increased training of staff and the education of parents and caretakers about the range of available alternatives when there is a crisis.

A second component of the emergency services program is the institution of a 24-hour crisis response capacity. Crisis beds will be identified and staffed so that children requiring a brief out-of-home stay can be housed in an apartment or house for a short time. In addition, case managers, outreach workers, and neighborhood liaisons will be available to provide crisis response services.

## Intensive Home-Based Services

The Baltimore City Family Preservation Initiative has been providing intensive home-based services for children and their families when the child is at imminent risk of out-of-home placement. Funds can be provided through the Partnership to purchase services from the Family Preservation Initiative so that their teams can be expanded and mobilized to prevent unnecessary hospitalizations in our target population. In addition, staff from the MACCC will provide home-based services on a somewhat less intensive basis than provided by the Family Preservation Initiative.

## Intensive Day-Treatment Services

This unit provides a treatment site for children not requiring hospitalization but requiring a level of therapeutic intensity not possible in a traditional outpatient setting. The integration of the day program with intensive after-school programs will facilitate the use of the program as a step-down unit following short periods of hospitalization or its use in conjunction with the crisis response and family preservation programs.

## Respite-Care Services

There is a critical need for both planned and crisis respite services for children in the target group and their families. The crisis residential settings that will be available may also be used to provide emergency respite services. The Mental Health Association has received funding from the State Mental Hygiene Administration to provide training for family-based respite services, and we will extend this training to families in the program. In addition, the neighborhood liaisons and other staff will be available to provide respite relief as part of the treatment plan.

## Therapeutic Foster-Care Services

Therapeutic foster-care services are already provided by the Department of Social Services. The EBMHP will review the existing capacities of the foster care system and expand the training and support services available to staff, foster families, and biological parents.

## Assistance in Transition to Adult Services

An advantage of the vesting of responsibility for planning of adult and child mental health services within a single lead agency is that this increases the capacity to integrate services for children and adults, to facilitate the transfers of children to adult services, and to provide services for children in the target population who have a parent with an SED or substance abuse problem. The EBMHP will explore the feasibility of modifying and expanding psychosocial rehabilitation services so that they are acceptable to and appropriate for use by teenagers. In addition, the supported employment programs that exist in the catchment area for adults will be brought into the planning process for developing services more appropriate for adolescents.

### Recreational Services

Funds from the EBMHP will support summer programs and after-school programs for children in the target population. Funding will also be used to support opportunities for participation in existing, community-based recreational activities for these children.

### Wraparound Funds

Clinicians and case managers have access to a pool of funds to provide for wraparound services. Use of these funds is coordinated by the MACCC, with criteria for using the funds included in the ISPs. The child, family members, clinicians, and community agencies have access to these funds through the child's case managers.

## Participation of Children With SED in Community Activities

We must improve the capacity of the family and the community to support the child, and we must increase the resiliency of the child and the family so that they are able to withstand the pressures and handicaps that accompany SED. Efforts to develop systems of services will meet with only limited success unless resources are focused both on services for the child and the family or caregiver, and on increasing the opportunities available in local communities for children with SED. There is still considerable stigma associated with mental illness. The Partnership plans to target this stigma by working with a variety of community agencies and organizations and by linking children who have SED with other children in recreational, educational, and community settings.

Mental health services must take into account the cultural preferences and characteristics of those who would use these services. Programs for children with SED and their parents or caregivers need to attend to the characteristics of the children and the communities in which they live. For example, several studies have found that African-Americans make less use of mental health services than whites, even when barriers related to income and availability are reduced or eliminated (Chung and Snowden 1990; Scheffler and Miller 1989; Vernon and Roberts 1982). Cultural differences exist concerning beliefs about mental illness and the expression and meaning of symptoms and behaviors (Kleinman and Good 1985). These differences in attitudes and behaviors must be taken into account when designing a system of services and supports.

In developing its continuum of services, the Partnership has worked with family members and community leaders to identify the aspects of service providers and services that facilitate the use of these services. Partnership collaborators from state and local agencies have initiated several programs to increase the cultural sensitivity of providers, including a contract with Morgan State University, a historically Black university, to provide conferences and seminars addressing multicultural competence in mental health and human services. The Baltimore City Department of Health and Mental Hygiene has focused special attention on efforts by local agencies to provide additional training to staff.

Because the East Baltimore Partnership is a family-focused and community-oriented program, cultural competence involves not only the technical competence of providers of clinical services, but also the competence of the Partnership to work with a diverse group of community agencies, organizations, and individuals to craft alternative support systems for children with very different needs and families with different orientations, expectations, and interests. Cultural competence requires knowledge of the local community and the needs of the residents of this community as well as an understanding of the agencies that provide services in this community.

The Partnership will continue to facilitate input from the local community by employing parents, by hiring local residents when possible, and by seeking feedback from parents and from local residents and organizations. The participation in the Partnership by a diverse group of community agencies will ensure that issues of cultural competence and gender appropriateness continue to be raised and dealt with in the context of the overall planning process.

# Summary

Although there is a consensus concerning the necessity for a seamless system of services in which children and their families or caregivers receive services and supports consistent with their needs, few communities have either the array of services needed or the mechanisms for increasing or decreasing services as needs change (Stroul and Friedman 1986). A dilemma facing planners and policy makers has been how to constitute a system that focuses on the individual child and family (Katz-Leavy et al. 1992) while allowing for continuity of care and linkages among providers. The EBMHP addresses these issues by using multiagency planning teams for the development of individualized treatment plans for the child and family and by using multiagency planning committees (including family members) to develop local policies that facilitate the implementation of the individualized treatment plans. Partnership staff work with families to facilitate parents and caregivers acting aggressively as case managers and case coordinators. By involving parents, children, and all agencies that provide services to the child in the crafting of treatment plans and the monitoring of progress, we expect that programs in individual agencies will become more responsive to the needs of the family and to other providers of services and supports.

As described earlier, the EBMHP has benefited enormously from efforts by the state and city to restructure existing organizational arrangements and strategies. Of particular importance is the ongoing effort in Baltimore to focus on the reinvigoration of local neighborhoods by coordinating activities of local government, neighborhood organizations, the business community, academic and health institutions, and local and national foundations. Under a multifaceted program that Mayor Kurt Schmoke has called "reinventing government," there is a concerted effort in East Baltimore to strengthen the community infrastructure. The EBMHP is actively involved in these efforts to ensure that children with SED and their families experience no barriers to benefiting from the increased housing, educational, recreational, and vocational opportunities that are created, and to work on problems related to the exposure to violence that have substantial implications for the children and families enrolled in the project. By linking individualized service planning with community efforts to improve the quality of life of residents, the EBMHP strives to develop a model for planning and delivering services to children with SED and their families.

# References

Chung FK, Snowden LR: Community mental health and ethnic minority populations. Community Ment Health J 26:277–291, 1990

Duchnowski AJ, Friedman RM: Children's mental health: challenges for the nineties. Journal of Mental Health Administration 17:3–12, 1990

England MJ, Cole RF: Building systems of care for youth with serious mental illness. Hosp Community Psychiatry 43:630–633, 1992

Friedman RM, Duchnowski AJ, Henderson EL: Advocacy on Behalf of Children with Serious Emotional Problems. Springfield, IL, Charles C Thomas, 1989

Katz-Leavy JW, Lourie IS, Stroul BA, et al: Individualized Services in a System of Care. Washington, DC, Georgetown University CASSP Technical Assistance Center, 1992

Kleinman A, Good B: Culture and Depression: Studies in the Anthropology and Cross-Cultural Psychiatry of Affect and Disorder. Berkeley, University of California Press, 1985

Knitzer J: Unclaimed Children: The Failure of Public Responsibility to Children and Adolescents in Need of Mental Health Services. Washington, DC, Children's Defense Fund, 1982

Scheffler RM, Miller AG: Demand analysis of mental health service use among ethnic subpopulations. Inquiry 26:202–215, 1989

Stroul B, Friedman RF: A System of Care for Severely Emotionally Disturbed Children and Youth. Washington, DC, Georgetown University CASSP Technical Assistance Center, 1986

Vernon SW, Roberts RE: Prevalence of treated and untreated psychiatric disorders in three ethnic groups. Soc Sci Med 16:1575–1582, 1982

Zirul DW, Lieberman AA, Rapp CA: Respite care for the chronically mentally ill: focus on the 1990s. Community Ment Health J 2553:171–184, 1989

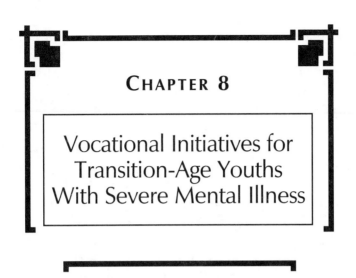

# CHAPTER 8

## Vocational Initiatives for Transition-Age Youths With Severe Mental Illness

**Judith A. Cook, Ph.D., Mardi L. Solomon, M.A.,
Diane Farrell, M.S., Matthew Koziel, B.A.,
and Jessica Jonikas, M.A.**

Throughout the 1980s there was increasing recognition of the underfunded, overly restrictive, fragmented system of mental health care for children and adolescents (Knitzer 1982; Stroul and Friedman 1986). Mental health services for this age group were characterized by overreliance on costly and unnecessary inpatient treatment (Weithorn 1988), lack of system coordination in creating a continuum of care (Saxe and Dougherty 1986), and failure to involve and support families of youths with severe emotional disturbances and behavior disorders (Collins and Collins 1990). As a result, the National Institute of Mental Health implemented the Children and Adolescent Service System Program (CASSP), to stimulate the development of a community-based system of comprehensive, coordinated care (Schlenger et al. 1992).

At the same time, the field of rehabilitation was questioning the effectiveness of special education services for youths with disabilities (Will 1983). The tremendous expenditure of tax dollars for public education of youths with special needs had yielded disappointing results (Will 1985). After years of special education services, youths exited high schools poorly prepared for transitions to employment or postsecondary education (Bellamy et al. 1985). Moreover, the field of vocational education had relied on overly restrictive models such as sheltered workshops, which offered piece-rate wages and limited opportunities for integration with nondisabled peers (Wehman et al. 1985). To address these issues, the U.S. Department of Education funded a series of model demonstration projects designed to facilitate the transition to work among youths with disabilities. A central feature of these programs was supported employment using a place-then-train approach (Wehman 1985) providing youths with jobs in integrated settings for minimum wage or above along with ongoing vocational support to maintain employment. After several studies had demonstrated the utility of this model, it was eventually followed by passage in 1990 of the Individuals with Disabilities Education Act or IDEA, which mandated the development of a transition plan by age 16 years for every youth in special education (Wermuth and Cook 1992).

Young adults (ages 16 through early twenties) with severe mental illness face illness-related obstacles, stigma, and poor service coordination resulting in poor chances of employment success (Cook et al. 1992). The earlier the age of first psychiatric hospitalization the poorer a young person's posthospital employment record and the higher his or her chances of rehospitalization (Beskind 1962; Bloom and Hopewell 1982; Pollack et al. 1968; Zigler and Levine 1981). The National Longitudinal Transition Study of students who exited special education programs (Wagner 1989) found that youths classified as emotionally disturbed had the highest percentage of high school dropouts and failing grades, the fourth lowest percentage of students pursuing postsecondary education (after multiply handicapped, deaf/blind, and mentally retarded), and the fifth lowest percentage of youths engaged in productive activity. The most recent findings from this study indicate that youths classified as emotionally disturbed had work experiences characterized by greater instability than all other disability groups (Wagner 1993). In a number of other follow-up studies of youths who received special education services in high school, those with emotional and behavioral difficulties had significantly lower rates of productive activity than comparison groups (Mithaug et al. 1985; Neel et al. 1988).

This chapter describes the services and client outcomes of a vocational program designed to address the multiple needs of this population in an integrated manner, using a community-based psychosocial rehabilitation context combined with supported employment.

# Program Description

## Setting

The Young Adult Program (YAP) for older adolescents at Thresholds in Chicago was based on the central tenet that the peer group is the primary agent of change for youths with psychiatric disorders (Farrell 1986). The psychosocial rehabilitation approach used since the YAP's inception stresses six major goals: vocational rehabilitation, educational achievement, development of strategies to manage symptomatology and divert hospitalizations, socialization and recreation, independent living, and maintenance of physical health (Dincin 1995). This model promotes consumer choice, individually tailored rehabilitation plans, a focus on strengths and wellness, psychoeducation about illness etiology and treatment, service delivery in integrated settings using natural supports, and membership for life (Barry 1982; Beard et al. 1982; Cook and Hoffschmidt 1993; Glascote et al. 1971; Mosher and Keith 1979; Paul and Lentz 1977). The YAP served as the foundation for the model program described in this chapter.

Youths attend an accredited day treatment school program in which they spend three mornings a week in small, academically oriented classes and two mornings working on the food or janitorial service crews to learn work readiness skills. In the afternoons youths participate in recreational activities, and individual and group sessions addressing such issues as grief, structured problem solving, stress management, and career development. Many youths reside in one of three community-based group homes or a network of supervised/supported apartments. While receiving vocational services, youths simultaneously receive training in independent living skills, medication management, individual therapy, and physical health services. Each youth's involvement in the program is coordinated by his or her case manager, who works in conjunction with multidisciplinary teams in treatment planning and implementation.

Prior to the new program's inauguration, Thresholds utilized a transitional employment placement (TEP) vocational model. The youngsters began on in-house crews, where they performed unpaid work in the agency two days per week learning basic, transferable work skills such as arriving at work on time, accepting supervision, and getting along with co-workers. After 4–8 months they progressed to their first paid group placement, with a community employer and an agency staff member called a job coach working alongside; placements were time-limited, requiring individuals to move on to a different position after about 6 months. Following successful completion of one or more group placements, youths moved on to a series of individual placements in which they were supervised directly by the employer and worked without the support of a job coach or other youths at the worksite. The final step was finding permanent competitive employment, which the youths located through employer-client matching or with the help of an agency Job Club, and which they held without workplace-based assistance.

## The Thresholds Supported Competitive Employment Program

In 1986, a program funded by the U.S. Department of Education, Office of Special Education and Rehabilitation Services, was inaugurated to add supported-employment services to those already available. The primary goal of the Supported Competitive

Employment Program (SCEP) was to synthesize the psychosocial model of psychiatric rehabilitation and the supported-employment model of vocational rehabilitation, in which vocational support is provided on an as-needed basis for as long as a youth needs or desires it. This was a departure from the previous "all or nothing" support philosophy in which youths either worked with a permanent job coach on a group placement or worked independently at an individual placement or competitive job with no on-site services (Cook et al. 1989). In the new program, job-support services were provided to youths at any stage of the rehabilitation process through the Mobile Job Support Worker (MJSW), who held a specially created staff position combining clinical and vocational expertise to provide immediate and mobile, on-the-job training, support, and advocacy. The new model also removed the time limits for holding agency placements. If a youth wanted to remain on a placement without changing to another position, this was arranged with the employer wherever possible. To increase the participation of community employers, the MJSW also engaged in assertive employer recruitment and education efforts, job finding and liaison services, and use of employers in a program advisory capacity. To encourage greater involvement of families, a Parent Advisory Board was established, attendance was encouraged at a Parents Support Group that met weekly at the agency, and outreach interviews were conducted with the parents of all new youths. Another major goal of the SCEP was the development and field testing of the On-the-Job curricular series focused on three problematic areas for employed youths with mental illness: social skills, stress management, and substance abuse.

The SCEP made MJSW services available to all youths who were employed, focusing especially on those youngsters who were having trouble on their jobs. This employed group consisted of 80 youths over the 3-year project period. Almost three-quarters (71%) were male; 66% were Caucasian, 28% African American, 5% Hispanic, and 1% other; and a quarter (26%) had secondary disabilities such as learning disabilities. The group averaged 19 years of age and 11.4 years of education at intake. Also at intake, youths had been psychiatrically hospitalized an average of 2 times; 44% had received a diagnosis of schizophrenia; and they averaged 22 total weeks as psychiatric inpatients, having spent 2.3% of their lifetimes in psychiatric hospitals.

After they entered the YAP, the average number of psychiatric hospitalizations for these youths was only .45. More than three-fourths of the young adults in this sample had some work experience before coming to the YAP, and held their longest jobs for an average of 34 weeks. Once in the YAP, it took the youths an average of almost 7 months before beginning job placements in the community. The young adults in this sample were involved in the YAP for an average of 1.5–2 years, and held an average of three jobs during their time in the program. The following sections describe the vocational and curricular components of the SCEP in which these clients participated along with case management issues that arose during service delivery.

### Case Management Issues

All turning points and life changes have the potential to elicit anxiety, but perhaps none so much as vocational growth (Viscott 1977). Employment means giving up the devalued yet familiar role of "mental patient" and taking on a new identity. The risks inherent in this process can be paralyzing given the compromised sense of mastery in many persons with mental illness along with impaired problem-solving abilities that impede risk-taking. An important component of this dilemma has been eloquently stated by Lamb (1979), who suggests that people with mental illness often mask their fear of failure by allowing others to see them as lazy and unmotivated rather than fearful or inadequate. It is essential to listen to youths as they express this anxiety and then help them break it down into manageable portions by encouraging the using of stress management and other coping skills.

The problem of stigma and its destructive effects on self-esteem and social interaction of persons with mental illness is well known (Link et al. 1991). Some of the concerns that are certain to come up for youths seeking employment include:

"What do I tell potential employers about my mental illness. Do I tell the truth? If I don't, how do I explain the gaps in my work record?" Once hired, youths worry about the reactions of their co-workers and supervisors to their consumer status or to potential disclosure of that status. As youths integrate into the work setting, issues never before encountered arise, such as the possibility of romance at the workplace or the need to ask for a raise or apply for a promotion. These are difficult concerns and case managers must reassure, educate, and support youths during this process. Targeted training in vocational social skills can help to prepare youths to cope with these issues.

Many young adults with psychiatric disorders find themselves accepting job situations that neither they nor their parents expected for them prior to the onset of their mental illness. Although every effort is made to accommodate youths' career aspirations, sometimes vocational or educational goals must be altered (Roussel and Cook 1987). Some youths are able to accept this, based on their awareness of their difficulties with pressure, problems interacting with others, and gaps in education and vocational preparation. In many cases, parents and siblings also will be able to accept this altered life course for their ill family member. Nonetheless, it may be difficult for other young adults to feel comfortable with their roles within the family structure if, for example, they have lower status jobs while their siblings are professionals. In individual counseling sessions, case managers need to be sensitive to this issue, and to listen to and understand the feelings associated with redefining vocational and other life goals in the struggle with severe mental illness.

Working with families at this juncture can be vital. Parents have their own sadness, fears, and losses to deal with in terms of their adolescents who have mental illness. Just as the adolescents have had to revise their expectations and hopes for themselves, parents have had to adjust to their own altered expectations for their children (Cook et al. 1994). Often this is difficult to accomplish, and professional intervention and support can aid the process. Parents need to grieve and this grief needs to be acknowledged and respected by professionals. To facilitate this process, a workbook was developed for parents of young adults with psychiatric disabilities who seek or hold community employment (Cook et al. 1991).

Separation can be as difficult for parents as for adolescents, and this is especially so in the case of adolescents with mental illness embarking on vocational careers. Parents fear that their children require protection and their genuine desire to provide that "cushion" of protection may in fact impede healthy attempts to separate and grow. It is important for case managers to convey the importance of separate and independent lives for people with mental illness, and to enlist parents' aid in helping their children to achieve this goal. Often, families require educational services to help them understand both the nature of mental illness and the nature of adolescence. This is particularly true for families from various cultures that have different ideas about the causes and meaning of mental illness than are accepted within typical psychosocial rehabilitation programs. Moreover, people from differing cultures may have a variety of views and expectations for all family members, regardless of the presence of mental illness. For instance, in some cultures women are not expected to work outside the home or to move away from their families until they are married, which often runs counter to the rehabilitation goals of employment and independent living. Case managers should convey a nonblaming message and attempt to build an alliance between the caseworker, the family, and the youth.

Case managers must be aware of their young clients' major concerns and priorities, because these may interfere with their ability to focus on vocational performance. Case managers must learn to wait until youths themselves are ready and then begin work toward vocational rehabilitation. This involves developing an awareness of where youths see the goal of employment in relation to other areas of their lives and how this may affect their job performance. Comprehensive case management must view nonvocational issues, such as the nature of social networks, loneliness, housing concerns, family problems, and financial difficulties, as an integral part of the ability to maintain vocational performance (Farrell 1992).

## Vocational Services

The greatest advantage of mobile job support is its tremendous flexibility in terms of when, where, and how support services can be provided. Sometimes this involves support at the workplace during the first few weeks of a new job. In other instances this entails assistance at job placements where youths have worked for a period of time but are now encountering difficulties. In still other cases youths need help dealing with a new supervisor or coping with job termination. Successful integration at the worksite also can create needs for support such as when a youth is promoted or seeks advancement within a company. Sometimes youths wish to keep their disability confidential because of the stigma attached to mental illness. In such cases the mobile nature of MJSW services makes it possible to meet young clients outside of work time to discuss job-related problems and formulate solutions.

In the SCEP program, MJSW job-development activities are designed to produce positions that correspond to youths' interests and that lay the groundwork for future jobs. The MJSW is the liaison with employers, teaching them about the needs of workers with psychiatric disability and teaching young workers about the needs of their employers. Many youths require individualized assistance in the job search process. This involves clarifying career goals and values, as well as learning and practicing specific job-seeking skills such as resume preparation and interviewing.

As youths become aware of the role of the MJSW, many are reassured by the knowledge that they can obtain help from a familiar staff member as they face the unknown. For some, the presence of the MJSW is enough to give them the security to work productively. Others see a visit from an MJSW as a reprimand for unsatisfactory work. Therefore, part of the planning process for a youth's support needs involves spending time with the MJSW away from the work setting. As the MJSW becomes a familiar resource to youths, they begin to define support visits as an expected and welcome part of most job placements.

Many youths need the greatest amount of support as they prepare for and begin a job, gradually needing less support as time passes. Youths who have difficulty waking early on their own are called or visited; many need direct assistance to learn the public transportation route to a new job, especially if it includes transfers or travel through unfamiliar areas. A careful orientation to such things as building layout, time-clock use, work and break schedules, the roles of various supervisors, and completing tax withholding and Federal I-9 forms often is necessary.

Once youths are established at their jobs, MJSWs gradually decrease the level of assistance, fading their support as needed. However, ongoing contact is maintained because it is better to check progress regularly rather than to wait for problems to arise. This also lets the youth know that the MJSW remains available and ready to give added support, especially during difficult periods. Without assistance, young workers may not take criticism constructively and may decompensate at work. In addition to finding new ways to approach vocational problems, the MJSW can reassure youths that they will not lose their jobs because of errors if they show some effort to improve their performance. With other individuals, however, the threat of job loss may be the only motivation that prompts them to change negative behaviors.

### Service Characteristics of MJSW Support

Throughout the 3-year program, MJSWs logged information about 297 different support events involving 41 clients. Eighty-four percent of the support events involved face-to-face interactions; phone calls accounted for 15% and nonroutine paper work 1%. The average number of support events per client was 7.2 (range 1–57). The MJSW spent an average of 43 minutes on each event, and an additional 33 minutes of travel time for the cases in which travel was required (185 of the 297 events or 62%). The majority of the support events were defined as routine, with only 26 (9%) classified as emergencies in which the youth was in immediate danger of hospitalization or of losing his or her job.

More than half (54%) of all support events occurred at a youth's current or potential worksite, sometimes in combination with other settings such as the surrounding neighborhood. Another frequent location was at the Thresholds agency (35%). In other cases, the MJSW met clients in public places or private homes, especially those youths who had not disclosed their psychiatric disability to employers and co-workers.

Regarding actors involved in the support events, more than half of all support instances included only the MJSW and the client (53%). A third of all support events (33%) included staff from the employing organization such as the youth's immediate supervisor, other supervisory staff, the firm's personnel manager, or the firm's liaison to the rehabilitation agency. In 8% of all events, the MJSW provided support to more than one client simultaneously, such as taking a small group of youths to visit a potential job site. There were also situations in which another YAP staff person, such as a job coach or case manager, would work with the MJSW to provide assistance to a client needing help.

The highest service utilizers were youths who were unemployed (28%), and those working individual placements (53%). Many youths sought MJSW assistance after quitting or being fired from a position, which often necessitated employer-client matching in order to find a setting that would better accommodate symptomatology or job skills limitations. Young adults employed at group placements did not require as much support (13%) because of the various supports built into the structure of the work arrangement (a permanent job coach at the job site and other clients working alongside). A significant amount of assistance was given to those making transitions from jobless to employed statuses and from a group work setting to an individual worksite. Youths employed independently also required relatively little support time (6%).

### The On-the-Job Curricular Series

The SCEP curricula were team taught by the MJSW and a certified special education teacher and were offered to all employed or recently employed youths. The social-skills curriculum encourages appropriate social behaviors and attitudes through use of guided discussion groups, role plays, exercises involving problem solving, and processing of clients' reactions to case studies that parallel their own experiences. Eighteen sessions one afternoon per week are devoted to developing appropriate working relationships with co-workers and supervisors (i.e., socialization at work, how to respond to questions about mental illness, overcoming withdrawal tendencies, understanding facial expressions and body posture, smoking etiquette, requesting raises and extra benefits, resolving conflicts, differentiating friendships from romantic interests, employee rights, and what to do when quitting or fired). The substance-abuse curriculum (10 sessions one afternoon per week) provides information about alcohol and drugs, how alcohol and drugs interact with the youths' illness and their prescribed medications, and how to effectively avoid using substances in social situations. Youths are encouraged to involve their supportive friends and families in the recovery process and to affiliate with support programs such as Alcoholics Anonymous and Dually-Diagnosed Anonymous. The stress-management curriculum (10 sessions one afternoon per week) uses group and individual discussions, case studies, role playing, problem-solving exercises, and questionnaires/rating scales targeting specific stressors and coping strategies. Youths are encouraged to make cassette tapes of relaxing music or self-enhancing statements to be played regularly. As in all curricula, participants keep a weekly journal documenting their stressful situations at work and their ability to apply the skills acquired in class.

# Program Evaluation

## Aggregate Hospitalization and Employment Outcomes

The proportion of youths hospitalized and the proportion employed were compared on a year-by-year basis for the 3 years preceding and the 3 years following SCEP implementation. As shown in Table 8–1, the proportion of youths hospitalized started at 18.2%, 3 years prior to the SCEP, and was 22.7% in the year immediately prior to SCEP inception, falling to 16.5% in the first year after program implementation and remaining at 17.9% in the third year after. The proportion employed, however, showed a clear trend toward increasing, beginning at 37.4%, 3 years before SCEP was established, and rising to 48.5% in the year before the program began. In the first year after implementation the percentage of youths employed rose to 56% and stayed there at 50.5% during the third year after SCEP inception.

By averaging proportions before and after implementation, the two aggregate outcomes can be compared. The average proportion hospitalized was lower after the SCEP began (18%) than before (21%), whereas the average proportion employed was higher after implementation (54%) as compared with before (43%) implementation. The fact that the hospitalization rate did not rise along with the employment rate suggests that employment is not connected with stress-related psychiatric relapse for youths with emotional difficulties.

**Table 8–1.**    Pre- and postprogram hospitalization and employment outcomes for youths with psychiatric disabilities

| Comparison dates | Hospitalized (%)[a] | Employed (%)[a] |
|---|---|---|
| Preprogram | | |
| 10/1/83–9/30/84 | 18.2 | 37.4 |
| 10/1/84–9/30/85 | 25.8 | 48.5 |
| 10/1/85–9/30/86 | 22.7 | 44.3 |
| Postprogram | | |
| 10/1/86–9/30/87 | 16.5 | 56.0 |
| 10/1/87–9/30/88 | 21.3 | 58.4 |
| 10/1/88–9/30/89 | 17.9 | 50.5 |

[a] Computed on the basis of the total number of youths served that year.

## Outcomes of MJSW Services

To address the question of whether receiving mobile job-support services was related to vocational success, we compared the vocational outcomes of youths, some of whom received MJSW services (55%) and some of whom did not (45%). The first step was to determine, through descriptive and correlational analyses, what characteristics (e.g., demographic, illness history, work history) differentiated these two groups. Correlation analysis revealed that younger adolescents were more likely then older ones to use MJSW services ($r = -.20, P < .05$). No other relationships were observed between receipt of MJSW services and client-level variables (such as gender, ethnicity, education, diagnosis, and secondary disability) or illness history characteristics (such as diagnosis, number of hospitalizations, number of weeks hospitalized, and proportion of lifetime hospitalized).

Three prior work-history variables were significantly related to receiving MJSW services. Youths were less likely to use services if they had some work experience prior to entering the program ($r = -.19, P < .05$). Youths were more likely to use MJSW services if they took a longer period of time before starting their first job ($r = .19, P < .05$). Finally, MJSW services were more likely to be used if youths held more jobs while in the SCEP ($r = .42, P < .001$). In addition, the longer youths were active in the program the more likely they were to receive MJSW services ($r = .53, P < .001$), making this latter factor an important control variable.

Next, employment outcomes of SCEP clients were calculated at three different time points: 6 months after entering the YAP program, 12 months after intake, and 6 months after beginning the first placement (which occurred at 14 months after intake on average). These measures (shown in Table 8–2) indicated that 38% were employed at 6 months, increasing to 56% employed at 12 months after intake, and 68% employed at 6 months after beginning their first jobs.

Next, the three employment outcome measures were correlated with receipt of MJSW services. At 6 months after intake, there was a nonsignificant negative relationship between receiving support and working; clients working at that time were less likely to receive MJSW services. At both 1 year after intake and 6 months after beginning the first placement, there was a positive and significant correlation between working and receiving mobile job-support services.

These results can be interpreted in light of the earlier finding that those individuals who began working most quickly were less likely to utilize MJSW services. Because it took the average young adult in this sample 7 months before beginning community employment, individuals who were working at 6 months tended to be the highest-functioning clients. In addition, youths working at 6 months after program entry were most likely to be in group placements where their need for MJSW support was lower because permanent job coaches were available.

Although the individuals who utilized support may have taken longer to begin work, once they started to work, MJSW support was associated with being employed 6 months later. This is noteworthy given that MJSW support was primarily, although

**Table 8–2.** Youths' employment status at three time points and relation to Mobile Job Support Worker services

| Time of assessment | % employed (*n* employed) | Correlation with MJSW services |
|---|---|---|
| 6 months after intake (*N* = 79) | 38 (30) | −.13 |
| 12 months after intake (*N* = 78) | 56 (44) | .32[*] |
| 6 months after first job (*N* = 76) | 68 (52) | .28[**] |

*Note.* Variations in *N* due to missing data for youths who left the program and whose employment status could not be verified. MJSW = Mobile Job Support Worker.
[a]Pearson correlation coefficient of MJSW services (0 = not received/1 = received) with employment status (0 = unemployed/1 = employed). Partial correlations (not shown) remained significant while controlling individually for gender, minority status, number of siblings, number of weeks at longest job ever held, time spent in psychiatric hospitals, and presence of a physical disability.
[*]$P > .05$. [**]$P < .01$.

not exclusively, directed to youths having difficulty. As we learned earlier, those receiving mobile job support were younger, had no prior work experience, and took longer to begin working. The fact that these youths are more likely to be employed at follow-up suggests that they may have closed the gap between themselves and their initially more successful peers.

The findings presented thus far demonstrate that receiving MJSW services is related to being employed at two out of three time periods following program entry. However, because youths were not randomly assigned to the two service conditions (mobile support and no mobile support), other features of the two groups may account for the relationships between mobile support and employment. The next phase of the analysis tested whether relationships between MJSW support and employment outcome variables remained significant when controlling for youths' background characteristics. To address this question, partial correlation coefficients (not shown) controlling for youths' background characteristics were computed for each of the three dependent outcomes and MJSW support. The relationships between support and working 1 year after intake and 6 months after beginning the first placement remained significant even when controlling (separately) for the effects of gender, minority status, physical disability, number of siblings, number of weeks at longest job ever held, and time spent in psychiatric hospitals.

The only control variable with an appreciable effect was program tenure, which diminished the relationship with employment at 12 months after intake but not at 6 months after beginning the first job, the last time point followed up. Here, controlling for tenure did not cause the coefficient to become nonsignificant; thus, youths at the latest follow-up time point were more likely to be employed if they had received MJSW support, regardless of program tenure.

The tenure finding is important, given that controlling for other variables had little impact on the association between mobile job support and employment. However, the association may have multiple meanings. The greater success of youths involved in the program longer may be due to their having received the new service as well as other program services (e.g., the on-the-job curricula, residential programming, individual and group therapy, medication management, and recreational activities). This interpretation assumes the program's effectiveness because the reasoning is that youths experiencing more programming do better. On the other hand, the MJSW-employment status relationship may simply be an artifact of the tendency for youths with long program tenure to have a greater likelihood of eventually getting a try at a job and receiving MJSW support. At 6 months after beginning employment, however, youths who received MJSW services did better regardless of tenure as well as all other background variables.

## Outcomes of the On-the-Job Curricula

As part of each of the three On-the-Job curricula, participants were evaluated with a pretest and a posttest to measure changes in social skills in the workplace (Waksman 1983), knowledge about addiction and recovery, and work-related stress (Golden 1986). Over the 3-year course of the SCEP, 50 youths took the social-skills curriculum, 28 took the substance-abuse curriculum, and 21 took the stress-management classes. In some cases, it was necessary to begin teaching the curricula before the final decisions had been made about the pretests and posttests. As a result, some youths who experienced the curricula were not tested. Of the 29 youths who received the social-skills curriculum after the pre- and posttests had been finalized, 22 completed tests and 7 did not complete tests for various reasons (e.g., leaving class to take a job, being rehospitalized, and leaving the program). Of the 19 who took the substance-abuse curriculum during the testing period, 15 completed one or both tests (11 completed both pre- and posttests) and 4 did not. Of the 21 youths who received the stress-management curriculum, 21 had at least 1 complete test and 12 completed both tests.

Overall, participation in all three curricula were associated with improvement in life areas related to course content: social skills, stress management, and substance use. Regarding social skills, paired $t$ tests computed between each youth's pre- and posttest scores (using ratings made by each youth's case manager) revealed that the mean for passive behavior fell from 17.3 to 13.8 ($t = -1.94, P < .10$) and for total social-skills deficits from 25.8 to 21.3 ($t = -1.72, P < .10$). The drop in ratings of aggressive behavior (from 8.5 to 7.5) was nonsignificant. Regarding the substance-abuse knowledge, the mean score of 79% correct rose to 83% correct; although this was an improvement in the anticipated direction, it was nonsignificant. On the other hand, there were significant reductions in the mean stress scores for youths on each of the 6 stress subscales (measuring stressors related to family, peers, school, emotional issues, developmental issues, and self). Paired $t$ tests also indicated that the total stress level declined significantly from a mean of 84 to a mean of 57 ($t = 3.00, P < .01$).

The final step in the analysis was to assess the presence of significant relationships between participating in each of the classes and being employed at a later point in time. Pearson correlation coefficients were computed between a variable measuring whether each curriculum was taken (none = 82; one = 19; two = 14; three = 5) and a dichotomous outcome variable assessing employment status at time of program termination or a cut-off date for clients who were still enrolled. As shown in Table 8–3, there were significant associations between taking each of the curricula and employment at program exit or its equivalent. Youths who experienced each class were more likely than those who did not to be working at follow-up. In addition, the actual number of classes taken by the youths was related to the dependent variable of later employment. In fact, the size of this latter correlation coefficient was the largest, suggesting the possible advantage of taking more than one of the curricula.

It is possible, however, that these significant relationships are spurious statistical artifacts of a true relationship between program tenure and employment success. Youths with poorer outcomes may have become discouraged and left the program

**Table 8–3.** Pearson correlations and partial correlations between receiving the curricula[a] and employment[b] at time of program exit or on January 31, 1990

| Curriculum | Correlation coefficient | Partial correlation (controlling for tenure[c]) |
|---|---|---|
| Substance abuse | .23[**] | .21[**] |
| Stress management | .31[***] | .32[***] |
| Social skills | .16[*] | .18[*] |
| Number of curricula | .32[***] | .31[***] |

[a]Coded as 0 = did not receive curriculum; 1 = received 70% of curriculum sessions.
[b]Coded as 0 = unemployed at closing or on 1/31/90 (if still active in program); 1 = employed.
[c]Tenure = number of days receiving program services.
[*]$P < .05.$ [**]$P < .01.$ [***]$P < .001.$

sooner, lowering the number of curricula in which they participated. Taking all three curricula could have been simply a by-product of remaining in the program longer because one was experiencing success. To test this possibility, partial correlation coefficients were computed controlling for length of time youths participated in the agency program (with an end point at termination or at time of follow-up assessment). As shown in the right-hand column of Table 8–3, results were virtually identical to the zero-order correlations. The positive association between participation in the curricula and later employment is not due to length of program tenure. Although the absence of a control group prevents us from making causal attributions, we can conclude that participating in one or more of the On-the-Job curricula was positively and significantly related to being employed in the community at follow-up. Not only did youths' scores on most of the pretest and posttest measures improve significantly over time, but taking each of the courses was significantly related to being employed at the time of leaving the program. Moreover, the greater the number of courses taken, the better the student's vocational outcome.

# Conclusions

The association between receiving MJSW support as well as SCEP curricula and subsequent employment suggests the need for individual tailoring of experiential vocational services along with focused didactic sessions. Altogether, these findings suggest that the psychosocial rehabilitation model can serve as an excellent context for implementing individualized supported-employment services. One of the strengths of the psychosocial approach is its comprehensiveness, which allows for developing unique rehabilitation plans from an "array of services" (Cook et al. 1992).

Although not currently popular given the emphasis on mainstreaming in education today (Shanker 1994), bringing youths with mental illness together in one program to serve as a reference group for growth and role modeling is a central part of this model's success. For service providers working within a mainstream school setting, our results at Thresholds suggest that bringing the psychosocial model into the public school curriculum and process may be beneficial in attempting to serve this population. The same may be true for providers of mental health services who operate in more traditional settings such as mental health centers or outpatient clinics. No matter what the organizational context, it is still possible to teach the On-the-Job curricula for stress management, social skills, and substance abuse avoidance, or provide case management sensitive to vocational issues to employed youths. Moreover, the mobile nature of MJSW services means that they can be provided in almost any type of organizational structure.

Providing services in the community and away from the school or rehabilitation agency was a priority in the SCEP. This approach was followed whenever possible by the MJSWs who delivered services in youth's work settings more than half of the time (54%). Many of the project members also were participating in a residential program for independent living, which involved moving from a neighborhood group home to a supervised apartment to an unsupervised residence to a privately rented apartment. In addition to community employment and community residence, leisure and recreational activities involved using the community to learn new social and problem-solving skills. The use of natural supports in settings aside from the vocational arena, such as residential and social, is a complementary mechanism to delivery of supported-employment services to youths with mental illness. These mechanisms are especially helpful because in the staff's experience, youths were highly sensitive to stigma and often resisted being labeled as "special" by their coworkers, family, or friends.

Analyses of case management issues and types of needed employment supports indicates that an integrated approach must be used with these youths. The intersection of age, disability, effects of medications, and stigma create a set of transition service needs unique to young adults with severe psychiatric disabilities. There has been prior documentation of service needs, gaps, resistance, and outdated legislation that hinders attempts to serve this population, who are especially vulnerable to "falling through the cracks" (Knitzer 1982; Stroul and Friedman 1986). The SCEP demonstrated that an integrated approach to case management and rehabilitation is associated with vocational success when the measure of success is community employment. This offers support for the suggestion that transition issues for these youths should be viewed in terms of their specific needs, keeping in mind the models used in successful programming for adults with mental illness.

Recent research indicates that youths with severe mental illness have significantly shorter job tenure than their adult counterparts (Cook 1992). It was clear from our analyses that the ongoing provision of support was needed by some, yet not all of the youths served in the program. Some young people chose to terminate services with the program once they had achieved their goal of community employment; others left before they were able to obtain a paid community job. However, others remained open in the program and took advantage of evening services for employed clients, became peer job coaches and job trainers, and participated in a Community Scholar Program (Cook and Solomon 1993) designed to help them secure college or postsecondary vocational training to improve job skills. Those who remained continued to use the MJSW as they sought to cope with new issues that arose at the workplace over time, or as they dealt with leaving one job and finding another. The longer they remained active in the program, the more likely they were to have taken the On-the-Job curricula, which were associated with employment at follow-up as well. It may be that those youths who achieved the highest levels of success were those who then needed the most support in order to maintain their jobs, as was found in a study of MJSW services to adults with mental illness (Cook and Razzano 1993).

The results of the SCEP for older adolescents are thought-provoking and action-inspiring. By applying some of the insights from this project to other service systems, an innovative model-building process is possible in most settings. With an imperative stemming from the unmet needs and relative neglect of this population, along with recognition of their great potential, we invite readers to join us in developing creative approaches to working with this group of young people.

# References

Barry P: Correlational study of a psychosocial rehabilitation program. Vocational Evaluation and Work Adjustment Bulletin 15:112–117, 1982

Beard J, Propst RN, Malamud TJ: The Fountain House Model of psychiatric rehabilitation. Psychosocial Rehabilitation Journal 5:47–53, 1982

Bellamy G, Wilcox B, Rose H, et al: Education and career preparation for youth with disabilities. Journal of Adolescent Health Care 6:125–135, 1985

Beskind H: Psychiatric inpatient treatment of adolescents: a review of clinical experience. Compr Psychiatry 3:354–369, 1962

Bloom R, Hopewell LR: Psychiatric hospitalization of adolescents and successful mainstream reentry. Exceptional Child 3:352–357, 1982

Collins B, Collins T: Parent-professional relationships in the treatment of seriously emotionally disturbed children and adolescents. Social Work 35:522–527, 1990

Cook JA: Job ending among youth and adults with severe mental illness. Journal of Mental Health Administration, 19:158–169, 1992

Cook JA, Hoffschmidt SJ: Comprehensive models of psychosocial rehabilitation, in Psychiatric Rehabilitation in Practice. Edited by Flexer RW, Solomon P. New York, NY, Butterworth-Heinemann, 1993, pp 81–97

Cook JA, Razzano L: Natural vocational supports for persons with severe mental illness: Thresholds Supported Competitive Employment Program, in Innovations in Mental Health Services. Edited by Stein L. San Francisco, CA, Jossey-Bass, 1993, pp 23–42

Cook JA, Solomon ML: The Community Scholar Program: an outcome study of supported education for students with severe mental illness. Psychosocial Rehabilitation Journal 17:83–97, 1993

Cook JA, Solomon ML, Mock L: What happens after the first job placement: vocational transitioning among severely emotionally disturbed and behavior disordered youth, in Programming for Adolescents with Behavior Disorders, Vol. IV. Edited by Braaten S, Rutherford R, Reilly R, et al. Reston, VA, Council for Children with Behavioral Disorders, 1989, pp 71–93

Cook JA, Jonikas JA, Solomon ML: Strengthening Skills for Success: A Manual to Help Parents Support Their Psychiatrically Disabled Youth's Community Employment. Chicago, IL, Thresholds National Research and Training Center, 1991

Cook JA, Jonikas JA, Solomon ML: Models of vocational rehabilitation for youth and adults with severe mental illness. American Rehabilitation 8:6–11, 1992

Cook JA, Lefley H, Pickett SA, et al: Age and family burden among parents of offspring with severe mental illness. Am J Orthopsychiatry 64:435–447, 1994

Dincin J: A Pragmatic Approach to Psychiatric Rehabilitation: Lessons From Chicago's Thresholds Program. San Francisco, CA, Jossey-Bass, 1995

Farrell D: Thresholds, a delivery system. Proceedings of the Schizophrenia Conference, Edmonton, Alberta, Canada, September, 1986

Farrell D: The missing ingredient: separate, specialized programming for adolescents with mental illness. Psychosocial Rehabilitation Journal 15:97–99, 1992

Glascote RM, Cumming E, Rutman ID: Rehabilitating the Mentally Ill in the Community: A Study of Psychosocial Rehabilitation Centers. Washington, DC, Joint Information Service, 1971

Golden B: Adolescent stress management. Paper presented at the 64th Annual Convention of the Council on Exceptional Children, New Orleans, LA, March, 1986

Knitzer J: Unclaimed Children: the Failure of Public Responsibility to Children and Adolescents in Need of Mental Health Services. Children's Defense Fund, Washington, DC, 1982

Lamb HR: Roots of neglect of the long-term mentally ill. Psychiatry 42:201–207, 1979

Link BG, Mirotznik J, Cullen FT: The effectiveness of stigma coping orientations: can negative consequences of mental illness labeling be avoided? J Health Soc Behav 32:302–320, 1991

Mithaug DE, Horiuchi CN, Fanning PN: A report on the Colorado statewide follow-up survey of special education students. Exceptional Children 51:397–404, 1985

Mosher LR, Keith SJ: Research on the psychosocial treatment of schizophrenia: a summary report. Am J Psychiatry 136:623–631, 1979

Neel RS, Meadows N, Levine P, et al: What happens after special education: a statewide follow-up study of secondary students who have behavioral disorders. Behavioral Disorders 13:209–216, 1988

Paul GL, Lentz RJ: Psychosocial Treatment of Chronic Mental Patients: Milieu vs Social Learning Programs. Cambridge, MA, Harvard University Press, 1977

Pollack M, Levenstein S, Klein DF: A three-year posthospital follow-up of adolescent and adult schizophrenics. Am J Orthopsychiatry 38:94–109, 1968

Roussel AE, Cook JA: The role of work on psychiatric rehabilitation: the Visiting Chefs Program. Sociological Practice 6:149–168 1987

Saxe L, Dougherty D: Children's Mental Health Needs: Problems and Services. Washington, DC, Office of Technology Assistance, U.S. Government Printing Office, 1986

Schlenger WE, Etheridge RM, Hansen DJ, et al: Evaluation of state efforts to improve systems of care for children and adolescents with severe emotional disturbances: the CASSP initial cohort study. Journal of Mental Health Administration 19:131–142, 1992

Shanker A: The fallacies of full inclusion. The Journal of the California Alliance for the Mentally Ill 5:13–15, 1994

Stroul B, Friedman R: A system of care for severely emotionally disturbed children and youth. National Institute of Mental Health, CASSP, Technical Assistance Center, Washington, DC, 1986

Viscott D: Risking. New York, Pocket Books, 1977

Wagner M: The Transition Experiences of Youth With Disabilities: A Report From the National Longitudinal Transition Study. Menlo Park, CA, SRI, 1989

Wagner M: Trends in postschool outcomes of youths with disabilities: findings from the National Longitudinal Transition Study of special education students. Interchange 12:2–4, 1993

Waksman S: Waksman Social Skills Rating Form (School Edition). Portland, OR, ASIEP Education Company, 1983

Wehman P: Supported competitive employment for persons with severe disabilities, in School-to-Work Transition for Youth with Severe Disabilities. Edited by McCarthy P, Everson J, Moon S, et al. Richmond, Virginia Commonwealth University, 1985, pp 167–182

Wehman P, Kregel J, Seyfarth J: Employment outlook for young adults with mental retardation. Rehabilitation Counseling Bulletin 29:90–99, 1985

Weithorn LA: Mental hospitalization of troublesome youth: an analysis of skyrocketing admission rates. Stanford Law Review 40:773–837, 1988

Wermuth TR, Cook JA: The impact of federal legislation on the transition of individuals with psychiatric disabilities from school to adult life. Community Support Network News 8:10–11, 1992

Will MC: OSERS Programming for the Transition of Youth With Disabilities: Bridges From School to Working Life. Washington, DC, Office of Special Education and Rehabilitative Services, 1983

Will MC: Opening remarks. J Adolesc Health Care 6:79–83, 1985

Zigler E, Levine J: Age of first hospitalization of schizophrenics: a developmental approach. J Abnorm Psychol 96:458–467, 1981

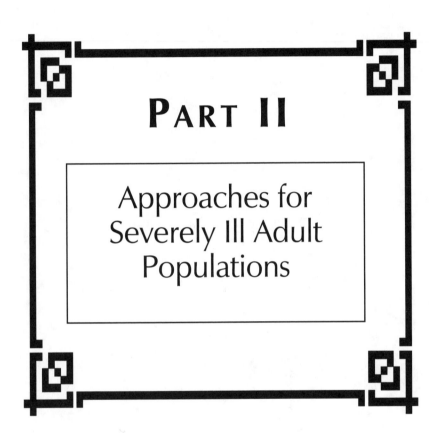

# PART II

## Approaches for Severely Ill Adult Populations

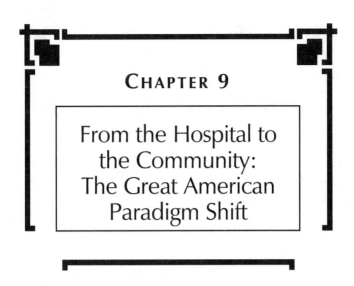

# CHAPTER 9

## From the Hospital to the Community: The Great American Paradigm Shift

**Neil Meisler, M.S.W., and Alberto B. Santos, M.D.**

One of the most important innovations in mental health services in this century was developed in the early 1970s by the staff of the Mendota Mental Health Institute in Madison, Wisconsin. These clinician-investigators facilitated a major prototype shift in the popular concept of the multidisciplinary-treatment-team approach. Through carefully controlled monitoring of outcomes and costs, they demonstrated significant advantages to shifting the team's work setting from the milieu of the psychiatric hospital to that of the natural community field. Over subsequent years the service approach that became known as Training in Community Living (TCL) or Program for Assertive Community Treatment (PACT) was identified as effectively addressing two key shortcomings that undermined the era of deinstitutionalization: service fragmentation and gaps in continuity of care. In this chapter we trace the development of the approach, describe its core elements, review the findings of systematic evaluations of its application in other circumstances

167

and settings, and discuss implications for mental health policy and future research.

## History and Early Studies

The service system evolved through a series of projects conducted on a research unit at one of Wisconsin's two state hospitals, Mendota Mental Health Institute in Madison. The research unit was established in 1966 by Arnold Ludwig, M.D., Director of Research at Mendota, with a mandate to innovate and evaluate progressive in-hospital approaches for long-stay patients with chronic schizophrenia to try to improve their hospital adjustment and facilitate their discharge. From 1966 to 1970, the unit's staff developed and evaluated several in-hospital interventions (e.g., use of peer pressure and behavioral therapy to improve social behavior, brief, intensive therapy, and mutual support). Each study lasted 6–8 months (Ludwig 1968; Ludwig and Marx 1968, 1969, 1970; Ludwig et al. 1971; Marx and Ludwig 1969). Improved patients would be discharged and followed through traditional office-based outpatient services provided at the Dane County Community Mental Health Center.

In 1970, Arnold Marx, M.D., was director of the research unit and Mary Ann Test, Ph.D., was associate director. Test and Stein (1992) reported that, in the spring of 1971, staff morale and enthusiasm seemed low. When queried during one of their routine brainstorming sessions in which research ideas were generated, staff reflected that they had been piloting in-hospital programs for 4 years, which resulted in a number of patients being discharged. However, although patients usually looked great at the time of discharge, many would be readmitted looking as if they had been living a horrible life in the community. It was as if no matter what was done with the patients in the hospital, it did not seem to help them live in the real world.

One staff person noted an exception to this experience. Discharged patients with whom the research unit social worker, Barbara Lontz, continued to work were not readmitted. The ensuing discussion revealed that Ms. Lontz assisted clients in getting established in their postdischarge living situation and then provided ongoing support—not just during workdays, but sometimes during evenings and weekends as well. She would help them to get familiar with stores and other resources in their neighborhoods. She would give her home phone number to the landlord and say, "If you have any problems, call me, any time during the day or night." She would ride the bus with the client to the mental health center to make sure he or she knew how to go down there to get medications. If her clients were referred to a sheltered workshop, she would go there with them, sitting side by side helping them to get comfortable and learn the work. In short, she did whatever needed to be done out on the client's turf to help the client make a successful adjustment to community living.

The idea for the next research project developed through that conversation. In an organized fashion, research unit staff would go into the community to facilitate the discharge and community adjustment of research unit patients. This step required the approval of the Hospital Executive Committee, which responded to the presentation by Drs. Test and Marx with a barrage of concerns. How would they supervise the staff in an open system? What about car insurance? What about liability if a patient under their care was hurt or hurt somebody? The only enthusiastic support they received at that meeting for this unusual proposal was from Leonard Stein, M.D., who had just succeeded Dr. Ludwig as Director of Research. Dr. Stein already had a longstanding interest in community care, and although he was new to his job as Director of Research, he was willing to take this risk.

Drs. Test, Marx, and Stein started working together on the ideas and very soon were able to develop a formal pilot study conducted between 1971 and 1972 (Marx et al. 1973). The unit chiefs of other wards at Mendota were asked to identify patients with high rates of hospital use who were definitely not ready for discharge to the community. These patients were randomly assigned to the research ward ($N = 41$) or were assigned to remain on their current treatment ward ($N = 20$). Patients assigned to the research ward were randomly assigned to a group that stayed on the research ward ($N = 20$) to further prepare them for community living, or to an experimental group ($N = 21$), whose members were discharged within 8 days of transfer to the research ward. Half the staff of the research ward were assigned to serve those who were discharged, doing the kind of hands-on work that Barbara Lontz had done with her discharged patients as well as extensive work with families, landlords, and community organizations. The experimental intervention was called Prevention of Institutionalization. The duration of the pilot study was 5 months. During this period, experimental-group clients spent an average of 6 days in the hospital, whereas clients in each control group spent an average of 100 days in the hospital. Experimental-group clients spent an average of 100 days living independently in apartments or rooming houses, whereas clients in the control groups spent an average of 10 and 15 days in independent housing. At the end of the 5 months, 17 of the experimental-group clients were living independently compared with 6 of the clients who were treated on the research ward and 3 of those who were treated on other wards. Nine of the experimental-group clients were employed part-time or full-time outside of a sheltered work setting compared with 3 in each of the control groups. There were no significant pretreatment and post-treatment within-group differences or between-group differences with regard to measures of symptomatology or self-esteem administered by independent raters who were blind to clients' treatment conditions.

In 1972, the inpatient research unit was closed and the staff, still under the auspices of Mendota Mental Health Institute, was relocated to a rented house in downtown Madison. The newly constituted community-based research unit was named the Program for Assertive Community Treatment (PACT). A second community treatment study was undertaken, which was named the Alternatives to Mental Hospital Study (Stein et al. 1975). An unselected group of patients (ages 18–62) presenting to the Mendota Mental Health Institute for admission were randomly assigned to the experimental intervention, called Training in

Community Living (TCL), or to a control group, which received short-term in-hospital treatment followed by aftercare, primarily in the Dane County publicly funded clinic. Most patients assigned to TCL were walked directly from the Mendota admissions suite by TCL staff who provided crisis stabilization and follow-up care in home- and community-based settings for a period of 12 months, after which they were transitioned over a period of 2 months to other service providers in Dane County. Experimental-group clients received the TCL intervention for 12 months; then they were gradually discharged (over 2 months) to the existing community programs in Dane County. After the 14-month treatment phase, experimental- and control-group clients were followed for an additional 14 months to measure the long-range effects of the TCL treatment condition. The client profile was as follows: mean age 31 years; 55% males to 45% females; 50% diagnosed with schizophrenia with the remaining half having a variety of diagnoses; average of 5 prior hospitalizations; and average total time in hospitals 14 months. At 4-month intervals, independent raters assessed the clients in both treatment conditions on measures of symptomatology, community adjustment, and self-esteem.

There were two key findings. First, during the 14-month treatment phase, persons assigned to the TCL program had significantly fewer hospital days, more independent living situations, more sheltered employment, more income from employment, more contact with friends, more satisfaction with their life situations, and less psychiatric symptomatology than those who received inpatient treatment followed by outpatient clinic care (Stein and Test 1980). A comprehensive economic cost-benefit study comparing the TCL with the traditional-care model revealed a small overall economic advantage in favor of the TCL model (Weisbrod et al. 1980). A study of the relative social costs of TCL versus the traditional model revealed that the significant gains made by the TCL patients were not at the expense of additional burden to family or community members (Test and Stein 1980). These findings were consistent with those of the pilot study.

The second major finding was not expected. Most of the differences in favor of the TCL approach were extinguished within 14 months of transfer from the PACT program to more traditional outpatient care (Stein and Test 1980). By the end of the 14-month posttreatment follow-up period, the only significant differences remaining between the TCL and control groups were in income from competitive employment and social groups attended.

> Now at first blush, that was a disappointing finding but on second thought I think we have to say it was the most important thing we learned in the study; up until this time, virtually all treatment programs for treatment with serious mental illness were time-limited programs and they were based on the notion of either curing people or preparing them to go on without significant help; the findings of this study provided evidence that TCL is an effective model of community treatment and rehabilitation for the revolving-door type of patients in the study. The study findings also suggested, however, that community treatment and rehabilitation may need to be long term and ongoing (Test and Stein 1992).

PACT has operated continuously since 1972. A group of PACT clients admitted between 1978 and 1985 comprise the experimental group in a 14-year prospective study (Test 1992; Test et al. 1985, 1992). The principal investigator, Mary Ann Test, and co-investigators William Knoedler and Deborah Allness, have been associated with PACT since its inception. Arnold Marx died in the mid-1970s. Leonard Stein left Mendota Mental Health Institute in 1975 to join the faculty at the University of Wisconsin Medical School Department of Psychiatry and to assume the position of medical director at the Dane County Mental Health Center. Mary Ann Test left Mendota Mental Health Institute in 1979 to join the faculty at the University of Wisconsin School of Social Work. William Knoedler has been the director of PACT since 1972. Deborah Allness, who joined PACT in 1972 and later became its co-director, left Mendota Mental Health Institute in 1986 to become the director of the Wisconsin Department of Health and Social Services Bureau of Community Mental Health. In that capacity between 1986 and 1990, she was instrumental in implementing statewide standards and Medicaid coverage for community-support programs based on the TCL model. William Knoedler and Deborah Allness have consulted in many states (including Michigan, Illinois, Indiana, Ohio, Idaho, Iowa, Rhode Island, Delaware, and South Carolina) and in Great Britain and Australia, assisting public mental health agencies and researchers in PACT replication efforts. PACT has hosted more than 400 visits of interested administrators, clinicians, researchers, and advocates.

In 1993, the American Public Health Association presented the distinguished Carl A. Taube Award for Outstanding Contribution to Mental Health Services Research, to Drs. Mary Ann Test, Leonard Stein, and Burton Weisbrod for their innovative research on TCL. Their research was the first to be implemented from the outset of the development of a new mental health service intervention and was the first to include a comparative evaluation of economic and social costs. Both because of their initial innovations and the long-term commitment of others involved in the implementation of PACT to the dissemination of the principles that underlie the TCL model, their research has had more impact on the provision of mental health services to persons with severe mental illness than any other intervention with empirically demonstrated effectiveness.

## Program Elements

This approach represents an integration of biological, psychological, and social interventions with innovations over traditional community mental health services in the organization and delivery of services (Table 9–1). TCL allows for the application of pharmacological and psychosocial treatments within an intensive field-based support system enabling most clients to live independently in their communities.

The approach directly addresses the multiple and complex needs of persons with severe mental illness in a pragmatic, flex-

**Table 9–1.**   Differences between TCL and traditional mental health care systems

| Service element | Traditional systems | TCL |
|---|---|---|
| Primary locus of care | Hospital, residential programs, day programs, offices | In the field (community, home, neighborhood, worksite) |
| Provider | Individual clinician for individual outpatients, multidisciplinary teams for inpatients. Treatment time highly variable. Outpatient caseloads high; inpatient caseloads low. Fragmented continuity of care across loci of care. | Generalist teams share a fixed caseload. Ratio of staff to clients, 1:10–15. Treatment time unlimited. Direct services continuously available. |
| Treatment approach | Specific individual and/ or group psychosocial therapies, and biological treatments provided mostly in a health care facility. Providers not held directly accountable for outcomes. | Medication monitoring and social support (help with housing, health, basic needs) in natural community environment. Providers held accountable for outcomes. |

ible, and comprehensive manner. The core of TCL is a treatment team, which assumes global responsibility for a group of clients. The treatment team is characterized by shared responsibility for clients and an intensive staff-to-client ratio. The ACT team's approach toward clients is assertive, emphasizing outreach and out-of-office interventions 24 hours a day, 7 days a week. To engage and retain persons in treatment, the team assumes a can-do attitude, using a comprehensive array of treatment, rehabilitative, and supportive interventions, as well as environmental modifications, to promote independent and productive functioning.

TCL operates as a self-contained program, incorporating core psychiatric, supportive, and rehabilitative services within the team, which serves as a fixed point of responsibility, accountable for clients' psychiatric and social welfare. The team focuses attention on specific client outcomes: reduced symptomatology and subjective distress; increased community tenure; enhanced satisfaction with life; and improved psychosocial functioning (Test 1992). Specific tasks include close psychiatric monitoring, including the taking of medications; facilitating the acquisition of basic resources (housing, entitlements, and general health care); support in dealing with life's daily problems, which can easily overwhelm clients; teaching and reinforcing essential skills in the natural environment (e.g., homemaking, financial management, communication, and employment); modifying pathological dependency relationships; and developing a supportive network among family and significant others, thus decreasing their stress and frustration in relating to the client (Stein and Test 1980).

The team traditionally includes a mix of disciplines (psychiatrist, nurses, social workers, rehabilitation therapists) who care for a shared caseload of up to 120 clients. Detailed psychosocial assessments and specific treatment plans are the core around which all interventions are organized in a weekly schedule for each client. The nature and frequency of client contact is determined by these, and by close monitoring of the individual's changing needs. Daily clinical rounds are held during which staff schedules are adjusted according to each client's present status. When a client is hospitalized or jailed, team members consult with the institution's staff and remain directly engaged with the client to facilitate resolution of the problems that contributed to the crisis episode.

## Research Support

Since the seminal controlled studies of the implementation of the TCL model (Marx et al. 1973; Stein and Test 1980; Stein et al. 1975), controlled studies have accompanied ACT program development in Australia and Great Britain as well as in several sites in the United States (see Table 9–2). None of these studies has included as comprehensive a set of measurement domains (hospitalization, independent living, symptoms, self-esteem, quality of life, criminal justice involvement, employment, economic cost-benefit, and social costs) as the TCL study by Weisbrod et al. (1980); nor have any demonstrated as clear a benefit of assertive community treatment over facility-based outpatient services across multiple domains. In these trials, the experimental treatment condition has ranged from close fidelity (Hoult et al. 1983; Muijen et al. 1992; R. Mulder, unpublished manuscript, August 1982) to loose fidelity (Bond et al. 1988, 1990; Jerrell and Hu 1989) to the TCL model. The following review, therefore, groups the studies into these two categories.

The TCL study (Weisbrod et al. 1980) and two randomized trials of ACT closely based on the TCL model (Hoult et al. 1983; R. Mulder, unpublished manuscript, August 1982), in which treatment costs were measured, demonstrated its cost-effectiveness. In each of these studies, as well as another that did not measure treatment costs (Muijen et al. 1992), the approach demonstrated improvements in community tenure. The two studies that compared the living arrangements of the two groups found that the E clients were more likely to be living independently (R. Mulder, unpublished manuscript, August 1982; Stein and Test 1980). All of these studies included a majority of patients with schizophrenia-related disorders. The one study that reported specifically and in detail about clients with schizophrenia (Hoult and Reynolds 1984) found significant differences in hospital use, satisfaction with treatment, and psychotic symptoms between E and control clients, with TCL having the advantage.

Regarding controlled studies of programs more loosely based on the TCL model, two found them to be more effective than office-based interventions in reducing hospital use (Bond et al. 1988, 1990), and one (Jerrell and Hu 1989) found comparable improvements in reduction of hospital use and comparable costs.

In all of the studies, with the exception of the one by Jerrell and Hu (1989), the control conditions were fairly standard, consisting of office visits for medication maintenance and counseling. In the study reported by Jerrell and Hu (1989), although control-group clients were assigned to outpatient clinics, which provided only medication maintenance and counseling in a staff-to-client ratio varying from 1:40 to 1:70, clients also had access to a generalist case manager program that provided community-based assistance with social, vocational, and housing needs and to a variety of social support and vocational rehabilitation programs operating parallel to the clinics.

The study by Jerrell and Hu (1989) had more mixed results than the others. Experimental-group clients received more clinical and case management contacts than control-group clients but the groups had comparably positive outcomes in regard to decreased inpatient service use. The reduction in inpatient use was less dramatic than in the case of the other studies that employed the TCL model. During the first three measurement intervals, the experimental group experienced improvements in psychosocial measures, whereas the control group did not; however, these differences were not evident at the end of the 2-year follow-up period. Total direct-care costs for the experimental group increased over the course of the study, whereas costs for the control group decreased by a comparable amount; however, there was no significant difference in total costs between the groups. This study would suggest comparability of benefit between ACT programs and comprehensive, but less coordinated, community mental health services. However, because the experimental condition varied from multiple core elements of the TCL model, the meaning of its findings is less clear.

There are several studies in progress in which the experimental conditions are the TCL model and the control conditions are community mental health centers that provide comprehensive, but less coordinated, services, including all 10 core elements of the federal Community Support Program systems model (Essock and Kontos 1995; Santos et al. 1993a, 1993b; Test 1992; Test et al. 1985). These studies may shed light on the effects of incorporating key principles of TCL (e.g., fixed point of accountability

**Table 9–2.** Outcomes of randomized trials

| Study | Site and years | Clinical and psychosocial outcomes |
|---|---|---|
| Marx et al. (1973) | Madison, WI[a] (1970–1972) | More effective (5-month trial) in reducing use of hospitals and ERs, in improving residential status, and in preserving occupational status |
| Weisbrod et al. (1980) | Madison, WI[a] (1974–1978) | More effective (12-month trial) in reducing use of hospitals, nursing homes, and law enforcement services; in improving residential status, and improving socialization, instrumental functioning, and symptom profiles |
| R. Mulder, unpublished MS., August 1982 | Grand Rapids, MI[b] (1982–1985) | More effective (30-month trial) in reducing use of hospitals and law enforcement services; and in improving instrumental functioning and residential status |
| Hoult and Reynolds (1983) | Sidney, Australia[a] (1979–1981) | More effective (12-month trial) in reducing use of hospitals and ERs; in improving instrumental functioning, symptom profile, residential status, and occupational activity |
| Bond et al. (1988) | 3 MHCs Indiana[b] (1986–1988) | More effective (6-month trial) in reducing use of hospitals in 2 of 3 sites |
| Jerrell and Hu (1989) | Santa Clara, CA[b] (1985–1988) | More effective in reducing use of hospitals and ERs. Positive changes in functioning and quality of life at 12 months not present at 24 months |

| Bond et al. (1990) | Chicago, IL[b] (1984–1987) | More effective (12-month trial) in reducing use of hospitals, and in improving instrumental functioning, satisfaction with life, and residential status |
| Muijen et al. (1992) | London, England[b] (1985–1990) | More effective (36-month trial) in reducing use of hospitals |
| Test et al. (1992) | Madison, WI[b] (1978–1990) | More effective (2-year follow-up) in reducing use of hospitals; in improving residential and mental health status |

[a]Subjects in acute phase of mental illness. [b]Subjects in stable phase of mental illness.

for care, assertive outreach, practical assistance, community-based contacts, support to social networks) within larger systems of care that incorporate a variety of programs and case management approaches. Preliminary results reported for two of these studies indicate advantage for TCL. A 14-year prospective study is comparing 7- to 10-year outcomes of clients with schizophrenic disorders randomly admitted as young adults early in the course of their illnesses to PACT or existing services in Dane County (Test 1992; Test et al. 1985). Findings after 2 years of treatment indicated that clients receiving TCL through PACT experienced significantly fewer hospitalizations and hospital stays and significantly more time living in independent arrangements than did clients receiving services in the comparison condition. The groups did not differ in the amount of time spent incarcerated or in homeless shelters, which was small in both cases.

An 18-month study in three Connecticut cities compared effects and costs of ACT programs, closely adhering to the TCL model, and case management by individual case management practitioners combined with access to comprehensive CMHC services (Essock and Kontos 1995). In both conditions, case management functions include assertive outreach and provision of direct assistance in the community. Preliminary results for a 6-month period early in the study indicated that ACT clients spent less time than control-group clients in inpatient settings or shelters.

# Dissemination

In addition to the dissemination of TCL throughout Wisconsin, there has been statewide, closely replicated dissemination of TCL in Michigan, Rhode Island, and Delaware (Meisler 1995; Plum and Lawther 1992). Programs with varying degrees of adherence to the TCL model are operating in many other states and in Canada, Australia, and Great Britain as well. A number of these programs have been implemented as research demonstration projects, making TCL the most empirically studied of all community mental health program approaches. A variety of names have been given to programs based on the TCL model, including mobile treatment teams (Detrick and Stiepock 1992), continuous treatment teams (CTT) (Torrey 1986), and assertive community treatment (ACT) (Taube et al. 1990).

The TCL approach also provided the foundation for the federal Community Support Program (CSP) systems model (Stroul 1989; Turner and TenHoor 1978). It incorporates all 10 of the services identified as essential within a community support system, as well as the recommended attributes of a community support system for service coordination at both system and client levels (see Table 9–3).

However, the CSP recommendations fell short of providing specific operational criteria. Therefore, there are now a variety of approaches in place across and within the states that use assertive case management principles. These can be differentiated by organization (e.g., freestanding case-management specialist programs, case managers within treatment programs, case management as a function of each member of a treatment team), orientation (e.g., service broker, peer/advocate, strengths facilitator, rehabilitation agent, network facilitator, clinician), intensity (e.g., client-to-staff ratios varying from 1:40 to 1:10), and availability (varying from weekdays to around the clock and from office-bound services to home- and community-based provision of assistance). These case management approaches have been described and differentiated as specific models in several reports (Chamberlain and Rapp 1991; Harris and Bergman 1993; Solomon 1992). The most prevalent approach in most states is the individual generalist case manager who provides outreach to keep clients engaged in mental health treatment and assists them in getting their needs met by mental health, welfare, health care, and rehabilitation systems (Intagliata 1982). The generalist case manager is not a treatment or rehabilitation agent and typically has a bachelor's level or less education in human services. The generalist approach fits the prevailing organization of community mental health services in the United States: outpatient clin-

**Table 9–3.**  Elements of community support systems and their origins in TCL

| Community support systems | TCL |
| --- | --- |
| I.   Philosophical principles<br>   A.  Services should have the following qualities:<br>     1. Be consumer centered<br>     2. Empower clients<br>     3. Be racially and culturally appropriate<br>     4. Be flexible<br>     5. Focus on strengths<br>     6. Be normalized and incorporate natural supports<br>     7. Meet special needs<br>     8. Be coordinated<br>   B.  Service systems should be accountable<br>II.  Service components<br>   A.  Client identification and outreach<br>   B.  Mental health treatments<br>   C.  Crisis response services<br>   D.  Health and dental care<br>   E.  Housing<br>   F.  Income support and entitlements<br>   G.  Peer support<br>   H.  Family and community support<br>   I.  Rehabilitation services<br>   J.  Protection and advocacy<br>   K.  Case management | I.   Organization and delivery of services<br>   A.  Core services team (continuous treatment team)<br>     1. Fixed point of responsibility (all needs)<br>     2. Primary provider of services<br>     3. Continuity of care and caregivers across functional areas and across time<br>   B.  Assertive outreach and in vivo treatment<br>   C.  Individualized treatment<br>     1. Between clients<br>     2. Within clients across time<br>   D.  Ongoing treatment and support<br>II.  Treatments and services provided<br>   A.  Direct assistance with symptom management<br>     1. Medications<br>     2. 24-hour crisis availability<br>     3. Brief hospitalization<br>     4. Long-term 1:1 clinical relationship |

*(continued)*

**Table 9–3.** Elements of community support systems and their origins in TCL *(continued)*

| Community support systems | TCL |
| --- | --- |
| | B. Facilitation of an optimally supportive environment<br>1. Assistance with meeting basic needs (housing, etc.)<br>2. Assistance with a supportive social environment<br>3. Assistance with a supportive family environment (psychoeducation) |
| | C. Direct assistance with instrumental functioning (work, social relations, activities of daily living)<br>1. In vivo skill teaching<br>2. In vivo support<br>3. Environmental modifications |

*Source.* Adapted from Stroul (1989) and Test (1992).

ics, day activity programs, psychosocial clubhouses, and supervised residential settings, which operate with a high degree of autonomy from one another, and in which clients are frequently involved in two or more programs concurrently. Generalist case managers have been added to these settings to provide outreach, linkage, monitoring, and advocacy functions. They work, more or less, as a member of a loose treatment team, with other professionals attending to clinical management, counseling, rehabilitation of the client, or all three.

Case management has also been organized within homogeneous or heterogeneous teams as discrete case management programs. Case management programs fall along a continuum in terms of orientation, intensity, and availability. At one end of the continuum is the generalist case manager program in which case managers work together as a unit within a comprehensive mental health agency or as a freestanding agency not affiliated with the mental health service program(s) in which the client is enrolled. Case managers work with clients on a solo basis to facilitate their access to, and appropriate use of, services across the mental health, health care, and social welfare systems. They also counsel clients to help them cope with the demands of daily living; and may provide some direct assistance in this regard, depending on the size and demand of their caseloads, which are typically 1:30 or greater.

Finally, at the other end of the continuum are TCL-like multidisciplinary treatment teams in which responsibility for case management is embedded within the function of each team member, who also performs one or more specialized roles within the team. Responsibility for case management for each client is also shared by multiple team members, although each client has a specific team member as a primary therapist/case manager. The multidisciplinary-treatment-team model contains a variety of disciplines necessary to provide a comprehensive array of psychotherapeutic, rehabilitative, and supportive services, minimizing the use of other mental health programs.

If the TCL model were superior to the prevailing structure of community support systems, the public policy implications for restructuring existing systems would be daunting. However, it may be that the approach and intensity of the TCL intervention has more to do with client outcome than with its structural characteristics. For example, positive findings similar to those reported above (Hoult and Reynolds 1984; Muijen et al. 1992; R. Mulder, unpublished manuscript, August 1982; Stein and Test 1980) have occurred in controlled clinical trials of family preservation using multisystemic therapy, an assertive case management approach to a variety of adolescent clinical problems (Borduin et al. 1990, in press; Brunk et al. 1987; Henggeler et al. 1986, 1990, 1991). Although team size and composition differ from one approach to another, they appear to have common elements to which their mutual success may be attributed.

First, they assume a social and ecological model of behavior. That is, they proceed from the assumption that the client's capacity to function in the community is linked both to his or her psychological and social characteristics and to key elements in the environment, such as family, work and school, and neighborhood. Moreover, the client's psychosocial characteristics and social environment are inexorably linked. Second, their treatment approaches are pragmatic, with an emphasis on action-oriented and well-specified interventions. Third, interventions are delivered in the client's natural environment. Such delivery of services reduces the frequency of missed appointments, facilitates the acquisition of assessment data that have greater ecological validity, and is conducive to a practical approach to the acquisition of skills and behavior change. Fourth, therapeutic goals are specific and intervention strategies are flexible. Essentially, staff are encouraged to do whatever it takes to attain specified treatment goals. Fifth, treatment-team members are held accountable for therapeutic outcomes. Outcomes are continuously monitored to allow rapid feedback regarding the viability of interventions and the possible need to alter or refine treatment plans. Thus, rather than being passive in the face of lack of progress by clients, staff are openly challenged in team meetings and supervisory sessions to seek creative solutions to intervene successfully with clients.

## Recommendations for Future Research

Although empirical study of the TCL model and its adaptations has been prolific, insufficient standardization of experimental and control interventions has limited the ability to generalize from the findings of multiple studies about how best to restructure local delivery systems to improve services for persons with severe mental illness. If there were a core of studies with very similar approaches, control conditions, and research methods, there would be more conclusive indications of its effectiveness. The work of Test and her colleagues in Wisconsin (Test et al. 1985, 1992) has proceeded in this direction, but most of the other studies have altered the experimental condition substantially from theirs, making comparison risky. Among the states that have implemented these programs, Rhode Island and Delaware have developed programs in accordance with the TCL model on a systematic, statewide basis (Meisler et al. 1995). Both have developed program standards for Medicaid certification of programs that operationally embody the specific characteristics of the TCL model. A set of program standards and a procedures manual would be useful steps toward standardizing the operationalization of the approach in future studies.

In addition to further validation through multiple-site replication, studies of specific characteristics of the model would be useful. These could help determine which characteristics are most essential and how to integrate them into local community mental health systems. For example, if the provision of assertive outreach and practical assistance were the defining characteristics of TCL's effectiveness compared with clinic-based medication and counseling services, modification of the prevailing community mental health system might prove less challenging than restructuring it into self-contained treatment teams. To date, the adaptations of TCL to various program initiatives have not been based on empirical evidence. More likely, they have been based on the resources available to staff the teams.

A third recommended research direction is additional study of application to specific subpopulations in the mental health system. The long-term study of persons with schizophrenic disorders who enter these programs early after the onset of their illness (Test 1992) is one such example. The study by Drake et al. (1993), which treated persons with dual diagnoses of schizophrenia and alcoholism, is another. There have been several positive evaluations of application to homeless populations in conjunction with federal demonstration grants at the Thresholds in Chicago, Connections in Wilmington, Delaware, and at the St.

Louis Mental Health Center. However, these have not been published and also were limited by the absence of controls or other methodological weaknesses limiting generalizability of the findings.

A fourth recommended direction for future research addresses the need to replicate the consistent finding by Test and colleagues of positive outcomes in the domains of independent living and employment. It is disappointing that few of the many programs that have been developed have reported significant employment outcomes. Vocational outcome should be incorporated as an explicit objective of programs in future research.

## Conclusions

The evident effectiveness of the TCL approach in engaging persons with severe mental illness in continuous community care, reducing their use of hospitals, and improving their capacity for independent living, makes it particularly timely with public and private sector payers seeking to limit the growth in health care expenditures. The recent trend of rapid national dissemination is likely to continue and accelerate. Nevertheless, rigorous empirical evaluation of all treatments and services, demonstrating clinical effectiveness and cost-effectiveness, is essential to ensure that reforms will be beneficial for clients. Such studies can help policy makers assess the role that specific programs should play in the overall mix of services, can assess the patient subgroups for which these programs are most effective, and can provide better overall assessment of a system's costs and benefits.

## References

Bond GR, Miller LD, Krumwied RD, et al: Assertive case management in three MHCs: a controlled study. Hosp Community Psychiatry 39:411–418, 1988

Bond GR, Witheridge TF, Dincin J, et al: Assertive community treatment for frequent users of psychiatric hospitals in a large city: a controlled study. Am J Community Psychol 18:865–872, 1990

Borduin CM, Henggeler SW, Blaske DM, et al: Multisystemic treatment of adolescent sexual offenders. International Journal of Offender Therapy and Comparative Criminology 34:105–113, 1990

Borduin CM, Mann BJ, Cone LT, et al: Multisystemic treatment of serious juvenile offenders: long-term prevention of violent offending. J Consult Clin Psychol 63:569–578, 1995

Brunk M, Henggeler SW, Whelan JP: A comparison of multisystemic therapy and parent training in the brief treatment of child abuse and neglect. J Consult Clin Psychol 55:311–318, 1987

Chamberlain R, Rapp CA: A decade of case management: a methodological review of outcome research. Community Ment Health J 27:171–188, 1991

Detrick A, Stieposk V: Treating persons with mental illness, substance abuse, and legal problems: the Rhode Island experience, in Innovative Community Mental Health Programs: New Directions for Mental Health Services. Edited by Stein LI. San Francisco, CA, Jossey-Bass, 1992, pp 65–77

Drake RE, McHugo GJ, Noordsy DL: Treatment of alcoholism among schizophrenic outpatients: 4-year outcomes. Am J Psychiatry 150:328–329, 1993

Essock SM, Kontos N: Implementing assertive community treatment teams. Hosp Community Psychiatry 46:679–683, 1995

Harris M, Bergman HC: Case Management for Mentally Ill Patients: Theory and Practice. Langhorne, PA, Harwood Academic Publishers, 1993

Henggeler SW, Rodick JD, Borduin CM, et al: Multisystemic treatment of juvenile offenders: effects on adolescent behavior and family interactions. Developmental Psychology 22:132–141, 1986

Hoult J, Reynolds I: Schizophrenia: a comparative trial of community oriented and hospital oriented psychiatric care. Acta Psychiatr Scand 69:359–372, 1984

Hoult J, Reynolds I, Charbonneau-Powis M, et al: Psychiatric hospital versus community treatment: the results of a randomized trial. Aust N Z J Psychiatry 17:160–167, 1983

Intagliata J: Improving the quality of community care for the chronically mentally disabled: the role of case management. Schizophr Bull 8:655–674, 1982

Jerrell JM, Hu T: Cost-effectiveness of intensive clinical and case management compared with an existing system of care. Inquiry 26:224–234, 1989

Ludwig AM: The influence of non-specific healing techniques with chronic schizophrenics. Am J Psychother 22:382–404, 1968

Ludwig AM, Marx AJ: Influencing techniques of chronic schizophrenics. Arch Gen Psychiatry 18:681–688, 1968

Ludwig AM, Marx AJ: The buddy treatment model for chronic schizophrenics J Nerv Ment Dis 148:528–541, 1969

Ludwig AM, Marx AJ: Companion therapy for hospitalized psychotics. Am J Psychiatry 10:182–190, 1970

Ludwig AM, Marx AJ, Hill PA: Chronic schizophrenics as behavioral engineers J Nerv Ment Dis 152:31–44, 1971

Marx AJ, Ludwig AM: Resurrection of the families of chronic schizophrenics: clinical and ethical issues. Am J Psychother 23:37–52, 1969

Marx AJ, Test MA, Stein LI: Extrohospital management of severe mental illness: feasibility and effects of social functioning. Arch Gen Psychiatry 29:505–511, 1973

Meisler N: Statewide dissemination of the training in community living program. Administration and Policy in Mental Health 23:71–76, 1995

Meisler N, Detrick A, Tremper R: Statewide dissemination of the training in community living model: the making of mental health policy. Administration and Policy in Mental Health 23:71–76, 1995

Muijen M, Marks I, Conolly J, et al: Home based care and standard hospital care for patients with severe mental illness: a randomized controlled trial. British Medical Journal 304:749–754, 1992

Plum TB, Lawther S: How Michigan established a highly effective statewide community-based program for persons with serious and persistent mental illness. Outlook 2:2–5, 1992

Santos AB, Hawkins GD, Julius B, et al: A pilot study of assertive community treatment for patients with chronic psychotic disorders. Am J Psychiatry 150:501–504, 1993a

Santos AB, Deci PA, Lachance KR, et al: Providing assertive community treatment for severely mentally ill patients in a rural area. Hosp Community Psychiatry 44:34–39, 1993b

Soloman P: The efficacy of case management services for severely mentally disabled clients. Community Ment Health J 28:163–180, 1992

Stein LI, Test MA: Alternatives to mental health hospital treatment, I: conceptual model, treatment program and clinical evaluation. Arch Gen Psychiatry 37:392–397, 1980

Stein LI, Test MA, Marx AJ: Alternative to the hospital: a controlled study. Am J Psychiatry 132:517–522, 1975

Stroul BA: Community support systems for persons with long-term mental illness: a conceptual network. Psychosocial Rehabilitation Journal 12:9–26, 1989

Taube CA, Morlock L, Burns BJ, et al: New directions in research on assertive community treatment. Hosp Community Psychiatry 41:642–647, 1990

Test MA: Training in community living, in Handbook of Psychiatric Rehabilitation. Edited by Liberman RP. New York, MacMillan, 1992, pp 153–170

Test MA, Stein LI: Alternative to mental hospital treatment, III: social costs. Arch Gen Psychiatry 37:409–412, 1980

Test MA, Stein LI: The history of assertive community treatment. Audiotape of paper presented at the Programs of Assertive Community Treatment (PACT) Research and Research Utilization Workshop, National Institute of Mental Health, Rockville, MD, December 1992

Test MA, Knoedler WH, Allness DJ: The long-term treatment of young schizophrenics in a community support program, in The Training in Community Living Model: A Decade of Experience. Edited by Stein LI, Test MA. San Francisco, CA, Jossey-Bass, 1985, pp 17–27

Test MA, Knoedler WH, Allness DJ, et al: Training in community living (TCL) model: two decades of research. Outlook 2:5–8, 1992

Torrey EF: Continuous treatment teams in the care of the chronic mentally ill. Hosp Community Psychiatry 37:1243–1247, 1986

Turner JC, TenHoor WJ: The NIMH community support program: pilot approach to a needed social reform. Schizophr Bull 4:319–349, 1978

Weisbrod BA, Test MA, Stein LI: Alternative to mental hospital treatment, II: economic benefit-cost analysis. Arch Gen Psychiatry 37:400–405, 1980

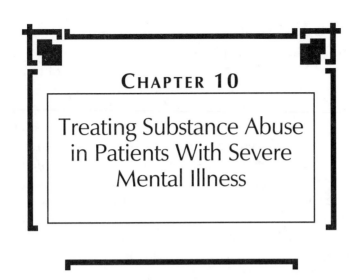

## CHAPTER 10

# Treating Substance Abuse in Patients With Severe Mental Illness

**Robert E. Drake, M.D., Ph.D., and Fred C. Osher, M.D.**

Substance use disorders are increasingly recognized as frequent co-occurring conditions that adversely affect the adjustment of persons with severe mental illnesses (Minkoff and Drake 1991). Approximately 50% of persons with severe mental disorders develop alcohol or other drug use disorders at some point in their lives, and the rate of dual diagnosis is even higher among those who are in clinical settings (Regier et al. 1990). Substance abuse among patients with severe mental illness is associated with a variety of problems, such as symptom worsening, violence, HIV infection, homelessness, rehospitalization, institutionalization, and suicide (Alterman et al. 1980; Bartels et al. 1993; Carey et al. 1991; Caton et al. 1994; Cournos et al. 1991; Drake et al. 1989, 1991c; Safer 1987; Yesavage and Zarcone 1983).

An earlier version of this paper was published in the *Journal of Nervous and Mental Disease*, 181:606–611, 1993. Used with permission of the publisher.

The rapidly developing literature on dual-diagnosis treatment reflects substantial progress since the original Alcohol Drug Abuse and Mental Health Administration reviews of treatment, training, and policy issues in the mid-1980s (Ridgely et al. 1986, 1987). Randomized clinical trials currently underway will add significantly to knowledge in this area. Nevertheless, current findings from a variety of clinical demonstrations and clinical research studies merit discussion at this time because many state and local mental health authorities are actively developing and implementing dual-diagnosis programs for severely mentally ill persons.

The authors' aim in this chapter is therefore to identify and clarify emerging treatment principles from current clinical research related to the treatment of substance use disorder among patients with severe mental illness. To develop these principles, we have surveyed the published clinical research, reviewed the 13 demonstration projects on young adults with serious mental illness and substance abuse problems funded by the National Institute of Mental Health (NIMH) between 1987 and 1990 (Mercer-McFadden and Drake 1995; Teague et al. 1990b), and drawn extensively from our work at the New Hampshire-Dartmouth Psychiatric Research Center.

## Principles of Treatment

We review nine principles: assertiveness, close monitoring, integration, comprehensiveness, stable living environment, flexibility and specialization, stages of treatment, longitudinal perspective, and optimism. These principles denote structural and clinical elements that underlie successful programs rather than specific clinical procedures or guidelines. Our review begins with the cross-sectional scope and intensity of services, and moves to their longitudinal pace and pattern.

### Assertiveness

Successful programs incorporate active interventions such as outreach in the community and assurance of practical assistance with basic needs as a precondition for effective, continuous engagement in treatment. Furthermore, they assertively address substance abuse as a central problem that destabilizes severe mental illness and interferes with rehabilitation.

People with dual disorders tend to be noncompliant with treatment (Drake and Wallach 1989; Osher et al. 1994; Safer 1987). They do not fit well into either mental health or substance abuse programs; they often appear unmotivated for treatment; and they are difficult to engage in outpatient treatment or rehabilitation programs (Ridgely et al. 1990).

Treatment therefore needs to be assertive and flexible, with an emphasis on outreach, practical assistance, and individualized educational efforts. Assertive interventions include meeting patients where they live, work, and pass time; accessing income entitlements and supports; providing medication management, skills training, and general assistance in the community; and working with family members, landlords, employers, and others who may be able to provide support. In addition, assertiveness often entails close monitoring, such as using payeeships, guardianships, or legal sanctions as inducements to engage in treatment (discussed below).

One common approach to assertive treatment involves interdisciplinary teams (often called assertive community treatment teams), and continuous treatment teams, which take full responsibility for a small but discrete group of patients with an explicit focus on engagement and stabilization (Test 1990; Torrey 1986). For example, continuous treatment teams in New Hampshire's community mental health centers combine assertive case management, mental health treatment, and substance abuse treatment (Drake et al. 1990b, 1991a)—an approach that has been successful in engaging dually diagnosed patients in long-term treatment (Drake et al. 1993a).

Once dually diagnosed patients are involved with a continuous treatment team (CTT), assertive approaches can also be used to connect them with substance abuse treatments. For example, among 240 dually diagnosed patients in one study, those randomly assigned to CTTs, which have low caseloads and provide extensive outreach, rather than standard case management services, were 6 times as likely to attend dual-diagnosis treatment groups (Teague et al. 1990a).

## Close Monitoring

Close monitoring refers to intensive supervision, which is sometimes provided with the patient's consent and at other times on an involuntary basis. Various forms of intensive supervision are often necessary to initiate and sustain early treatment. For people who are not psychiatrically disabled, close monitoring improves outcomes for the treatment of alcoholism (Moos et al. 1990), cocaine addiction (Higgins et al. 1991), and narcotics dependence (Vaillant 1966). Close monitoring may be even more important for patients whose lives are ravaged by two chronic illnesses with the resultant clinical instability, functional impairments, lack of insight, poor judgment, self-destructiveness, and demoralization.

Disability often renders dually diagnosed persons dependent on several systems—mental health, welfare, legal, criminal justice, housing, and family—which can provide a range of options for close monitoring. For example, when public entitlements are being used for alcohol and other drugs, legal procedures such as payeeships and protective guardianships can help dually diagnosed persons to manage their funds. For patients who have engaged in crimes or dangerous behaviors, substance abuse treatment can sometimes be included in the conditions of probation, parole, outpatient commitment, or conditional discharge from the hospital. Pharmacological treatments, such as antipsychotic medications and disulfiram, and urine drug tests can also be mandated and supervised by staff (Nikkel and Coiner 1991; Osher and Kofoed 1989). In addition, mental health systems often have available a continuum of supervised living situations (Bebout and Harris 1992) and day treatment settings (Carey 1989a), in which close monitoring can be provided as needed.

Clinicians' experiences across a range of programs indicate

that these methods of close monitoring—ranging from voluntary to involuntary—are key components of dual-diagnosis treatment (Mercer-McFadden and Drake 1995). Patients themselves often report ambivalence regarding monitoring—they fear losing independence but recognize that some external controls may be necessary and helpful. As they recover from substance abuse disorders, patients typically need less intensive supervision and steadily move toward genuine independence.

## Integration

Combining mental health and substance abuse interventions in a concurrent and coordinated fashion is referred to as integrated treatment (Minkoff and Drake 1991). For historical reasons, the mental health and substance abuse systems are quite separate. Extruding patients from each system because of the co-occurrence of other disorders remains common (Ridgely et al. 1990). For example, active alcohol abuse frequently results in exclusion from psychiatric treatment centers, and active psychosis prevents admission to alcohol treatment units. Treating only one disorder or treating the two disorders sequentially also generally fails because the overlooked disorder frequently undermines treatment of the targeted disorder. For example, patients who are actively drinking and using drugs show poor compliance with prescribed antipsychotic medications (Drake et al. 1989).

Concurrent, parallel treatment in the two systems—another common approach to dual diagnosis—often results in fragmented, contradictory, and inadequate care. Parallel treatment is problematic for several reasons: it places on the patient the burden of integrating two systems with disparate philosophies, treatments, and clinicians; it allows each system to continue to provide a standard form of treatment and to resist specific modifications for special populations; and it maximizes the potential for miscommunications and contradictory recommendations (Galanter et al. 1988; Kline et al. 1991; Ridgely et al. 1990; Wallen and Weiner 1989). For persons ambivalent about their commitment to any treatment plan, separate and at times contradictory plans encourage noncompliance. Too often, the patient in parallel treatment becomes lost between the two treatment systems.

Integrated treatment programs, in which the same clinicians provide mental health and substance abuse treatments in the same setting, have been demonstrably effective, at least in open clinical trials (Drake et al. 1996). Kofoed et al. (1986) treated 32 dually diagnosed patients in a group setting and found that those who remained in treatment for a year (34%) had a reduced rate of hospitalization. Hellerstein and Meehan (1987) found that 10 substance-abusing schizophrenic patients who participated in a weekly outpatient dual-diagnosis group reduced their days in the hospital during 1 year of treatment. Ries and Ellingson (1989) found that 12 of 17 dually diagnosed patients (70.6%) who attended drug and alcohol discussion groups while in the hospital were abstinent a month after discharge. Bond et al. (1991) found that 19 young adults with major mental illness and substance use disorder who were treated in a dual-diagnosis group for 18 months reduced their use of marijuana, although not of alcohol and other drugs. Drake et al. (1993a) found that 11 of 18 schizophrenic patients with alcohol-use disorders (61%) achieved stable remission from alcohol-use disorders during 4 years in an integrated treatment program that included assertive case management and substance abuse treatment groups. Durrel et al. (1993) followed 84 patients with severe mental illness in intensive case management for 18 months or longer. Among the 51% ($n = 43$) who were also substance abusers, two-thirds showed reduced substance abuse at follow-up.

Substance abuse treatment can be integrated into most community mental health programs as a core component at a relatively low cost (Bartels and Drake 1991). The substance abuse treatment can be provided on an individual basis by clinical case managers or CTTs and in groups by the same staff. The expense of initiating such a program involves little more than educating and supporting the clinical staff while they develop skills for treating dual disorders.

## Comprehensiveness

Comprehensive treatment programs address not just the specific manifestations of a disorder but a wide range of skills, activities, relationships, and supports associated with recovery. Substance abuse treatment for persons who do not have a dual diagnosis is most effective when it is broad-based and comprehensive (McLellan 1992; Miller 1990). Living context, relationships, and vocational and interpersonal skills are critically related to engagement in treatment (Higgins et al. 1991) and to long-term recovery (Moos et al. 1990). Persons with problems related to substance abuse typically need structure, such as new relationships and activities, in their lives (Vaillant 1988). Long-term follow-up studies indicate that recovery typically occurs during intervals of increased structure rather than during episodes of intensive treatment (Vaillant 1983).

The need for broad-based, comprehensive treatment is even more evident in people who have co-occurring severe mental illness because they tend to be deficient in the skills, relationships, supports, and living contexts that are associated with stable recovery from substance abuse (Mercer-McFadden and Drake 1995). Mental health programs organized according to the community support system model (Stroul 1989) have an advantage over other programs that would need to create extensive new services or link their services with outside agencies in a parallel treatment model. In a dual-diagnosis program, each of the service components may need to be modified in correspondence with the complexities of dual diagnosis. For example, family psychoeducation must include information on not only mental illness but also substance abuse and dual diagnosis (Ryglewicz 1991).

## Stable Living Environment

Dually diagnosed persons need to have access to a range of housing options that provide safety, freedom from alcohol and drugs, support, and companionship. The living situation critically affects recovery from alcoholism for persons who are not psychiatrically impaired as well; the posttreatment environment predicts outcomes more strongly than the treatment environment across a range of inpatient and residential alcohol-treatment programs (Moos et al. 1990). Persons with severe mental illness, especially in urban areas, tend to reside in drug-infested neighborhoods and settings with large numbers of homeless persons (Belcher 1989; Drake et al. 1989, 1991b). The toxicity of the living environment, including the easy access to drugs, may explain why dually diagnosed individuals in urban areas are often attracted to the hospital as a safer living environment (Drake and Wallach 1992). Clinicians who work with homeless, dually diagnosed persons observe that active treatment and recovery are difficult, if not impossible, without access to decent housing (Drake et al. 1991b).

A significant proportion of these patients do well while in hospitals or residential treatment settings, but have difficulty transferring gains or skills for maintaining abstinence to the community. For example, Bartels and Thomas (1991) found that 17 of 46 patients (37%) admitted to a dual-diagnosis residential program had no difficulty maintaining abstinence for 3 months, but all relapsed soon after discharge to their usual community living situation. Conversely, dually diagnosed patients who achieved and maintained stable recovery in several studies typically resided in supportive housing situations in the community (Bartels et al. 1993; Mercer-McFadden and Drake 1995). For example, in a Washington, DC, study of 168 homeless, dually diagnosed patients, the vast majority of those achieving stable abstinence lived in structured, congregate living settings (Drake et al. 1993b).

## Flexibility and Specialization

Since dual-diagnosis treatment differs from traditional substance abuse and mental health treatments, successful administrators and clinicians modify previous beliefs, learn new skills, and try new approaches empirically; they become dual-diagnosis specialists (Mercer-McFadden and Drake 1995; Minkoff and Drake 1991). Clinicians with a background in substance abuse treatment alter previous approaches based on basic information about treating major mental illness. For example, confrontation and other intensive, emotionally charged interventions are often ineffective and increase the risk of dropout or relapse of psychiatric symptoms in this population; effective treatments proceed slowly and gently, with a low level of affect, a high level of structure, and attention to psychotic vulnerability (Carey 1989b; Fariello and Scheidt 1989). At the same time, mental health clinicians alter their approaches in accordance with basic facts about drugs of abuse and addictive behaviors. They learn to discern cognitive changes that are due to drugs rather than to mental illness, to monitor drug use with laboratory tests, to be aware of behaviors and interventions that reinforce (or enable) substance abuse, and to help their patients develop skills to achieve and maintain abstinence.

## Stages of Treatment

Substance abuse can be conceptualized as a chronic, relapsing disorder that is to some extent independent of the co-occurring mental illness, and that is treatable in a program oriented toward rehabilitation and recovery (Minkoff 1989). Like the treatment of major mental illness, substance abuse treatment proceeds in stages. Osher and Kofoed (1989) conceptualized four stages—engagement, persuasion, active treatment, and relapse prevention—which refer to overlapping processes: developing a trusting relationship, or working alliance, with the patient (engagement); helping the patient to perceive the adverse consequences of substance use in his or her life and to develop motivation for recovery (persuasion); helping the patient to achieve stable recovery, whether that is controlled use or abstinence (active treatment); and helping the patient to maintain a stable recovery (relapse prevention).

A stage model of treatment serves mainly heuristic purposes because treatment rarely proceeds in a linear pathway. Patients typically cycle back and forth between engagement and persuasion early in treatment and may also relapse from active treatment or relapse prevention stages. The stage model does, however, guide clinicians in planning and deciding what interventions are appropriate at a particular point in time. For example, because many of these patients do not perceive their substance use as problematic (Drake et al. 1990a; Test et al. 1989), insisting on abstinence when they are in the engagement or persuasion stage of treatment often drives them away from treatment.

### Engagement

Many dually diagnosed persons are not involved in regular outpatient treatment and must first be attracted to a program. These patients are often engaged in treatment by offering them practical assistance; for example, aid in obtaining food, clothing, housing, entitlements, jobs, or medications, or help during crises. For homeless or isolated, highly symptomatic individuals, outreach must often be persistent and assertive over time.

Help with engagement often comes from other sources such as family members, public guardians, or the criminal justice system. For example, participation in outpatient treatment can be mandated as a condition of probation, parole, or conditional discharge as a means to avoid further institutionalization.

### Persuasion

When dually diagnosed clients become engaged in mental health treatment, they tend to be in a premotivational state with respect to their substance abuse. That is, they do not yet recognize or acknowledge that substance abuse is a problem or they do not express an interest in substance abuse treatment. Clinical work at this stage involves helping them to gradually develop awareness of the negative consequences of using alcohol and other drugs by observing and reviewing the effects of many episodes of substance use over time (Kofoed and Keys 1988; Noordsy and Fox 1991), often in the context of crisis intervention and stabilization (Fariello and Scheidt 1989; Nikkel and Coiner 1991). The goal of persuasion is to have the patient embrace the need for long-term, abstinence-oriented treatment (Kofoed and Keys

1988; Miller and Rollnick 1991; Stark and Kane 1985).

In individual meetings and in groups, clinicians (often aided by peers in a group format) help the patient to make connections between substance use and problems in living, to recognize the discrepancy between current life adjustment and aspirations, and to develop confidence in the possibility of becoming abstinent and living a more satisfying life. Stabilizing psychiatric symptoms and making progress in some areas of life are often preconditions to developing motivation for active substance abuse interventions, but progress in the persuasion stage can also be made during crises and hospitalizations, when the consequences of abuse are often salient and enforced abstinence improves judgment. As Miller and Rollnick (1991) suggest, the clinician's approach during this stage is empathic, nonconfrontational, and supportive of self-efficacy.

### Active Treatment

Once the patient accepts the need to achieve and maintain abstinence, a variety of active change strategies can be offered. These interventions, which are matched with the patient's needs and preferences, include psychoeducational, medical, behavioral, familial, social, and vocational strategies. All are aimed at developing the attitudes, skills, and supports needed to remain sober. Stable abstinence typically develops over time, following setbacks and attempts at controlled use, as the patient acquires a larger and more effective repertoire of active change strategies. Some patients will initially want to use these strategies to reduce their substance use; research data (Drake and Wallach 1993; Drake et al. 1989) and their own experiences with controlled use are used to move them toward adopting abstinence as a goal. Developing a culture of abstinence is an integral part of the milieu of dual-disorder programs (Osher and Kofoed 1989).

Among the variety of active change strategies, behavioral interventions, which involve identifying, practicing, and reinforcing specific skills, are particularly helpful to persons with severe mental disorders. This work can often be done in a group format

(Noordsy and Fox 1991). Other commonly used active interventions include structured activities, family involvement to provide positive reinforcement for abstinence, social skills training, behavioral treatments for anxiety, and the use of disulfiram. Self-help groups such as Alcoholics Anonymous (AA) and Narcotic Anonymous are recommended for all patients during this stage. Some patients are able to make use of these groups; however, those with schizophrenic disorders have a particularly difficult time developing a long-term attachment to these groups (Noordsy et al. 1996). By contrast, most dually disordered patients are able to make use of dual-disorder groups in the mental health center (Drake et al. 1993a).

### Relapse Prevention

Stable abstinence does not signify the end of substance abuse treatment, especially for people with mental illness, who may have a lifetime vulnerability to psychoactive substances. Once stable abstinence is achieved, however, treatment shifts to monitoring for risk factors and prodromes, which often precede relapses, in order to prevent them. Particular interventions, which again depend on individual preferences, range from regular contact with a case manager to involvement in specific substance abuse treatments, such as AA or groups in the mental health center for recovering persons.

Relapses are expected and should be anticipated so that the reactions to them by staff, family, and patients are not extreme. Relapse can be used as a learning experience that reminds the patient of vulnerability and perhaps of cognitive, behavioral, or social factors that will continue to represent risks until they are modified. A return to former behaviors rather than a brief episode of use may indicate return to an earlier stage of treatment and a need for further active interventions.

## Longitudinal Perspective

Substance abuse is a chronic, relapsing disorder. The need for a longitudinal perspective in viewing severe mental disorders such as schizophrenia (Group for the Advancement of Psychiatry 1992) applies equally to substance use disorders (Vaillant 1983). Treatment occurs continuously over years rather than episodically or during crises. Progress can be observed and measured after years rather than weeks or months. For example, the 11 schizophrenic patients with alcoholism who became stably abstinent in our pilot program in New Hampshire did so after an average of 2 years of treatment (Drake et al. 1993).

Standard substance abuse treatment in the United States has been criticized for concentrating service resources at the beginning phase of treatment in a brief but intensive and expensive model, such as the 28-day inpatient treatment model, with minimal follow-up care (Holder et al. 1991). Most controlled studies do not show that intensive inpatient treatment for alcoholism is superior to outpatient treatment (Holder et al. 1991; McLellan et al. 1992; Miller and Hester 1986). Longitudinal research also demonstrates that recovery from alcoholism (Vaillant 1983) or narcotics addiction (Vaillant 1966) usually occurs over years.

Experience with dually diagnosed patients also supports the need for a long-term perspective. Stable recovery from substance abuse does not typically occur in the first year of treatment, perhaps because most patients are in the persuasion stage and are not yet ready for active treatment (Lehman et al. 1993). The majority of these patients are unable to benefit from intensive residential substance abuse treatment. For example, we found that nearly two-thirds of the 46 dually diagnosed patients admitted to an intensive, 90-day, residential treatment program left prematurely (Bartels and Thomas 1991). Of the 11 schizophrenic patients with alcoholism who became stably abstinent in another study, none did so in conjunction with an inpatient substance abuse admission, whereas all recovered gradually in the context of outpatient dual-diagnosis treatment (Drake et al. 1993a).

## Optimism

Patients, families, and treatment providers need to have hope for recovery. Demoralization among patients and their families occurs almost inevitably as part of adjusting to a chronic illness (Frank 1974; Smyer and Birkel 1991). People with dual disorders are particularly likely to become discouraged and hopeless about the future—a state often misconstrued and labeled as poor motivation. Defining motivation as a fixed attribute can result in blaming the patient for treatment failure, whereas conceptualizing motivation as a psychological state emphasizes that motivation can be influenced by various psychological and behavioral strategies (Miller 1985).

Treatment of chronic illness inevitably addresses demoralization (Frank 1974). As patients begin to trust their caregivers and to experience some improvement, their attitudes typically change. They develop some hope for the future, greater expectations for themselves, and more wishes and demands for treatment. They therefore appear to be more motivated. Families go through parallel stages in adjusting to their relatives' chronic illnesses (Tessler et al. 1987). Clinicians also tend to be pessimistic about treating dual disorders.

Observations of successful dual-diagnosis treatment programs indicate that patients, families, and caregivers achieve and maintain a hopeful attitude toward recovery (Mercer-McFadden and Drake 1995). For example, rather than extruding or rejecting patients who appear to be unmotivated, clinicians recognize that motivation appears naturally during the persuasion stage of treatment. Several mechanisms can serve to enhance and maintain clinicians' optimism. In New Hampshire, the dual-diagnosis teams from across the state meet monthly for peer supervision and training sessions. These meetings serve not only to increase knowledge and skills but also to develop a secure identity for team members as dual-diagnosis specialists.

# Conclusions

Despite the lack of controlled clinical trials, our review of demonstration programs and clinical research has identified several emerging principles of dual-diagnosis treatment. These elements are common to successful dual-diagnosis programs: an assertive style of engagement, techniques of close monitoring, integration of mental health and substance abuse treatments, comprehensive services, supportive living environments, flexibility and specialization of clinicians, stage-wise treatment, a long-term perspective, and optimism.

# References

Alterman AI, Erdlen FR, McLellan AT, et al: Problem drinking in hospitalized schizophrenic patients. Addict Behav 5:273–276, 1980

Bartels SJ, Drake RE: Dual diagnosis: new directions and challenges. California Journal of the Alliance for the Mentally Ill 2:6–7, 1991

Bartels SJ, Thomas WN: Lessons from a pilot residential treatment program for people with dual diagnoses of severe mental illness and substance use disorder. Psychosocial Rehabilitation Journal 15:19–30, 1991

Bartels SJ, Teague GB, Drake RE, et al: Service utilization and costs associated with substance abuse among rural schizophrenic patients. J Nerv Ment Dis 181:227–232, 1993

Bebout RR, Harris M: In search of pumpkin shells: residential programming for the homeless mentally ill, in Treating the Homeless Mentally Ill. Edited by Lamb HR, Bachrach LL, Kass FI. Washington, DC, American Psychiatric Press, 1992, pp 159–181

Belcher JR: On becoming homeless: a study of chronically mentally ill persons. Journal of Community Psychology 17:173–185, 1989

Bond GR, McDonel EC, Miller LD, et al: Assertive community treatment and reference groups: an evaluation of their effectiveness for young adults with serious mental illness and substance abuse problems. Psychosocial Rehabilitation Journal 15:31–43, 1991

Carey KB: Treatment of the mentally ill chemical abuser: description of the Hutchings day treatment program. Psychiatr Q 60:303–316, 1989a

Carey KB: Emerging treatment guidelines for mentally ill chemical abusers. Hosp Community Psychiatry 40:341–342, 349, 1989b

Carey MP, Carey KB, Meisler AW: Psychiatric symptoms in mentally ill chemical abusers. J Nerv Ment Dis 179:136–138, 1991

Caton CL, Shrout PE, Eagle PF, et al: Risk factors for homelessness among schizophrenic men: a case-control study. Am J Public Health 84:265–270, 1994

Cournos F, Empfield M, Horwath E, et al: HIV prevalence among patients admitted to two psychiatric hospitals. Am J Psychiatry 148:1225–1230, 1991

Drake RE, Wallach MA: Substance abuse among the chronic mentally ill. Hosp Community Psychiatry 40:1041–1046, 1989

Drake RE, Wallach MA: Mental patients' attraction to the hospital: correlates of living preference. Community Ment Health J 28:5–11, 1992

Drake RE, Wallach MA: Moderate drinking among people with severe mental illness. Hosp Community Psychiatry 44:780–782, 1993

Drake RE, Osher FC, Wallach MA: Alcohol use and abuse in schizophrenia: a prospective community study. J Nerv Ment Dis 177:408–414, 1989

Drake RE, Osher FC, Noordsy DL, et al: Diagnosis of alcohol use disorder in schizophrenia. Schizophr Bull 16:57–67, 1990a

Drake RE, Teague GB, Warren RS: New Hampshire's dual diagnosis program for people with severe mental illness and substance use disorder. Addiction and Recovery 10:35–39, 1990b

Drake RE, Antosca L, Noordsy DL, et al: New Hampshire's specialized services for people dually diagnosed with severe mental illness and substance use disorder, in Dual Diagnosis of Major Mental Illness and Substance Disorder. Edited by Minkoff K, Drake RE. San Francisco, CA, Jossey-Bass, 1991a, pp 57–67

Drake RE, Osher FC, Wallach MA: Homelessness and dual diagnosis. Am Psychol 46:1149–1158, 1991b

Drake RE, Wallach MA, Teague GB, et al: Housing instability and homelessness among rural schizophrenic patients. Am J Psychiatry 148:330–336, 1991c

Drake RE, McHugo GJ, Noordsy DL: A pilot study of outpatient treatment of alcoholism in schizophrenia: four-year outcomes. Am J Psychiatry 150:328–329, 1993a

Drake RE, Bebout RR, Quimby E, et al: Process evaluation in the Washington, D.C. dual diagnosis project. Alcoholism Treatment Quarterly 10:113–124, 1993b

Drake RE, Mueser KT, Clark RE, et al: The course, treatment, and outcome of substance disorder in persons with severe mental illness. Am J Orthopsychiatry 66:42–51, 1996

Durell J, Lechtenberg B, Corse S, et al: Intensive case management of persons with chronic mental illness who abuse substances. Hosp Community Psychiatry 44:415–416, 428, 1993

Fariello D, Scheidt S: Clinical case management of the dually diagnosed patient. Hosp Community Psychiatry 40:1065–1067, 1989

Frank JD: Persuasion and Healing. New York, Schocken Books, 1974

Galanter M, Castenada R, Ferman J: Substance abuse among general psychiatric patients: place of presentation, diagnosis, and treatment. Am J Drug Alcohol Abuse 142:211–235, 1988

Group for the Advancement of Psychiatry: Beyond Symptom Suppression: Improving Long-Term Outcomes of Schizophrenia. Washington, DC, American Psychiatric Press, 1992

Hellerstein DJ, Meehan B: Outpatient group therapy for schizophrenic substance abusers. Am J Psychiatry 144:1337–1339, 1987

Higgins ST, Delaney DD, Budney AJ, et al: A behavioral approach to achieving initial cocaine abstinence. Am J Psychiatry 148:1218–1224, 1991

Holder H, Longabaugh R, Miller WR, et al: The cost effectiveness of treatment for alcoholism: a first approximation. J Stud Alcohol 52:517–540, 1991

Kline J, Bebout R, Harris M, et al: A comprehensive treatment program for dually diagnosed homeless people in Washington, D.C., in Dual Diagnosis of Major Mental Illness and Substance Disorder. Edited by Minkoff K, Drake RE. San Francisco, CA, Jossey-Bass, 1991, pp 95–106

Kofoed LL, Keys A: Using group therapy to persuade dual-diagnosis patients to seek substance abuse treatment. Hosp Community Psychiatry 39:1209–1211, 1988

Kofoed LL, Kania J, Walsh T, et al: Outpatient treatment of patients with substance abuse and coexisting psychiatric disorders. Am J Psychiatry 143:867–872, 1986

Lehman AF, Herron JD, Schwartz RP: Rehabilitation for young adults with severe mental illness and substance use disorders: a clinical trial. J Nerv Ment Dis 181:86–90, 1993

McLellan AT, Metzger D, Alterman AI, et al: How effective is substance abuse treatment—compared to what? In Advances in Understanding the Addictive States. Edited by O'Brien CP, Jaffe J. New York, Association for Research in Nervous and Mental Disease, 1992, pp 232–252

Mercer-McFadden C, Drake RE: A review of 13 NIMH demonstration projects for young adults with severe mental illness and substance abuse problems. Rockville, MD, Center for Mental Health Services, Substance Abuse and Mental Health Services Administration, 1995

Miller WR: Motivation for treatment: a review with special emphasis on alcoholism. Psychol Bull 98:84–107, 1985

Miller WR, Hester RK: Inpatient alcoholism treatment: who benefits? Am Psychol 41:794–805, 1986

Miller WR, Rollnick S: Motivational Interviewing. New York, Guilford, 1991

Minkoff K: An integrated treatment model for dual diagnosis of psychosis and addiction. Hosp Community Psychiatry 40:1031–1036, 1989

Minkoff K, Drake RE (eds): Dual Diagnosis of Major Mental Illness and Substance Disorder. San Francisco, CA, Jossey-Bass, 1991

Moos RH, Finney JW, Cronkite RC: Alcoholism Treatment: Context, Process, and Outcome. New York, Oxford Press, 1990

Nikkel R, Coiner R: Critical interventions and tasks in delivering dual diagnosis services. Psychosocial Rehabilitation Journal 15:57–66, 1991

Noordsy DL, Fox L: Group intervention techniques for people with dual disorders. Psychosocial Rehabilitation Journal 15:67–78, 1991

Noordsy DL, Schwab B, Fox L, et al: The role of self-help programs in the rehabilitation of persons with severe mental disorders and substance use disorders. Community Ment Health J 32:71–86, 1996

Osher FC, Kofoed LL: Treatment of patients with psychiatric and psychoactive substance abuse disorders. Hosp Community Psychiatry 40:1025–1030, 1989

Osher FC, Drake RE, Noordsy DL, et al: Correlates and outcomes of alcohol use disorder among rural outpatients with schizophrenia. J Clin Psychiatry 55:109–113, 1994

Regier DA, Farmer ME, Rae DS, et al: Comorbidity of mental disorders with alcohol and other drug abuse: results from the Epidemiologic Catchment Area (ECA) study. JAMA 264:2511–2518, 1990

Ridgely MS, Goldman HH, Talbott JA: Chronic mentally ill young adults with substance abuse problems: a review of the literature and creation of a research agenda. Baltimore, MD, University of Maryland Mental Health Policy Studies Center, 1986

Ridgely MS, Osher FC, Talbott JA: Chronic mentally ill young adults with substance abuse problems: treatment and training issues. Baltimore, MD, University of Maryland Mental Health Policy Studies Center, 1987

Ridgely MS, Goldman HH, Willenbring M: Barriers to the care of persons with dual diagnoses: organizational and financing issues. Schizophr Bull 16:123–132, 1990

Ries RK, Ellingson T: A pilot assessment at one month of 17 dual diagnosis patients. Hosp Community Psychiatry 41:1230–1233, 1989

Ryglewicz H: Psychoeducation for clients and families: a way in, out, and through in working with people with dual disorders. Psychosocial Rehabilitation Journal 15:79–89, 1991

Safer DJ: Substance abuse by young adult chronic patients. Hosp Community Psychiatry 38:511–514, 1987

Smyer MA, Birkel RC: Research focused on intervention with families of the chronically mentally ill elderly, in The Elderly with Chronic Mental Illness. Edited by Light E, Lebowitz B. New York, Springer, 1991, pp 111–130

Stark MJ, Kane BJ: General and specific psychotherapy role induction with substance-abusing clients. Int J Addict 20:1135–1141, 1985

Stroul BA: Community support systems for persons with long-term mental illness: a conceptual framework. Psychosocial Rehabilitation Journal 12:9–26, 1989

Teague GB, Drake RE, McKenna P, et al: Implementation analysis of continuous treatment teams for dually diagnosed clients. Presented at the NIMH Community Support Program conference, Washington, DC, June, 1990a

Teague GB, Schwab B, Drake RE: Evaluating programs for young adults with severe mental illness and substance use disorder. Arlington, VA, National Association of State Mental Health Program Directors, 1990b

Tessler RC, Killian LM, Gubman GC: Stages in family response to mental illness: an ideal type. Psychosocial Rehabilitation Journal 10:3–16, 1987

Test MA: The training in community living model: delivering treatment and rehabilitation services through a continuous treatment team. Madison, WI, Mental Health Research Center, 1990

Test MA, Wallish L, Allness DJ, et al: Substance use in young adults with schizophrenic disorders. Schizophr Bull 15:465–476, 1989

Torrey EF: Continuous treatment teams in the care of the chronic mentally ill. Hosp Community Psychiatry 37:1243–1247, 1986

Vaillant GE: A twelve-year follow-up of New York narcotic addicts, IV: some characteristics and determinants of abstinence. Am J Psychiatry 123:573–584, 1966

Vaillant GE: The Natural History of Alcoholism. Cambridge, MA, Harvard University Press, 1983

Vaillant GE: What can long-term follow-up teach us about relapse and prevention of relapse in addiction? Br J Addict 83:1147–1157, 1988

Wallen MC, Weiner HD: Impediments to effective treatment of the dually diagnosed patient. J Psychoactive Drugs 21:161–168, 1989

Yesavage JA, Zarcone V: History of drug abuse and dangerous behavior in inpatient schizophrenics. J Clin Psychiatry 44:259–261, 1983

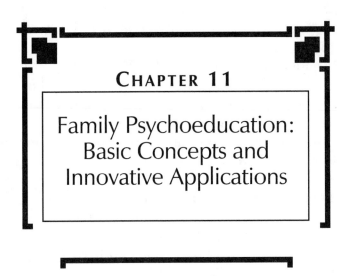

# CHAPTER 11

## Family Psychoeducation: Basic Concepts and Innovative Applications

**William R. McFarlane, M.D.**

The idea of working with the families of the severely mentally ill (SMI) in order to affect the course of the illness goes back at least as far as the early 1950s when Bateson first formulated the notion of the "double bind" and Jackson attempted to translate this theoretical construct into a treatment (Bateson et al. 1956). The family therapy that evolved from this source was unfortunately rooted in the notion that families had in some way caused the illness of their relative and that the illness itself was rather more a metaphor for trouble in the family than a biological reality. The treatment attempted to induce the family, through a variety of means, to change its behavior toward the patient while simultaneously allowing the patient to get out of a dysfunctional role. These efforts were dismally unsuccessful. Families naturally resented the notion that they had caused the illness and patients were unable to simply shed their symptoms regardless of how clearly the supposed link between their illness and the family's dynamics was articulated. Predictably, family therapy as an organized body of theory and practice began to move away from the treatment of schizophrenia when success continued to elude it.

Yet living with an illness such as schizophrenia is difficult and confusing for patients and families alike. A well-functioning family under these circumstances has to possess the available knowledge about the illness itself, and coping skills specific to this disorder, skills that are counterintuitive and only nascent in most families. It is unrealistic to expect families to understand such a mystifying condition and to know what to do about it naturally. Given that perspective, the most adaptive family will be the one that has access to information, with the implication that the treatment system is a crucial source of that information. As to coping skills, many families have developed methods of dealing with positive and negative symptoms, functional disabilities, and the desperation of their ill relatives through painful trial and error. These successes, however, are few and far between. Therefore, a critical need is that families have access to each other to learn of other families' successes and failures and to establish a repertoire of coping strategies that are closely tailored to the disorder.

## Family Psychoeducation

It took more than 10 years to revive an interest in involving families in the treatment of persons with SMI, and then that interest emerged with an entirely different conceptual framework. Investigators began to recognize the crucial role families played in outcome after a schizophrenic episode had occurred and endeavored to engage families collaboratively, sharing illness information and suggesting behaviors that promote recuperation as well as coping strategies to reduce their sense of burden (Anderson et al. 1980; Falloon and Liberman 1983; Goldstein et al. 1978; Leff et al. 1983). The group of interventions that emerged became known as family psychoeducation. This approach recognizes that schizophrenia is a brain disorder that is usually only partially remediable by medication and that families can have a significant effect on their relative's recovery. Thus, the psychoeducational approach shifted away from attempting to get families to change their "disturbed" communication patterns toward educating families and persuading them that how they behave toward the patient can facilitate or impede recovery. For example, a family might interfere with recuperation if in their natural enthusiasm to promote and support progress they create unreasonable demands and expectations.

Psychoeducation typically includes formal training sessions for families, in an effort to teach them as much as is currently known about the illness and to encourage their continued involvement with the treatment of their relative. For example, families are taught about negative symptoms of schizophrenia—that long periods of lethargy, anhedonia, passivity, and social withdrawal typically follow an episode of more active, positive symptoms. With such knowledge families can better create a more low-key convalescent environment within which the patient can more naturally recuperate from a major psychotic episode. Clinicians work collaboratively with families in resolving difficulties that are naturally generated by the illness. Research on the psychoeducational model, in particular the work of Anderson and Hogarty, Falloon, Leff, and Goldstein, has led to a set of basic assumptions that underlie its application; these are outlined in Table 11–1.

The psychoeducational approaches have been remarkably effective in reducing rates of illness relapse when rigorously evaluated in experimental outcome studies; the results of these studies are unusually consistent, and point to a valid, reliable, and quite robust main effect (Falloon et al. 1985; Goldstein et al. 1978; Hogarty et al. 1986; Leff et al. 1985, 1989; McFarlane 1990; McFarlane et al. 1995a, 1995b; Tarrier et al. 1988).

## Single-Family Psychoeducational Model

The basic single-family psychoeducational model consists of four treatment stages—joining, survival skills training/workshop,

**Table 11–1.**  Psychoeducation: basic assumptions

Schizophrenia has a clear and demonstrable biological component. Numerous recent studies strongly support this perspective (DeLisi et al. 1983; Stevens 1982; Weinberger et al. 1986).

Schizophrenia is a chronic illness that is characterized by episodes of up to 2 years in duration. During this time either positive and negative symptoms of the illness, or both, may be in evidence, which diminish slowly in the absence of stress (Hogarty and Ulrich 1977).

The specific deficit in schizophrenia is one involving attention, arousal, and underfunctioning of the dorsolateral prefrontal cortex, such that the patient's ability to gate stimuli adequately is impaired (Tecce and Cole 1976).

Families can have an influence on this biological process such that they are either able to protect the patient from further relapses into illness or they appear to inadvertently exacerbate them (Vaughn and Leff 1976).

Familial behaviors can be most parsimoniously described as "natural" responses to a difficult situation, and do not indicate anything about the level of functioning in the family (Leff and Vaughn 1985).

Living with an ill relative has negative consequences for the family (Johnson 1986).

The illness itself has a negative impact on the social support networks of both patient and family (Beels 1981).

reentry, and social/vocational rehabilitation—which roughly correspond to the phases of an episode of schizophrenia, from the acute phase through the slow recuperative and rehabilitation phases (Anderson et al. 1986). These phases apply to the clinical approach used in single- and multifamily versions.

### Joining

This stage refers to a way of working with families that is characterized by collaboration in attempting to understand and relate to the family. The joining phase is typically three to five single-family sessions in both single- and multifamily approaches. The goal of this phase is to establish a working alliance, to acquaint oneself with any family issues and problems that might contribute to stress either for the patient or for the family, to learn about the family's strengths and resources in dealing with the illness, and to create a contract with mutual and attainable goals. Joining, in its most general sense, continues throughout the treatment, because it is always the responsibility of the clinician to remain an available resource for the family as well as to be their advocate in dealing with any other clinical or rehabilitation system necessitated by the illness of their relative. To foster this relationship, the clinician demonstrates genuine concern for the patient, acknowledges the family's loss and grants family members sufficient time to mourn, is available to the family outside of the formal sessions, avoids treating family members as patients or blaming them in any way, helps to focus on the present crisis, and serves as a source of information about the illness.

### Survival Skills Training/Workshop

In this treatment stage, the family is invited to attend workshop sessions conducted in a formal, classroomlike atmosphere. Biological, psychological, and social information about schizophrenia and its management are presented through a variety of formats, such as videotapes, slide presentations, lectures, discussion periods, and question and answer periods. Information about the way in which the clinician and the family will continue to work together is also presented. Typically 8 hours in length, the workshop is attended by several families at a time. The opportunity to interact with other families in similar situations greatly enhances the power of this portion of the intervention. The families are also introduced to the guidelines for management of the illness. These consist of a set of behavioral instructions for family members, which integrates the biological, psychological, and social aspects of the disorder with recommended responses that help maintain a home environment that minimizes relapse-inducing stress (see Table 11–2 ).

**Table 11–2.** Family guidelines for the management of schizophrenia

Here's a list of things everyone can do to help make things run more smoothly:

1. Go slow. Recovery takes time. Rest is important. Things will get better in their own time.
2. Keep it cool. Enthusiasm is normal. Tone it down. Disagreement is normal. Tone it down, too.
3. Give each other space. Time out is important for everyone. It's okay to reach out. It's okay to say no.
4. Set limits. Everyone needs to know what the rules are. A few good rules keep things clear.
5. Ignore what you can't change. Let some things slide. Don't ignore violence.
6. Keep it simple. Say what you have to say clearly, calmly, and positively.
7. Follow doctor's orders. Take medications as they are prescribed. Take only medications that are prescribed.
8. Carry on business as usual. Reestablish family routines as quickly as possible. Stay in touch with family and friends.
9. No street drugs or alcohol. They make symptoms worse.
10. Pick up on early signs. Note changes. Consult with your family clinician.
11. Solve problems step by step. Make changes gradually. Work on one thing at a time.
12. Lower expectations, temporarily. Use a personal yardstick. Compare this month to last month.

*Source.* Adapted from Anderson et al. 1986.

### Reentry

Twice-monthly meetings focus on planning and implementing strategies to cope with the vicissitudes of a person recovering from an acute episode of schizophrenia. Major content areas include medication compliance, helping the patient avoid the use of street drugs, alcohol, or both, the general lowering of expectations during the period of negative symptoms, and an increase in tolerance for these symptoms. Two special techniques are introduced to participating members as supports to the efforts to follow family guidelines (Falloon and Liberman et al. 1983): formal problem solving and communications skills training. The application of either one of these techniques characterizes each session. Further, each session follows a prescribed, task-oriented format or paradigm, designed to enhance family-coping effectiveness and to strengthen the alliance between the family and the clinician.

### *Social and Vocational Rehabilitation*

Approximately a year following an acute episode, most patients begin to show signs of a return to spontaneity and active engagement with those around them. This is usually the sign that the negative symptoms are lifting and the patient can now be challenged more intensively. The focus of this phase deals more specifically with the rehabilitative needs of the patient, addressing the two areas of functioning in which there are the most common deficits: social skills, and their ability to get and maintain employment. The sessions are used to role-play situations that are likely to cause stress for the patient if entered into unprepared. Family members are actively used to assist in various aspects of this training endeavor. Additionally, the family is assisted in rebuilding its own network of family and friends, which has usually been weakened as a consequence of the presence of schizophrenia in one of its members. Regular sessions are conducted on a once- or twice-monthly basis, although more contact may be necessary at particularly stressful times.

## Multiple-Family Psychoeducational Model

This section describes an innovative treatment approach, the psychoeducational multiple-family group (McFarlane 1990), which brings together aspects of family psychoeducation and multiple-family behavioral approaches. As such, it is a second-generation treatment model that incorporates the advantages of each of its sources, diminishes their negative features, and leads to a number of synergistic effects that appear to enhance efficacy. Building on the psychoeducational family approach of Anderson et al. (1986), the model has attempted to reflect contemporary understanding of schizophrenia from biological, psychological, and social perspectives, on the assumption that an effective treatment should address as many known aspects of the illness as possible, at all relevant system levels.

Unlike the recent origins of psychoeducation, however, multiple-family group work arose nearly 3 decades ago in attempts by Laqueur et al. (1964) and Detre et al. (1961) to develop psychosocial treatments for hospitalized patients with schizophrenia. Unlike family therapy during its early period, the emphasis was more pragmatic than theoretical. Indeed, the first reported successful experience with the modality emerged serendipitously from a need to solve ward management problems. In the process, Laqueur (personal communication, September 1974) noted improved ward social functioning in patients who insisted on attending a group organized for visiting relatives. Detre et al. (1961) started a multiple-family group in order to encourage cooperation between resident psychiatrists and social workers on an acute inpatient service but found a high level of interest in the group among patients and family members alike, as well as improvements in social functioning among patients, and in family communication and morale. From these beginnings, the modality has grown steadily; most of the focus has continued to be on the major psychiatric disorders (Benningfield 1980; O'Shea 1985; Strelnick 1977).

Many clinicians have observed that specific characteristics of the multiple-family group have remarkable effects on a number of social and clinical management problems commonly encountered in schizophrenia (Lansky et al. 1978; McFarlane 1983). A critical goal of psychoeducation and family behavioral management is to reduce family expressed emotion and thereby to reduce the risk of psychotic relapse (Leff and Vaughn 1985). The multiple-family group approach goes beyond the focus on expressed emotion, because families attempting to cope with schizophrenia inevitably experience a variety of stresses, which secondarily put them at risk of manifesting exasperation and discouragement as natural reactions (Johnson 1990).

The common observation that many families containing a member with schizophrenia seem more socially isolated has been partially confirmed by studies of social networks (Anderson et al. 1984; Brown et al. 1972; Garrison 1978; Hammer 1963, 1978; Lipton et al. 1981; Pattison et al. 1979; Potasznik and Nelson 1984; Tolsdorf 1976). Isolation of the family assumes significance when one considers the functions of a social network. Hammer (1981) has emphasized social and instrumental support, access to other people and resources, mediation of information, the placing of demands, and the imposition of constraints, all of which are essential to developing skills for coping with a chronic mental disability. Lack of social support markedly increases vulnerability to ordinary stressors in both medical and psychiatric illness, whereas moderate network size and density interact to predict low relapse rates (Dean and Lin 1977; Dozier et al. 1987; Steinberg and Durell 1968). Although the lifetime risk of schizophrenia is about the same the world over, its course is more benign in developing, nonindustrialized cultures with a more permeable village social structure (World Health Organization 1979). Thus, the social support available to the family may be one of the critical factors determining outcome; the lack of it appears to make everyone, especially the person with schizophrenia, more vulnerable to stress. Where social support is not available, the treatment context may have to provide it.

With respect to the issue of stigma, although the available studies are in some conflict (Freeman and Simmons 1961; Lamb and Oliphant 1978; Rabkin 1974; Yarrow et al. 1955), the conclusion can reasonably be drawn that a patient's family members do not automatically feel stigmatized but often behave as if they do, and that friends and relatives do tend to avoid them as if they are stigmatized. Thus, many families may be isolated and stigmatized, and may feel so as well, in combinations that may be complex and variable. These problems produce strains that are likely to lead to exasperation, a sense of abandonment, and eventually demoralization. These effects on the family are likely to interfere with their capacity to support the ill member and to assist in rehabilitation.

Multiple-family groups address these issues directly by increasing the size and complexity of the social network, by exposing a given family to other families like themselves, by providing a forum for mutual aid, and by providing an opportunity to hear the experiences of other adults who have had similar experiences and found workable solutions. In addition, psychoeducational multiple-family groups reiterate and reinforce the information learned at coping-skills workshops. Coupled with formal problem solving (Falloon and Liberman 1983), the group experience serves to enhance the family's available coping skills for the many problems encountered in the course of the patient's recovery and rehabilitation.

The psychoeducational multiple-family group has been designed to counter family isolation and stigma, while incorporating the clinical methods that have been shown to alleviate expressed emotion and foster extended remission. The general character of the approach can be summarized as consisting of three components, roughly corresponding to the phases of the group. In the first phase, the content of the model follows that of Anderson et al. (1986), with its emphasis on single-family joining in a collaborative alliance with family members, conducting a multifamily educational workshop, and focusing on preventing relapse for a year or so after discharge from an acute hospitalization. Unlike the single-family psychoeducational approach, the format for treatment after the workshop is a multifamily group. The second phase involves moving beyond stability to gradual increases in patients' community functioning, a process that uses problem solving based on multiple-family groups as the primary means for accomplishing social and vocational rehabilitation. This occurs, roughly, during the second year of the multiple-family group. The third phase consists of deliberate efforts to mold the group into a social network that can persist for an extended period and that can satisfy family and patient needs for social contact, support, and ongoing clinical monitoring. This format is also an efficient context in which to continue psychopharmacological treatment and routine case management. Expansion of the families' social networks occurs through problem solving, direct emotional support, and out-of-group socializing, all involving members of different families in the group. The multifamily group treatment approach is briefly described below, and in detail in a treatment manual that is available from the author.

**Engagement and family education.** The intervention begins with a minimum of three engagement sessions, in which the patient's primary clinician meets with the individual family unit, usually without the patient present. These are accompanied by separate meetings with the patient. For both philosophical and practical reasons, we establish treatment plans based on the patient's and family's stated goals and desires. When five to eight families have completed the engagement process, the clinicians, usually including the patients' psychiatrist, conduct an extensive educational workshop, again usually without patients. The biomedical aspects of schizophrenia are discussed, after which the clinicians present and discuss guidelines for the family management of both clinical and everyday problems in managing the illness in the family context.

**The ongoing psychoeducational multiple-family group.** The first meeting of the ongoing psychoeducational multifamily group follows the workshop by 1 or 2 weeks; its format includes a biweekly meeting schedule, 90-minute session length, leadership by two clinicians, and participation by 5–8 patients and their families. From this point forward, patients are strongly encouraged to attend and actively participate. The multifamily group's primary working method is to help each family and patient to apply the family guidelines to their specific problems and circumstances. This work proceeds in phases, the timing of which is linked to the clinical condition of the patients. The actual procedure uses a multiple-family group-based problem-solving method adapted from a single-family version by Falloon and Liberman (1983). Families are taught to use this method in the multiple-family group as a group function. It is the core of the multiple-family group approach, one that is acceptable to families, is remarkably effective, and is tuned to the low-intensity and deliberate style that is essential to working with the specific sensitivities of people with schizophrenia.

The first phase concentrates on problems being experienced by the patient as he or she begins to reenter the world outside the protection of the hospital or clinic. A central goal during this phase is prevention of relapse, achieved primarily by limiting functional expectations and demands and artificially reducing the level of stimulation and stress in the social environment. That is, the family is recruited to institute a relatively simple low-demand and low-intensity milieu at home to the degree possible without totally disrupting family life. Beyond that general approach, the multifamily group maintains remission by systematically applying the group problem-solving method, case-by-case, to difficulties in implementing the family guidelines and fostering recovery. The rehabilitation phase should be initiated only by patients who have achieved clinical stability by successfully completing this community reentry phase.

As stability increases, the multiple-family group functions in a role unique among psychosocial rehabilitation models: it operates as an auxiliary to the in vivo social and vocational rehabilitation effort being conducted by the clinical team. The central emphasis during this phase is the involvement of both the family and the group in helping each patient to begin a gradual, step-by-step resumption of responsibility and socializing. The clinicians continue to use problem solving and brainstorming in the multiple-family group to identify and develop jobs and social contacts for the ill group members, to help individual patients obtain job placement, and to find new ways to enrich their social lives.

In the current model for multiple-family group sessions, a stable membership of from five to eight families meets with two clinicians on a biweekly basis 2 years or more following the onset of an episode of schizophrenia. In most instances, the decision to have a given patient attend is based upon his or her mental status and susceptibility to the stimulation such a group may engender. The format of the sessions is closely controlled by the clinician, following a standard paradigm (see Table 11–3). This structure serves to reduce the likelihood that the sessions will turn into emotional potboilers or nonproductive gripe sessions, which, given the nature of the illness, would not be rehabilitative for the patient or helpful to families. The task of the clinicians, particularly at the beginning, is to adopt a warm tone and businesslike approach that promotes a calm group climate oriented toward learning new coping skills and engendering hope.

Each session of the multiple-family group begins and ends with a period of purely social chat, facilitated by the clinicians, the purpose of which is to give the patients and even some families the opportunity to recapture and practice any social skills they may have lost due to their long isolation and exposure to high levels of stress. Following the socializing, the clinicians spe-

**Table 11–3.** Time structure of psychoeducational multifamily group sessions

| | |
|---|---|
| Socializing with families and patients | 15 minutes |
| A go-around, reviewing | |
| ■ The week's events | |
| ■ Relevant biosocial information | |
| ■ Applicable guidelines | 20 minutes |
| Selection of a single problem | 5 minutes |
| Formal problem solving | |
| ■ Problem definition | |
| ■ Generation of possible solutions | |
| ■ Weighing pros and cons of each | |
| ■ Selection of preferred solution | |
| ■ Delineation of tasks and implementation | 45 minutes |
| Socializing with families and patients | 5 minutes |
| Total: 90 minutes | |

cifically inquire as to the status of each family and offer advice based on the family guidelines or direct assistance, when it can be done readily. A single problem that has been identified by any one family is then selected and the group as a whole participates in problem solving. This problem is the focus of an entire session, during which all members of the group contribute suggestions and ideas. Their relative advantages and disadvantages are then reviewed by the affected family, with some input from other families and clinicians. Typically, the most attractive of the proposed solutions is reformulated as an appropriate task for trying at home and is assigned to the family. This step is then followed by another final period of socializing.

### Research on Multiple-Family Group Treatment

Early studies on multiple-family group treatment were quasi-experimental or impressionistic (Berman 1966; Falloon 1981; Lansky 1978; Levin 1966; Lurie 1972). The positive effects reported in these uncontrolled studies are consistent with those measured in more recent experimental studies conducted by the author and described below:

**The Bergen County, New Jersey, study.**      Schizophrenic or schizoaffective subjects hospitalized for an acute episode of psychosis ($N = 41$), were randomly assigned to one of three conditions: psychoeducational multiple-family group, single-family psychoeducational treatment without interfamily contact, and dynamically oriented multiple-family therapy (McFarlane et al. 1995a). Medication was used in all cases; dosage was determined by the staff psychiatrist for the patients and was set at lowest effective dose levels. At 4 years after discharge, the psychoeducational multiple-family group had a significantly longer time to first relapse than psychoeducational single-family treatment (Cox's coefficient/SE = 2.09; $P = .01$). Final 4-year relapse rates were 50% for group 1, 76.5% for group 2, and 57.1% for group 3. These data suggest a specific and independent multiple-family group effect that appears to prevent or forestall relapse.

**The New York State study.** The sample consisted of schizophrenic, schizoaffective, or schizophreniform subjects ($N = 172$)
from six public psychiatric facilities, who were randomly assigned
to 2 years of treatment with a standard-dose medication strategy
plus either the psychoeducational multiple-family group or psychoeducational single-family treatment approach (McFarlane et
al. 1995b). Relapse rates (using criteria based on the Brief Psychiatric Rating Scale) at 1 year were 19% for group 1, and 28.6%
for group 2; the relapse rates at 2 years were 28% and 42%, respectively (80% of the sample completed the treatment protocol).
Controlling for medication compliance, this was a statistically
significant difference ($P < .05$). Rates of clinically significant relapse (cases that met criteria for 7 days) were 15.7% versus 26.8%,
respectively. The multiple-family group effect, an annual clinically significant relapse rate of under 10%, compares quite favorably with expected relapse rates of about 40% using
medication alone or with supportive individual therapy (Hogarty
et al. 1979). Among Caucasian subjects, a subgroup with the
highest level of severity, there was a marked difference in relapse,
again favoring the multiple-family group format: 17% versus 59%
at 2 years, using the more rigorous criteria. For subjects discharged after index episode with low positive symptoms (BPRS
mean item score $\leq 2, N = 96$), there was no difference in relapse
rate between treatment modalities (32.7% in multiple-family
groups vs. 31.8% in single-family treatment). However, for subjects who were symptomatic at discharge (BPRS $> 2, N = 76$),
19% of the multiple-family group cases relapsed, whereas 51%
of the cases assigned to single-family treatment relapsed. A Cox's
analysis showed that, for patients discharged in a partially remitted state, being assigned to multiple-family group treatment
meant a risk of relapse only 28% of that of single-family treatment
($\chi^2_{(2)} = 12.51$, $P < .01$; $\beta$(treatment) $= -1.28$, SE $= 0.46$,
$P < .01$). This higher-symptom subgroup accounts almost entirely for the difference in relapse outcomes between multiple-
family group and single-family treatment. That is, in the
highest-risk subsample, the multiple-family group relapse rates
were actually lower than in more well-stabilized patients, whereas

the opposite effect was observed in single-family treatment. There was little difference in relapse rates between the modalities in minority patients. Mean number of hospital admissions for the entire sample for 2 years prior to the study were reduced to one-third by the end of the 2 years. There was a significant increase in full- or part-time competitive or sheltered employment for the entire sample (from 17.3%, 2 months prior to the test treatments, to 29.3% during the 18- to 24-month period in treatment; $\chi^2 = 7.63$, $P = .001$). However, the between-group differences (16% multiple-family group vs. 8% single-family treatment) were not statistically significant. Further, because the multiple-family group approach requires one-half the staff time of single-family treatment, the cost-benefit ratio (1:2.5) strongly favors the multiple-family group format. The cost-benefit ratio between multiple-family group and prior treatment, comparing hospitalization costs before and during treatment, is 1:34. Finally, both psychosocial interventions had a strong effect on medication compliance, as assessed by the treating psychiatrists, averaging close to 90% for the entire sample across the 2 years.

### Merging Multiple-Family Psychoeducation and Assertive Community Treatment

We have also had considerable experience in merging multiple-family group psychoeducation strategy with the Assertive Community Treatment (ACT) service system approach. More recently, the combined approach has been applied as a method for vocational rehabilitation. On-the-job training, high counselor contact, and individualized placement planning, all key components of ACT rehabilitation, have been shown in uncontrolled studies to yield better placement ratios (Knoedler 1979; D. Vandergoot, unpublished manuscript, February 1983; Worral and Vandergoot 1982; Zadny and James 1979). In one study (Field et al. 1978), a comparison between ACT "supported employment" and sheltered workshop placement did not yield significantly different competitive employment rates. In general, however, it appears that higher levels of vocational adjustment can be achieved through direct advocacy and job coaching, bypassing conventional rehabilitation programs (Drake et al. 1994).

However, as a method that relies extensively on existing community resources and direct therapeutic support by a team of clinicians, ACT has shown a complicated relationship to the client's family. Initially, ACT promoted "constructive separation" of the patient from his or her family during crisis episodes. Further, patients were encouraged to live away from the family home and restrict their contact with family members, who usually were not included in the treatment effort. More recently, ACT proponents have made more of an effort to include family members, but not systematically and not as an integral part of the patient's rehabilitation. On the other hand, the family psychoeducational interventions have their limitations. Our studies have consistently shown that approximately 14% of study patients experienced repeated relapses and rehospitalizations without observable effects from family intervention. Also, because the psychoeducational model is not linked to a more comprehensive service system, patients are referred to conventional vocational rehabilitation services. Some families, although involved and motivated, may simply be too burdened to devote the necessary energy to an intensive rehabilitation effort. Further, neither ACT nor single-family psychoeducation significantly expand the patient's or the family's social network, as is the case with a multifamily group.

We therefore hypothesized that combining ACT with psychoeducational multiple-family group treatment might lead to enhanced outcomes, compared with ACT or psychoeducation alone, because they compensate for each other's deficiencies. We term the combined approach *family-aided assertive community treatment* (FACT). It fosters coordination between important people and social forces that influence a given patient. Thus, the FACT approach consists of a merging of interrelated elements of ACT (see Chapter 9) with those of the psychoeducational multiple-family group as outlined below.

■ Integration of the patient into the natural community milieu

- Rehabilitation services provided in the natural community environment
- Relapse prevention strategies and around-the-clock access to crisis intervention
- Expectation of gradual increase in patient responsibilities with team support
- Supportive guidance and education of community members about patient's disability
- Goal-oriented and flexible team approach with shared caseloads
- Family engagement and education, and patient goal setting
- The ongoing psychoeducational multifamily group
- Family-based goal setting
- Creating a compendium of potential jobs
- Individualized job finding

During the initial engagement sessions the clinician meets with the family alone. The cohort of patients due to join the psychoeducational multifamily group meets together for nine sessions beginning in tandem with the psychoeducational workshop for families. These meetings are like classes, in which the team teaches the patients how to set a goal, how to decide on the steps necessary for its achievement, and how to deal with barriers that might impede success.

When five to eight families have completed the joining process, the FACT team conducts the educational workshop, again usually without patients. In this presentation, we also closely follow Anderson's format, except that we present the biomedical aspects of schizophrenia by showing a standardized videotape and have added new guidelines and other components specifically geared to the vocational rehabilitation phase.

Following the workshop is the first meeting of the ongoing psychoeducational multifamily group; its format includes a biweekly meeting schedule, 90-minute session length, leadership by two FACT clinicians, and participation by six to nine patients and their families. Patients are strongly encouraged to attend and actively participate. The multifamily group is conducted in a manner similar to that described previously.

We emphasize the patient's perceived desires for their vocational and social lives as the nucleus of work by both the FACT team and the families in the multifamily group. Thus, the initial and crucial step is getting a sense of the patient's previous work history and his or her interests either in continuing a career already started or in changing directions. This occurs in the initial sessions held with the patient alone and in the joint patient-family sessions. However, the rehabilitation phase in FACT should be initiated only by patients who have achieved clinical stability by successfully completing this community reentry phase. As stability increases, the multifamily group functions as an auxiliary to the in vivo vocational rehabilitation effort being conducted by the clinical team. The clinicians continue to use group-based problem solving and brainstorming to identify and develop jobs, to help individual patients obtain job placement, or to enrich their social lives.

Family-based goal setting inevitably involves some reduction or postponement of previously held vocational goals, and because those goals are often held as strongly by family members as by patients themselves, the process and outcomes of the goal-setting classes are reported into the multifamily group as a regular part of each session. This allows each family to express doubts and reservations, opinions, or possibly support, so that the final result of goal setting is something that has been ratified by the patient's own family in the public arena of the multifamily group. Further, the other families in the group are aware of each patient's intentions, making the vocational progress of the group's patients the project of the entire group, which, in turn, helps to define a positive group identity. Reciprocally, the families' ideas, opinions, and information can be taken back to the goal-setting class and incorporated into patients' rehabilitation aims.

After the group completes the goal-setting process, several group meetings are spent on developing a list of possible job opportunities among the members of the group's families and their extended kin. Potential jobs may be located in the homes or businesses of group members, in those of relatives and friends outside the group, in their workplaces, or in those of their kin. In this way, patients may work at jobs with members of other families in the group and/or their extended kin. Jobs known to group members may also be identified by simple informal connections, chance encounters (for instance, seeing help-wanted signs), or through deliberate inquiry and community advocacy.

Ultimately, families, in collaboration with the team and local family advocacy associations, may create jobs for the patients through community action. In general, such jobs are potentially less stressful, because they are embedded within the social network of the multifamily group and involve social connections that are inherently more familiar to the patients. To a large degree, we have modeled this approach after the usual methods—involving networks and personal connections—by which a mentally healthy individual obtains a job or job leads (Granovetter 1974, 1979; Roessler and Hiett 1983; Vandergoot 1976). Family members may be asked to gather additional information on job possibilities between meetings, but actual job development is carried out by the team clinicians.

After the completion of a job-opportunity compendium, the vocational or social rehabilitation process for each patient is broken into steps that are attempted sequentially. The achievement of the next rehabilitative step, usually employment, is raised as a focus in the problem-solving portion of the multifamily group. The members of the group and their extended kin are polled for sources of jobs, job leads, and even possibilities for job development, with specific reference to one particular patient in the group. In this brainstorming process, various ideas are generated from participants in the multifamily group. These suggestions are then reviewed by the patient and the patient's family and a final plan is developed. This usually involves job preparation, job development, coaching, planning, and problem solving, all carried out in the field by the FACT team. The results of these efforts are then reported back to the team during rounds, during treatment planning, and during the next multiple-family group. If necessary, the entire process is repeated if initial results were disappointing.

**Research on FACT.** The FACT research project began in 1987, sponsored by the New York State Office of Mental Health and the New York State Alliance for the Mentally Ill. The FACT project used a two-cell experimental design: one combined the ACT treatment method with psychoeducational multifamily group (FACT); the other was ACT treatment with limited single-family crisis intervention (ACT). This design tested ongoing family participation in a multifamily group as a primary treatment factor. The sample consisted of 72 patients at three community mental health centers in New York State. Patients were selected according to the following criteria: diagnosis (DSM-III-R schizophrenia, schizophreniform, and schizoaffective disorders), associated complicating factors (homelessness, treatment noncompliance, substance abuse, criminal charges, suicidality), family availability, and age (18–45). Analysis of baseline psychiatric and demographic data indicated that no differences existed between cohorts.

Hospitalizations declined from a pretreatment mean of 1.85 hospitalizations per patient in the 2 years prior to treatment to a mean of 1.37 hospitalizations per patient during the 2 years of treatment ($t_{(52)} = 2.89$, $P < .01$), without significant differences between FACT and ACT. We found no difference in employment activity between the two cohorts at intake (11% of FACT patients were engaged in employment activity vs. 6% of TCL patients, $t(66) = 0.62$, n.s.). A repeated-measures MANOVA (multivariate analysis of variance) of data collected at 4-month intervals found that employment activity showed an increase in the first 4 months of treatment ($F(1, 52) = 8.54$, $P < .01$) and that patients were able to maintain this level for nearly the duration of the project. The maximum level of employment activity was 33%, achieved at the 20-month assessment point. After achieving this peak level, activity dropped off in the last 4 months of treatment, down to 17% ($F(1,52) = 9.18$, $P < .01$). We compared employment activity between FACT and ACT. At 12 months FACT was superior to ACT in number of patients employed at any job, whether full-time, part-time, in a sheltered workshop, or as a volunteer (37.0% vs. 15.4%), and in competitive employment (16.0% vs.

0%). Averaged over the full 2 years, there was a significant result in favor of FACT for sheltered work (18% of the FACT sample over 2 years vs. 6% of the ACT sample; $t(51) = 1.99$, $P = .05$) and no difference for nonsheltered activity (patients showed an average of 10% nonsheltered work activity regardless of family involvement).

## Conclusion

The paradigms presented in this chapter for the treatment of schizophrenia are educationally oriented, clinical management models, which optimally align with and support the family. Psychoeducation is a powerful tool for the avoidance of future relapse and significant improvement in the quality of life for patients and their families. The merging of psychoeducation with a multifamily group experience in the context of assertive community treatment represents state-of-the-art use of powerful and well-established models of treatment, uniquely developed and suitable for alleviating the psychiatric and personal catastrophe that is schizophrenia. Because they promote repetition and structure, they are gradually effective in promoting the restitution and rehabilitation of the afflicted person, the relief of family burden and suffering, and the rebalancing of family relationships.

Throughout, the aim is that the multifamily group become something of a task force, in which individuals share experiences, information, planning, and the creation of new ideas and options, especially in the difficult area of vocational rehabilitation. The professional team's job is then to take these possibilities and attempt to realize them. The assumptions are that all aspects of the patient's network should be brought to bear on the effort toward employment and that expanding that network through the natural connections in a multifamily group can gain each patient access to a greatly expanded pool of potential jobs and opportunities. This total process is a major contributor to the higher employment rates achieved to date in our experimental clinical trials of the FACT approach.

Training in family intervention varies between approaches, but for the psychoeducational, long-term clinical management approaches, clinicians will require intensive workshop-style training and some supervision to fully realize the potential of the model. The psychoeducational multifamily-group approach has been described in a treatment manual, which has been used to train a large cadre of practitioners in New York State (McFarlane et al. 1993). Recent trainees have almost universally been able to initiate successful multiple-family groups, if the administrative elements have supported their efforts.

The outcome data available and continuing to emerge suggest that these eminently teachable and practical approaches may be the most cost-effective psychosocial treatment yet developed for chronic and severe psychiatric disorders. These studies provide the following evidence.

- A multifamily-group version of psychoeducation yields significantly fewer relapses than the single-family form and markedly fewer relapses in partially remitted patients.
- There is a significant increase in employment in both forms of psychoeducational family treatment and a trend toward superiority for the multifamily-group format.
- FACT yields better vocational outcome than ACT alone.

Ultimately, however, the most persuasive recommendation for this type of work is that it allows the family and patient to move this devastating illness off to a corner of their lives and proceed to live a bit more as their neighbors and friends do, something that until now has been all but impossible for most families.

# References

Anderson CM, Hogarty GE, Reiss DJ: Family treatment of adult schizophrenic patients: a psychoeducational approach. Schizophr Bull 6:490–505, 1980

Anderson CM, Hogarty GE, Bayer T, et al: Expressed emotion and social networks of parents of schizophrenic patients. Br J Psychiatry 144:247–255, 1984

Anderson CM, Hogarty GE, Reiss DJ: Schizophrenia and the Family. New York, Guilford, 1986

Bateson G, Jackson DD, Haley J, et al: Toward a theory of schizophrenia. Behav Sci 1:251–264, 1956

Beels CC: Social support and schizophrenia. Schizophr Bull 7:58–72, 1981

Benningfield AB: Multiple family therapy systems. Advances in Family Psychiatry 2:411–424, 1980

Berman KK: Multiple family therapy: its possibilities in preventing readmission. Mental Hygiene 50:367–370, 1966

Brown GW, Birley JLT, Wing JK: Influence of family life on the course of schizophrenic disorders: a replication. Br J Psychiatry 121:241–258, 1972

Dean A, Lin N: The stress-buffering role of social support. J Nerv Ment Dis 165:403–416, 1977

DeLisi LE, Schwartz CC, Targum SD, et al: Ventricular brain enlargement and outcome of acute schizophrenic disorder. J Psychiatr Res 9:169–171, 1983

Detre T, Sayer J, Norton A, et al: An experimental approach to the treatment of the acutely ill psychiatric patient in the general hospital. Connecticut Medicine 25:613–619, 1961

Dozier M, Harris M, Bergman H: Social network density and rehospitalization among young adult patients. Hosp Community Psychiatry 38:61–64, 1987

Drake RE, Becker DR, Biesanz JC, et al: Rehabilitative day treatment vs. supported employment, I: vocational outcomes. Community Ment Health J 30:519–532, 1994

Falloon IRH, Liberman RP: Behavioral family interventions in the management of chronic schizophrenia, in Family Therapy in Schizophrenia. Edited by McFarlane WR. New York, Guilford, 1983, pp 141–172

Falloon IRH, Liberman R, Lillie F: Family therapy for relapsing schizophrenics and their families: a pilot study. Fam Process 20:211–221, 1981

Falloon IRH, Boyd JL, McGill CW, et al: Family management in the prevention of morbidity of schizophrenia. Arch Gen Psychiatry 42:887–896, 1985

Field G, Allness D, Knoedler W, et al: Employment training for chronic patients in the community. Paper presented at the annual meeting of the American Psychological Association, Toronto, Canada, August, 1978

Freeman H, Simmons O: Feeling of stigma among relatives of former mental patients. Social Problems 8:312–321, 1961

Garrison V: Support systems of schizophrenic and non-schizophrenic Puerto Rican women in New York City. Schizophr Bull 4:561–596, 1978

Goldstein MJ, Rodnick E, Evans J, et al: Drug and family therapy in the aftercare of acute schizophrenics. Arch Gen Psychiatry 35:1169–1177, 1978

Granovetter MS: Getting A Job: A Study of Contacts and Careers. Cambridge, MA, Harvard University Press, 1974

Granovetter MS: Placement as brokerage—information problems in the labor market for rehabilitated workers, in Placement in Rehabilitation. Edited by Vandergoot D, Worrall J. Baltimore, MD, University Park Press, 1979

Hammer M: Influence of small social networks as factors on mental hospital admission. Human Organization 22:243–251, 1963

Hammer M: Social supports, social networks, and schizophrenia. Schizophr Bull 7:45–57, 1981

Hammer M, Makiesky-Barrow S, Gutwirth L: Social networks and schizophrenia. Schizophr Bull 4:522–545, 1978

Hogarty GE, Ulrich RF: Temporal effects of drug and placebo in delaying relapse in schizophrenic outpatients. Arch Gen Psychiatry 34:297–301, 1977

Hogarty GE, Schooler NR, Ulrich RF: Fluphenazine and social therapy in the aftercare of schizophrenic patients. Arch Gen Psychiatry 36:1283–1294, 1979

Hogarty GE, Anderson CM, Reiss DJ, et al: Family psychoeducation, social skills training and maintenance chemotherapy in the aftercare treatment of schizophrenia. Arch Gen Psychiatry 43:633–642, 1986

Johnson DJ: The family's experience of living with mental illness, in Families as Allies in Treatment of the Mentally Ill. Edited by Lefley HP, Johnson DJ. Washington, DC, American Psychiatric Press, 1990, pp 31–64

Knoedler WH: How the Training in Community Living program helps patients work. New Directions for Mental Health Services 2:57–66, 1979

Lamb HR, Oliphant E: Schizophrenia through the eyes of families. Hosp Community Psychiatry 29:803–806, 1978

Lansky MR, Bley CR, McVey GG, et al: Multiple family groups as after-care. Int J Group Psychother 29:211–224, 1978

Laqueur HP: Mechanisms of change in multiple family therapy, in Progress in Group and Family Therapy. Edited by Sager CJ, Kaplan HS. New York, Brunner/Mazel, 1972

Laqueur HP, LaBurt HA, Morong E: Multiple family therapy, further developments. Int J Soc Psychiatry 10:69–80, 1964

Leff J, Vaughn CE: Expressed Emotion in Families. New York, Guilford, 1985

Leff JP, Kuipers L, Berkowitz R, et al: A controlled trial of social intervention in the families of schizophrenic patients: two year follow up. Br J Psychiatry 146:594–600, 1985

Leff JP, Kuipers L, Berkowitz R: Intervention in families of schizophrenics and its effect of relapse rate, in Family Therapy in Schizophrenia. Edited by McFarlane WR. New York, Guilford, 1983, pp 173–187

Leff J, Berkowitz R, Shavit N, et al: A trial of family therapy vs a relatives group for schizophrenia. Br J Psychiatry 154:58–66, 1989

Levin EC: Therapeutic multiple family groups. International Journal of Psychotherapy 19:203–208, 1966

Lipton FR, Cohen CI, Fischer E, et al: Schizophrenia: a network crisis. Schizophr Bull 7:144–151, 1981

Lurie A, Ron H: Socialization program as part of aftercare planning. General Psychiatric Association Journal 17:157–162, 1972

McFarlane WR: Multiple family therapy in schizophrenia, in Family Therapy in Schizophrenia. Edited by McFarlane WR. New York, Guilford, 1983, pp 141–172

McFarlane WR: Multiple family groups in the treatment of schizophrenia, in Handbook of Schizophrenia, Vol 4. Edited by Nasrallah HA. Amsterdam, The Netherlands, Elsevier, 1990, pp 167–189

McFarlane WR, Dunne E, Lukens E, et al: From research to clinical practice: dissemination of New York State's Family Demonstration Project. Hosp Community Psychiatry 44:265–270, 1993

McFarlane WR, Link B, Dushay R, et al: Psychoeducational multiple family groups: four-year relapse outcome in schizophrenia. Fam Process 34:127–144, 1995a

McFarlane WR, Lukens E, Link B, et al: Multiple family groups and psychoeducation in the treatment of schizophrenia. Arch Gen Psychiatry 52:679–688, 1995b

O'Shea MD: Multiple family therapy: current status and critical appraisal. Fam Process 24:555–582, 1985

Pattison EM, Llama R, Hurd G: Social network mediation of anxiety. Psychiatric Annals 9:56–67, 1979

Potasznik H, Nelson G: Stress and social support: the burden experienced by the family of a mentally ill person. Am J Community Psychol 12:589–607, 1984

Rabkin J: Public attitudes toward mental illness: a review of the literature. Schizophr Bull 10:9–33, 1974

Roessler RT, Hiett A: Strategies for increasing employer response to job development surveys. Rehabilitation Counseling Bulletin 26:368–370, 1983

Steinberg HR, Durell JA: A stressful social situation as a precipitant of schizophrenia. Br J Psychiatry 114:1097–1105, 1968

Strelnick AH: Multiple family group therapy: a review of the literature. Fam Process 16:307–325, 1977

Stevens JR: Neuropathology of schizophrenia. Arch Gen Psychiatry 39:1131–1139, 1982

Tarrier N, Barrowclough C, Vaughn C, et al: The community management of schizophrenia: a controlled trial of a behavioral intervention with families to reduce relapse. Br J Psychiatry 153:532–542, 1988

Tecce JJ, Cole JO: The distraction-arousal hypothesis, CNV and schizophrenia, in Behavioral Control and Modification of Psychological Activity. Edited by Mostofsky DI. Englewood Cliffs, NJ, Prentice-Hall, 1976, pp 162–219

Tolsdorf CC: Social networks, support and coping: an exploratory study. Fam Process 15:407–417, 1976

Vandergoot D. A comparison of two mailing approaches attempting to generate the participation of businessmen in rehabilitation. Rehabilitation Counseling Bulletin 20:73–75, 1976

Vaughn CE, Leff JP: The influence of family and social factors on the course of psychiatric illness: a comparison of schizophrenic and depressed neurotic patients. Br J Psychiatry 129:125–137, 1976

Weinberger DR, Berman KR, Zec RF: Physiologic dysfunction of dorsolateral pre-frontal cortex in schizophrenia. Arch Gen Psychiatry 43:114–135, 1986

World Health Organization: Schizophrenia: An International Follow-up Study. Chichester, Wiley, 1979

Worrall JD, Vandergoot D: Additional indicators of non-success: a follow-up report. Rehabilitation Counseling Bulletin 26:88–93, 1982

Yarrow M, Schwartz C, Murphy H, et al: The psychological meaning of mental illness in the family. Journal of Social Issues 11:33–48, 1955

Zadny JJ, James LF: Job placement in state vocational rehabilitation agencies: a survey of technique. Rehabilitation Counseling Bulletin 22:361–378, 1979

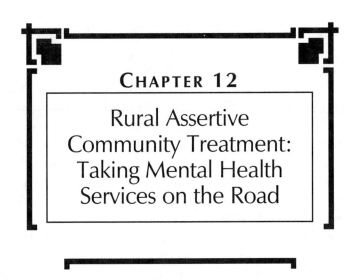

# CHAPTER 12

## Rural Assertive Community Treatment: Taking Mental Health Services on the Road

**Kerry R. Lachance, M.A., L.M.S.W., Paul A. Deci, M.D., Alberto B. Santos, M.D., Nancy M. Halewood, R.N., and J. Mark Westfall, M.D.**

In many rural parts of the nation, mental health workers gamely venture out, day after day, along networks of winding roads and dirt paths, in search of the familiar landmarks—the gnarled tree near the brick pile, the white post immediately following the county line—that will lead them to the homes of their clients. The idea of taking mental health services to the clients is not new. Mental health professionals have long recognized a need for outreach to rural areas. What is not known is the value of such services in terms of their cost-effectiveness. In this chapter we describe a pilot study and introduce a controlled clinical trial designed to address this question.

## The Experimental Intervention

The experimental intervention in this project was developed through the authors' experience with the urban-based Training in Community Living Model (see Chapter 9). Although controlled studies of this approach have largely been limited to urban areas, significant dissemination to rural areas has occurred. For example, the state mental health authority of Wisconsin supported the flexible, widespread dissemination of Assertive Community Treatment (ACT) throughout rural Wisconsin, which was reported as positive both in terms of clinical outcome and reduction in hospital costs (Test et al. 1985). In addition, the state mental health authorities of Oregon and Michigan have implemented similar rural programs (personal communication, J. Donald Bray and Thomas Plum, September 1992). The setting of this study is rural South Carolina. The population is predominantly African-American and poor, with high levels of illiteracy, poor health, and limited or nonexistent transportation and telephone services. Many are without basic sanitation, running water, electricity, and indoor toilets. Patients typically are unable to follow complicated procedures or complete application forms required for governmental entitlements and other public benefits. Although the state mental health authority operates a network of mental health centers organized by counties, individuals from rural areas frequently enter the mental health system by commitment through the courts and are hospitalized in centralized facilities. When discharged back to their rural areas, they are often lost to follow-up, and remain untreated until their need for services necessitates emergency attention.

The program named Rural Outreach, Advocacy, and Direct Services (ROADS) was developed by the Charleston/Dorchester Community Mental Health Center in 1988, to target individuals with chronic psychotic disorders who are high users of centralized inpatient facilities. Clinical services are provided by a multidisciplinary team for a shared caseload of patients. The staff spends most of their time in the rural communities monitoring medication effects and compliance, facilitating access to basic resources, and developing and educating each patient's indigenous community support network about the patient's illness and its treatment. When necessary, the team provides financial management and other individualized services such as the use of sign language for deaf patients. The nature and frequency of staff contacts are determined by each patient's individual needs. The absence of a time limit to the service allows for long-term and continuous clinical care and assessment rather than brief episodic care and crisis intervention. Two community health nurses with extensive backgrounds in home health care and social work and a part-time psychiatrist comprised the original ROADS clinical team. Gradually, with additional federal funding from the Center for Mental Health Services, the ROADS team expanded to include two social workers, two additional registered nurses, and a full-time secretary.

On a typical day, ROADS staff travel in teams of two in state-owned vans, carrying perhaps a change of clothes, a pair of "mud shoes," a first-aid kit, and other assorted items. Too frequently they get caught in the rain or must trek through a washed-out dirt road. Lunch boxes, fresh water, and a couple of rolls of toilet paper are also essential in the remote rural areas because restaurants and public restrooms are not always conveniently available. In dramatic contrast to a more traditional office-based setting in an urban area, the call of the open road and other characteristics of rural living make rural mental health work especially appealing to the ROADS team.

The psychiatrist provides direct services for 2 full days a week, and is available by telephone the remainder of the week. The psychiatrist visits patients in their homes, usually accompanied by one of the other ROADS staff, and is directly responsible for the pharmacological treatment of the patients as well as for their overall clinical management. In addition to providing direct clinical services, the psychiatrist provides clinical and administrative input into the program and continuing education to the team members on an ongoing basis. This occurs formally during the weekly team meeting but more often it occurs informally during interactions with staff and patients in the field. The psychiatrist also supervises the clinical experiences of third-year psychiatry residents as they rotate for a year with the ROADS programs. Below are offered three case vignettes to illustrate the work of the team.

Mr. M is a 32-year-old single African-American male living 45 miles from Charleston on a rural coastal island. He was hospitalized for evaluation and treatment after a home visit from the mental health center's emergency psychiatry team, prompted by a report by a neighbor that he had not been seen for several years but supposedly was still in the family home. Mr. M lived in a small four-room shack with electricity but without running water, toilets, or window screens. He had barricaded himself in one bedroom, wired the door shut, covered the windows, and used a hole in the floor for a toilet. He began doing this several years earlier, because, he said, "I got into trouble if I came out." He had previously worked as a farm laborer and socialized with family and friends but then became very paranoid and bizarre, resulting in his self-imposed isolation. He did not bathe and did not change clothes during those years. He always wore several layers of clothing, in spite of the intense summer heat, and had impaired circulation in his extremities because of the tightness of his clothing. He left his room only occasionally at night when no one else was awake. He refused to allow others to enter his room but he accepted food and drink through a partially opened door. Emergency involuntary psychiatric admission was arranged. Mr. M was diagnosed with chronic schizophrenia, paranoid type, and was started on an intramuscular long-acting neuroleptic every 4 weeks. On medication he became much less paranoid, more communicative, less isolated, and his auditory persecutory hallucinations were diminished. He was discharged to the local mental health center and was expected to return there for his injections and follow-up care. However, he failed to show for his appointments due to his lack of motivation for treatment, lack of transportation, lack of insight into his illness, and lack of support for treatment from his family. He was referred to the ROADS program.

The ROADS team slowly developed a relationship with Mr. M and his family. ROADS visited him at least once a week and administered his injections monthly. The ROADS psychiatrist visited him at home because he still refused to travel. ROADS focused on improving his environment and hygiene, arranging through other social services and volunteer agencies for running water in the house, an outhouse, a refrigerator, mattresses, roof repairs, and window screens. ROADS helped him obtain Medicaid and a disability income. They worked with his family on basic hygiene and food preparation, including convincing the family to not let their chickens run free in the house. Mr. M's environment was clearly pathological for him, particularly in view of the fact that his alcoholic father had attempted to kill him on four occasions because of his frustration with Mr. M and his unwillingness to work. However, Mr. M strongly resisted efforts to be relocated, even with other family members who lived nearby, because, he said, "This is home and it is the only home I've ever known." Mr. M still lives with his family. He now sits out with his family in the living room and walks around in the yard. He eats with the family and takes baths about weekly, although he still prefers to wear layers of clothes. On medications he is without any hallucinations and his paranoia is minimal. He and his family appreciate the improvements in their living conditions and increase in family income due to ROADS.

Mr. S is a 59-year-old African-American male who lives on a rural island off the South Carolina coast. He was referred to the mental health center at the age of 50 after being discharged from the state hospital. He had been committed to the hospital on an emergency basis for disorganized behavior, which included throwing rocks at cars, attempting to set furniture on fire, and threatening harm to his family. He was delusional and hallucinatory. He was found to have a history of psychiatric treatment in another state, was diagnosed with chronic schizophrenia, paranoid type, and started on an oral neuroleptic. The mental health center followed Mr. S after discharge and continued to treat him with traditional outpatient services. The patient was noncompliant with appointments and oral medication. He was hospitalized twice more in the following year and a half for psychotic episodes. He was found to have an alcohol abuse problem that compounded his illness and his ability to comply with treatment. He was eventually referred to the ROADS program.

The ROADS team began to see Mr. S at his home or place of occasional employment on a weekly basis. The reasons for lack of compliance became much more clear. Mr. S lived alone in a small cinder block house on a rural sea island 30 minutes from the mental health center in Charleston. He had no mode of transportation. He had no running water, no bathroom facilities indoors or out, and no appliances. An outdoor water well that he had dug himself was contaminated, and doors and windows were heavily damaged following multiple break-ins. He worked occasionally at a nearby shrimp dock and frequently spent his money on alcohol or had it stolen by others who took advantage of his disorganized mental state.

A working relationship with Mr. S was slow to establish. He continued to be noncompliant and required further hospitalizations. He continued to use alcohol, which typically led to an increase in his psychotic symptoms and often resulted in physical altercations. Over time the ROADS team learned his early signs of decompensation and were able to intervene. For example, pieces of metal roofing strewn across a dirt driveway (in a yard already full of trash and metal) meant Mr. S was becoming more paranoid and trying to ward off evil, and might do well with an increase in his neuroleptics even though he might deny worsening symptoms in an interview. ROADS also found support for Mr. S in his own environment, such as the owner of the shrimp docks where Mr. S worked on occasion. The owner would give Mr. S his oral medication at work and inform the team if he felt Mr. S was not doing well. Eventually a working relationship was established and Mr. S allowed the ROADS staff to administer intramuscular neuroleptics, which he had previously refused. He became less guarded, which allowed the ROADS staff to be of even more assistance. ROADS arranged for a financial manager to receive and distribute Mr. S's income. The ROADS staff rallied support from local churches, missionaries, and Mr. S's employer to donate time and money to help improve Mr. S's living situation. He received running water, indoor plumbing, new floors, doors, and windows, and new appliances. Mr. S himself was able to contribute also, having actually saved up money through his financial manager. Mr. S is enjoying his new surroundings. His drinking frequency has decreased and his work frequency has increased. His nutrition and hygiene have improved with his new facilities.

He is appreciative of the increase in living standard he has achieved with the help of the ROADS program.

Mr. G is a 61-year-old African-American with schizophrenia and polysubstance abuse. Originally from a rural island off the coast of South Carolina, he lived in New York for much of his adult life but returned to South Carolina at the age of 59. His sister, who lives in South Carolina and had lost contact with him years ago, reestablished contact with him after seeing him on national television among the homeless in New York. She arranged for his relocation to South Carolina. She offered assistance but was met with disorganized and violent behavior by her brother. Mr. G lived out of an abandoned car, wandering the rural highways on foot. He was unable to care for himself, going long periods of time without bathing or changing clothes. He ate very poorly and lost a considerable amount of weight. He was suspicious of everyone, including his family. On one occasion he threatened his sister with a baseball bat. At that point he was committed for psychiatric care at the state hospital. He was stabilized on an intramuscular neuroleptic after 3 months in the hospital and discharged to live with his sister. She lives in a small house with her husband on a rural coastal island 30 minutes from Charleston. Her husband worked during the day, and she did not leave the house very often due to her age and lack of transportation. Mr. G also had no transportation and although stabilized on medication, his marked negative symptoms left him with no insight into his illness and no initiative to pursue treatment. Simply to attend monthly appointments at the mental health center for his neuroleptic injection was a task loaded with hurdles too numerous to surmount. Had he been relegated to that treatment setting, he would most probably have fallen out of treatment and back into a psychotic state. Mr. G was referred to the ROADS program.

The ROADS team began to see him once a week at his sister's house, administering his neuroleptic injection once a month. Mr. G continued to remain stable regarding his positive symptoms, with no overt delusions, hallucinations, or paranoia. Mr. G and his family were pleased with his improvement. However, he continued to have significant negative symptoms of schizophrenia. He would spend all day withdrawn in the house, either sitting or pacing. He had paucity of speech, no initiative, and flat affect. He gave no direct eye contact. His hygiene was only fair. The next focus of the ROADS team was to help him obtain services and improve the quality of his daily living. They first helped Mr. G obtain Medicaid and a disability income. Next they concentrated on helping Mr. G become more interactive with his environment, while the ROADS psychiatrist worked to optimize Mr. G's medication. Mr. G was thought to have akinesia secondary to his neuroleptic. With the ROADS staff seeing Mr. G weekly, the physician felt comfortable aggressively managing the medication by decreasing the dosage. Mr. G tolerated a decrease in his neuroleptic to half the original dose. His akinesia improved. As the staff formed a relationship with Mr. G, they were able to encourage him to be more interactive with his environment. Mr. G still lives with his sister and has not had a relapse of overt psychotic symptoms. He occasionally sits outside in a lounge chair the ROADS staff helped him obtain. He rides a bicycle and takes walks with staff. He occasionally goes fishing in a nearby creek. Overall he continues to be impaired by negative symptoms but he and his sister's quality of life have clearly improved since first coming to the ROADS program.

# Comparing Urban and Rural TCL Programs

Differences in implementation of the Training in Community Living (TCL) system (Test 1991) in rural versus urban areas are based on inherent differences between rural and urban life in regard to mobility, accessibility, communications, health expectations, attitudes toward treatment, means of transportation, and basic community resources (Bachrach 1977; Boyer and Elkin 1989; Wagenfeld 1990). Table 12–1 highlights differences between customary mental health services, and urban and rural TCL. Such differences affect the manner in which TCL is delivered and its desired outcomes achieved.

For example, pay telephones, automobile service stations, and other resources that one takes for granted in urban settings are not readily available in rural settings. Cellular phones, important tools of urban community teams, do not work reliably in remote areas. The daily service route therefore requires thoughtful planning. Staff travel in teams of two and leave behind a detailed itinerary at a central office. In locations where staff are very familiar with patients and their families and neighbors, one team member may be dropped off at a client's home while the partner visits a nearby site. The urban TCL practice of providing total care insures that the range of patient needs are addressed through direct services. However, because of the long travel distances involved in serving rural patients, staff are unable to provide all services directly. Therefore, to develop a comprehensive total-care package for each patient, available community resources are mobilized, trained, and coordinated. When possible, family members or neighbors are engaged in the treatment plan, assisting with administering or delivering daily medication, transporting clients to appointments, and lending support during emergencies.

Because residential and vocational alternatives are more limited in rural areas, independent living and employment do not receive the emphasis found in urban TCL programs. The team does, however, focus on goals related to productive, personally satisfying daytime activities such as hobbies, increased involvement with family, volunteer work, and use of available community resources.

The urban TCL practice of a daily team meeting, daily contact with unstable patients, and direct emergency service availability 24 hours a day is impractical in rural areas because of the travel distances involved. Instead the rural team meets twice a week and is available after hours for telephone consultation with emergency personnel from the Charleston/Dorchester Community Mental Health Center and police department. During regular workdays, staff members spend time with support systems, including family members, neighbors, and others to make provisions for potential after-hours crises. The indigenous support persons are educated about alternatives in these instances. In addition to the option of contacting the local sheriff, support persons learn that they can contact ROADS personnel in the morning and receive rapid assistance. When patients and their

**Table 12–1.** Differences between standard systems, urban TCL, and a rural TCL application

| Service element | Standard systems | Urban TCL | Rural TCL application |
|---|---|---|---|
| Provider | Individual clinician | Team | Team (more nurses) and community volunteers |
| Consumer | Individual patient | Shared caseload | Shared caseload |
| Clinical staff/patient ratio | 1:50 | 1:10–12 | 1:10–12 |
| Caseload composition | Variable | Fixed and limited | Fixed and limited |
| Team communications | Infrequent | Daily meeting | Twice weekly |
| Staff availability | Traditional office hours | 24 hours/day, 7 days/week | Daytime only[a] |
| Treatment site | In the clinic or hospital | In the field | In the field |
| Rehabilitation | In vitro | In vivo | In vivo |
| Treatment approach | Focused (psychotherapy, medication) | Flexible and individualized | Flexible and individualized |
| Frequency of contact | 1–3 months in most cases | 1–3 days/week (daily for 25%) | Weekly[b] |
| Family contact | Occasional | Frequent (weekly in most cases) | Coincides with home visit |

| | | | |
|---|---|---|---|
| Medication compliance | Responsibility of patient and family | Responsibility of staff, can be monitored daily by staff if needed | Responsibility shared by staff, patient, family, neighbors, etc. |
| Housing arrangements | Responsibility of patient and family | Responsibility of staff | Responsibility shared by staff, patient, family, neighbors, etc. |
| Case management function | Broker of services | Service provider | Both provider and broker |
| Housing expectations | Gradual approach from supported to independent living | Maximize independence from beginning, drop back if necessary | Most live with family[c] |
| Resource mobilization (i.e., general health care) | Slight effort | Considerable effort | Extensive effort |

[a]24-hour telephone availability—team takes responsibility for arranging emergency protocols. [b]Difference in frequency due to differences in means of transportation and distances from services. [c]Expectation to increase satisfaction with current housing situation by improving role functioning.

environment are properly evaluated and monitored through regular and consistent home visits during the day, timely interventions can be made and many emergencies avoided.

Regarding the professional backgrounds of the ROADS team members, nurses were hired initially, rather than social workers or bachelor's level mental health counselors, because community health nurses can perform numerous social work functions, but social workers and mental health counselors are not licensed to provide essential nursing functions such as administering and monitoring medication. Nursing job descriptions include traditional social work, vocational rehabilitation, and home health duties, thus preserving the critical TCL service element of the multidisciplinary team. Later, when funding expanded, the rural team was able to hire social workers with backgrounds in community mental health.

The numerous administrative responsibilities of staff in their role of "keeper of the medical record" involve managing documentation according to agency requirements (i.e., making sure that consent forms are signed, treatment plans developed, physicians' signatures on treatment plans secured, prescriptions signed, services received by the patient documented, billing submitted, etc). Because of the inordinate amount of travel time involved, these duties are difficult to manage efficiently. Ideally, large sections of the medical records, such as assessment and progress notes, can be dictated by staff during routine travel and transcribed by clerical support staff the following day.

Staffing a program such as ROADS can be problematic. The demands of the job, including excessive travel and the absence of the in-office camaraderie more common in traditional settings, make staff recruitment and retention difficult. On the other hand, we have found that certain mental health professionals seem especially well-suited for the rural work. A background in home health care, a love of the outdoors, and a distaste for the limits of office-bound work contribute to a good worker–setting match. Of everything we have learned in the years of involvement with the ROADS project, this is by far the most important: quality staff is the critical variable in a successful program.

# Pilot Data

Patients ($N = 23$) were ages 18–65, 74% men and 87% African-American. They had a principal DSM-III-R (American Psychiatric Association 1987) diagnosis of schizophrenia ($n = 17$; 74%), schizoaffective disorder ($n = 3$; 13%), and bipolar disorder ($n = 3$; 13%). A majority of patients ($n = 14$; 61%) was also identified as abusing drugs or alcohol. They had histories of high rates of use of centralized psychiatric hospital services or persistent and largely untreated symptomatology. Several individuals had no significant history of psychiatric hospitalization but had long histories of untreated psychosis with accompanying disabilities. State Management Information System (MIS) and hospital records were reviewed to determine the number of hospital days for a period prior to assignment to ROADS (5 years), and for the period after assignment (the patients had participated in the program from 4 to 26 months at the time of final assessment).

The mean rate of psychiatric hospital use (number of inpatient days per year) decreased from 45 to 10 days per year per patient. This observed mean reduction of 35 days per year (a 78% reduction) was highly statistically significant ($t = 3.63$, $P = .001$). The average length of stay per admission decreased by 42 days (75%), from 56 to 14 days ($t = 2.55$, $P = .009$). The average number of admissions per year per patient decreased by 64%, from 1 to 0.4 admissions ($t = 3.33$, $P = .002$). A detailed trend analysis was conducted for the 5-year period pre-enrollment to detect a decreasing trend in number of hospitalizations. No decreasing trend was detected ($P > .95$) (Santos et al. 1993).

An examination of inpatient and outpatient costs and total mental health care costs for the 23 patients in the pilot study revealed the following results. At $250 per day, public hospital-based care for these patients prior to their enrollment in the ROADS program was estimated at $11,250 per patient per year and during the ROADS program at $2,500 per patient per year. The cost of outpatient services for an adult patient followed in the traditional outpatient system is estimated to be $1,200 per year compared with $4,000 per year for the 23 patients during the period of the study. Total mental health care cost for inpatient and outpatient care prior to the start of the ROADS program was about $12,450 per patient per year; during the ROADS pilot study the overall direct mental health care cost was estimated at $6,500. This represents a 52% reduction in the total cost of mental health care. In South Carolina, most of the ROADS teams' work is now reimbursable through Medicaid, and these revenues can support the majority of recurring personnel costs.

At this time, a prospective randomized controlled trial, which assesses the costs and effectiveness of ROADS in comparison with the standard system, is underway. In addition to inpatient service use, the hypotheses being tested center on expected changes in mental health status, level of functioning, quality of life, overall use of services, and costs. Costs will be measured for health and mental health service use, family burden, jail, police and court use, and maintenance (such as Supplemental Security income [SSI] and Social Security disability income [SSDI]).

# References

American Psychiatric Association: Diagnostic and Statistical Manual of Mental Disorders, 3rd Edition, Revised. Washington, DC, American Psychiatric Association, 1987

Bachrach LL: Deinstitutionalization of mental health services in rural areas. Hosp Community Psychiatry 28:669–672, 1977

Boyer PA, Elkin B: Rural chronically mentally ill. Human Services in the Rural Environment 12 (special issue), 1989

Santos AB, Deci PA, Lachance KR, et al: Providing assertive community treatment for severely mentally ill patients in a rural area. Hosp Community Psychiatry 44:34–39, 1993

Test MA: Training in community living, in Handbook of Psychiatric Rehabilitation. Edited by Liberman RP. New York, McMillan Press, 1992, pp 153–170

Test MA, Knoedler WH, Allness DJ: The long-term treatment of young schizophrenics in a community support program, in The Training in Community Living Model: A Decade of Experience. Edited by Stein LI, Test MA. San Francisco, CA, Jossey-Bass, 1985, pp 17–27

Wagenfeld MO: Mental health and rural America: a decade review. Journal of Rural Health 6:507–522, 1990

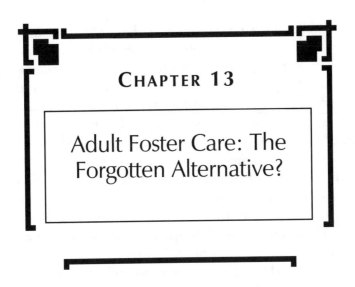

CHAPTER 13

## Adult Foster Care: The Forgotten Alternative?

**Paul A. Deci, M.D., and Gail N. Mattix, M.S.W.**

The practice of accepting mentally ill people into private homes can be traced back to the thirteenth century (Carling 1984) and, beginning with that period, spread widely throughout Europe. Dorothea Dix, credited with bringing the concept to the United States, was first introduced to adult foster care (AFC) during the 1800s while on a visit to Scotland, where mentally ill persons were placed on farms and contributed to the household by helping out with the farm chores (Oktay 1987). In the United States during the Depression, many states began to establish AFC programs on a large scale. The Veterans Administration (VA) began the first and only national AFC program in 1951, eventually serving between 12,000 and 15,000 people (Oktay 1987). AFC received renewed interest and expansion in the 1960s as the result of changes in state commitment laws, the advent of new psychotropic medications, and negative media exposure of conditions in some state hospitals (Rubin 1990), as well as in response to deinstitutionalization

(Blake 1989; Oktay 1987). By the 1970s, with the expansion of community-based services, many states moved away from the use of AFC as planners and program developers became partial to publicly financed halfway houses, group homes, and apartment programs (Carling 1984; McCoin 1989; Rubin 1990). However, the onslaught of mentally ill patients being discharged from the institutions resulted in a dramatic increase in board-and-care and nursing home facilities (Rubin 1990), often with the number of beds far exceeding the regulated limit of 30 persons per household (Beyer et al. 1984). In effect, a "transinstitutionalization" occurred, whereby custodial care was shifted from the state hospital to mini-institutions in the community known as residential care facilities (Searight and Handal 1987). In 1984, renewed interest in AFC led to an NIMH-sponsored Workshop on Family Foster Care and a resource guide on family-oriented service approaches (Carling 1984). In an optimal setting, AFC is available as part of a continuum of residential options in the context of a comprehensive treatment and rehabilitation service system, which offers opportunities for social activities using companions and available community resources. Ideally, only one adult enters a community household owned or rented by the reimbursed AFC provider as his own home, and lives like a member of the household (Lakin et al. 1989). This model of adult foster care is known as Homeshare.

Responsibilities of the AFC providers include completing initial and ongoing training, integrating the consumer into their household and assuming an active role in teaching independent living skills, protecting the consumer's confidentiality, being responsible for daily medication management and safe storage of medications, receiving scheduled and unannounced home visits by the case manager, and attending monthly *network meetings*— staff-facilitated groups that give support to providers and that aid in problem solving.

One clinical case manager from the sponsoring agency is assigned for every 10 consumers to provide intensive services. Responsibilities include coordinating preplacement and trial visits, providing ongoing guidance to the provider to follow through on goals, broadening consumers' interests and experiences in the community, ensuring follow-up for psychiatric assessment and medication monitoring, being available by beeper during the consumer's transition from the hospital and for emergencies, serving as a liaison between the consumer's natural family and the AFC provider, and maintaining necessary documentation. Respite services are available to cover a provider's annual leave and hourly or overnight respite needs. These services also provide a backup home when a client needs to move. Respite providers must complete the same screening and training requirements as other providers. The AFC provider's stipend is suspended when respite services exceed the 2-week-per-year limit.

The case manager is backed up by a team, which includes a program supervisor, a secretary, and other case managers who share responsibility for various tasks related to the recruitment and screening of providers, selection of consumers, and coordination of clinical services and supports. Also included as part of the team are the AFC providers as well as *assisting neighbors* and *companions*. Assisting neighbors are reimbursed for assisting consumers in developing and/or enhancing their skills by spending several hours each week providing individual and group activities that enhance the quality of their lives in the community. Companions are community volunteers who spend up to 4 hours each week assisting consumers to identify, plan, and participate in leisure and recreational activities, mostly during the evenings and on weekends (a stipend is provided to cover the cost of activities). Every effort is made to strengthen ties to natural family and to increase use and enjoyment of community services and opportunities. Companions, providers, and staff often involve their friends and families with the program (personal communication, W. Turkel, Community Enterprises, Inc., March 1992).

When recruiting providers, it is more helpful to look for a positive attitude and values orientation than specific credentials. Nurturing skills are usually more important than factors such as age, gender, or marital status. Interviewing applicant providers in their homes allows the recruiter to determine the physical capacity of the residence and to observe interactions with children and other family members. The recruiter is also able to explore carefully the applicant's motivation for wanting to become a provider and be assured that no rules will be set for the consumers that will not apply equally to all household members (Carling 1984). Applicant providers often screened out include those dependent upon AFC for their principal source of income, those with criminal convictions, those with unsupportive family members, those with conflicting attitudes or unhelpful beliefs, and those who want to be "therapists."

Recruitment is often most successful by word of mouth among current providers. Other recruitment strategies include newspaper, radio, and television advertisements, posters, and church and organizational newsletters. It is important to note that the specific recruiting strategies employed will often determine the type of provider who applies (Carling 1984).

All AFC and respite providers are expected to participate in training sessions to receive overview information (i.e., provider, staff, and consumer expectations and responsibilities), as well as the following additional information.

- Information about the major mental illnesses and their treatment
- Information to help the providers understand consumers' self-image and problematic behavior, thus assisting in the development of a supportive provider/consumer relationship
- Information on how to assist the consumers to develop increasingly more independent daily living and community living skills
- Information on the needs of special groups, such as geriatric and young adult populations
- Information on the importance of maintaining the consumers' physical and mental health (i.e., medications, sleep, personal habits, nutrition, and exercise are discussed, including how to check for signs and symptoms of illness and injury and how to get help in an emergency)

■   Information for providers on the importance of maintaining
their own emotional and physical health through stress reduction strategies and techniques for getting organized
(Manual for Family Care Program, n.d.)

AFC financing is possible through Supplemental Security income (SSI), Social Security disability income (SSDI), Medicaid,
or other state general funds available to the consumer. An outside
third party is often sought to provide financial management services for consumers. The provider stipend to cover expenses for
room and board is based on difficulty of care. Payments are ex-
cludable from gross income per Internal Revenue Code Section
131. Pertinent and applicable portions of the code section include
Section 131 (a), (b) (1), and (c) (1). Providers are given a copy of
the code and are advised to consult their tax preparer. AFC
providers are required to maintain adequate coverage under
their homeowner's and automobile insurance policies. Formal
contracts outlining standardized agreements between the agency
and the provider to cover all contingencies—including conflict
resolution and termination—as well as regular monitoring are
essential to assure safe and healthful settings, as well as to promote a high level of quality in service delivery (Carling 1984).
Program success often lies in a clear understanding of the roles
and responsibilities of each program participant (staff, companions, consumers, and providers).

It is difficult to obtain a contemporary picture of the use of
AFC in the United States; federal standards for model design,
operations, and reporting of information do not exist. A 1989
survey identified 5,214 psychiatrically disabled adults in foster
care in the states outlined in Table 13–1 (Lakin et al. 1989). Several agencies, including the NE Georgia Community Mental
Health Center, Community Enterprises, Inc., in Massachusetts,
and the South Carolina Department of Mental Health, include
transitional, crisis, and long-term living arrangements. South-
west Denver (Colorado) Community Mental Health Services, Inc.
operates a crisis stabilization program that alternates the use of
providers with average lengths of stay at around 10 days (Brook

**Table 13–1.** Adult foster care programs for psychiatrically disabled adults

| State | Agency name | Program name |
|---|---|---|
| Georgia | Fulton Co. Health Dept. | The Supportive Living Program |
| | NE Georgia CMHC | Family Support Homes |
| Indiana | Indiana DMH | Community Living Program |
| Massachusetts | Community Enterprises, Inc. | Project AIM/Homeshare |
| Michigan | Kent County CMH Board | Foster Care |
| | Washtenaw CMH Board | Foster Care |
| New Jersey | SERV Centers of NJ | Home Care Program |
| New York | Pilgrim Psychiatric Center | Family Care Program |
| North Carolina | | American Home Program |
| South Carolina | Charleston/Dorchester CMHC | Homeshare |
| | Coastal Empire CMHC | Homeshare |
| | Columbia Area CMHC | Homeshare |
| | Lexington County CMHC | Homeshare |
| | Orangeburg CMHC | Homeshare |

et al. 1976). Another variation is living with a roommate who is a designated provider. In self-directed households, a home-sharing experience is provided for four to six psychiatrically disabled adults who might not otherwise be able to live successfully in the community. This home-sharing alternative can provide a permanent home for individuals who require long-term care and can support or serve as a transitional home for those who may eventually live independently. A self-governing process is conducted by household members and encompasses all aspects of shared living and program direction. Community people are recruited and trained as providers to reside in the household as peers. Staff members visit frequently but there is no professional on-site coverage. The role of staff and volunteers is one of facilitation and engagement. Opportunities are offered but it is the responsibility of the household members to choose among available options. The self-directed household model may also be extended to individuals who live in their own apartment with a community roommate. The goal for self-directed household members is to become progressively self-sufficient over time (personal communication, W. Turkel, Community Enterprises, Inc., March 1992). No matter which home-sharing arrangement a consumer chooses, the assigned case manager does not change. Previously established trusting relationships and continuity in care are the primary ingredients necessary for ensuring successful community living.

Very little research has been published on AFC. Although there are a few uncontrolled evaluations dating back to the 1940s (Cunningham et al. 1969; Lee 1963; Linn 1987; Linn et al. 1977, 1980, 1982; Molholm and Barton 1941; Simon et al. 1968; Ullmann and Berkman 1959a, 1959b, 1959c; Ullmann et al.1958), these studies generally do not describe the number of clients served in each home and include homes serving three or more clients. When the literature is reviewed exclusively for studies of programs serving one or two adults with serious mental illnesses in family homes, there is only one relevant study.

Linn et al. (1977) conducted a randomized, controlled, multiple-site trial in which they evaluated the clients' social functioning and foster-care home characteristics for 210 male veterans (75% with a diagnosis of schizophrenia). Social functioning at 4 months after hospital discharge increased for clients placed in foster homes, which served only one or two clients, had less than 10 people living in the household, and had children in the home (Linn et al. 1980). Two studies examined foster-care sponsors and concluded that the typical sponsor is a middle-aged woman who had caretaking experience with her family and little formal education or work experience (Beatty and Seeley 1980; Van Putten and Spar 1979). Dubin and Ciavarelli (1978) studied foster-care homes with one to six clients and concluded that the providers were motivated by factors other than money, such as feelings of loneliness or a desire to perform a community service. There is a clear need for controlled research on AFC in different settings and with different types of clients in order to better establish its role in the spectrum of community support and residential services. For example, the definition of traditional AFC as put forth by Carling (1984), McCoin (1987), and Otkay (1987) includes three or more individuals in a residential care facility, small group home, or family-type setting. These facilities are usually regulated by a state and/or federal governmental agency. Private homes having one or two consumers living in the household are not subject to such regulations. The provider household is supported by a stipend that reimburses for daily living and difficulty-of-care costs. A better understanding of the effect of program design and operation may help to develop standards that will guard against the practice of serving large numbers of clients in crowded institutional environments, which offer little or no opportunity for rehabilitation.

# References

Beatty LS, Seeley M: Characteristics of operators of adult foster homes. Hosp Community Psychiatry 31:774–780, 1980

Beyer J, Buckley J, Hopkins P: A model act regulating board and care homes: guidelines for the states. Washington, DC, U.S. Department of Health and Human Services, 1984

Blake R: The anarchy of adult foster care policy. Adult Residential Care Journal 3:93–106, 1989

Brook BD, Cortes M, March R, et al: Community families: an alternative to psychiatric hospital intensive care. Hosp Community Psychiatry 27:195–197, 1976

Carling PJ: Developing family foster care programs in mental health: a resource guide. Proceedings of the National Institute of Mental Health workshop on family foster care for "chronically mentally ill" persons, Washington, DC, October 1984

Cunningham MK, Botwink W, Dolson J, et al: Community placement of released mental patients: a five year study. Social Work 14:54–61, 1969

Dubin WR, Ciavarelli B: A positive look at boarding homes. Hosp Community Psychiatry 29:593–595, 1978

Lakin KC, Hayden MF, Hill BK, et al: Utilization of adult foster care services in the United States. Adult Residential Care Journal 3:145–159, 1989

Lee DT: Family care:selection and prediction. Am J Psychiatry 120:561–566, 1963

Linn MW: Adult foster care: good patients and good homes. Adult Foster Care Journal 1:124–134, 1987

Linn MW, Caffey EM, Klett CJ, et al: Hospital vs community (foster) care for psychiatric patients. Arch Gen Psychiatry 34:73–83, 1977

Linn MW, Klett CJ, Caffey EM: Foster home characteristics and psychiatric patient outcome. Arch Gen Psychiatry 37:119–132, 1980

Linn MW, Klett CJ, Caffey EM: Relapse of psychiatric patients in foster care. Am J Psychiatry 139:778–783, 1982

Manual for Family Care Program. Albany, NY, New York State Office of Mental Health, n.d.

McCoin JM: Adult foster care: old wine in a new glass. Adult Foster Care Journal 1:21–41, 1987

McCoin JM: Toward a social movement for adult residential care. Adult Residential Care Journal 3:161–180, 1989

Molholm HB, Barton WE: Family care: a community resource in the rehabilitation of mental patients. Am J Psychiatry 98:33–41, 1941

Oktay JS: Foster care for adults, in Encyclopedia of Social Work. Edited by Minihan A. Silver Spring, MD, National Association of Social Workers, Inc., 1987, 634–638

Rubin JS: Adult foster care for people with chronic mental illness. Adult Residential Care Journal 4:5–20, 1990

Searight HR, Handal PJ: Psychiatric deinstitutionalization and social policy: implications for foster care. Adult Foster Care Journal 1:7–20, 1987

Simon SH, Heggested W, Hopkins J: Some factors relating to success and failure of male chronic schizophrenics on their first foster home placement. Community Ment Health J 4:314–318, 1968

Ullmann LP, Berkman VC: Efficacy of placement of neuropsychiatric patients in family care. Arch Gen Psychiatry 1:273–274, 1959a

Ullmann LP, Berkman VC: Judgements of outcome of home care placement from psychological material. J Clin Psychol 15:28–31, 1959b

Ullmann LP, Berkman VC: Types of outcome in family care placement of mental patients. Social Work 4:72–78, 1959c

Ullmann LP, Berkman VC, Hamister RC: Psychological reports related to behavior and benefit of home care placement. J Clin Psychol 14:254–259, 1958

Van Putten T, Spar JE: The board and care home: does it deserve a bad press? Hosp Community Psychiatry 30:461–464, 1979

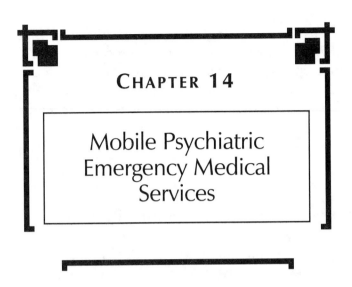

# CHAPTER 14

## Mobile Psychiatric Emergency Medical Services

Joseph J. Zealberg, M.D., Susan J. Hardesty, M.D.,
Neil Meisler, M.S.W., and Alberto B. Santos, M.D.

Consider a family needing help with their son, who has become suspicious and irritable, retreating to the basement, which he refuses to leave. They call their family physician and several area mental health providers, who invite them to come in for help. The local Emergency Medical Service (EMS) advises the family to call the police. The police make a house call, consider the son odd but in control, and recommend that the family contact an attorney to petition for judicial commitment. Eventually the son leaves the house and begins breaking windows on parked cars. Police respond, restrain him in handcuffs, and transport him to. . . .

To serve these and other patients who do not have ready access to available resources, clinicians will need to employ more flexible service delivery models (Factor et al. 1988; Lamb 1984; Mechanic and Aiken 1987). Clearly, many communities need emergency psychiatric medical services in the field or the equivalent of a psychiatric EMS (Cohen 1990; Gillig et al. 1990; Goldberg 1973). Compared with the usual procedure of detention by law enforcement officials and transportation to various facilities for evaluation and treatment, a mobile psychiatric EMS offers many advantages. In this chapter we illustrate the nature of psychiatric EMS and overview programs currently in operation throughout the United States.

## Potential Benefits of Mobile Psychiatric EMS

Many patients experiencing acute psychiatric symptoms resist the efforts of family and police to take them to a clinic or hospital. If they comply, the wait in the emergency room can increase their anxiety and agitation; if released from the facility, they may be unable or unwilling to obtain prescribed medication or attend scheduled appointments. A patient who becomes increasingly agitated in an unfamiliar facility may distort the natural clinical presentation and be less able to provide accurate historical information than when he or she is calm. A mobile team of mental health professionals is better able to assess in the natural surroundings (Andreoli et al. 1992; Blansjaar and Bruna 1990), begin treatment immediately, and enlist the help of support systems. The outreach response may decrease tensions, preventing the use of force and subsequent involuntary judicial process (Chiu and Primeau 1991). Additionally, the service flexibility allows the establishment of more favorable working alliances and can implement more rational and continuous care arrangements to ensure better 1- to 2-year outcomes (Andreoli et al. 1992).

Police officers are often the first to respond to crisis calls from homes or other sites in the community (Bengelsdorf and Alden 1987; Bonovitz and Bonovitz 1981; Matthews 1970). One study estimated that 50% of police calls involve family crises or potential psychiatric problems (Bard and Berkowitz 1967). Their role often includes emergency assessment of family crises, violence, substance abuse, unusual behavior, or altered mental states as well as the apprehension and transportation of mentally ill persons. In New York City the number of emotionally disturbed persons brought to municipal hospital emergency rooms by police increased by 1600% from 1976 to 1988 (Crisis in Mental Health, New York, 1989). Clearly, police officers are asked to accept an inordinate amount of responsibility in handling psychiatric crises, often with a minimum of training and knowledge.

Psychiatric EMS can help develop effective liaisons between law enforcement and mental health organizations to improve care and increase safety and security for officers and service providers. For example, techniques used with criminals (i.e., hostage negotiations) are often ineffective with psychotic patients. Periodic meetings with law enforcement officials, reclarification of mutual responsibilities and expectations, and review of critical situations are all necessary in maintaining efficient collaboration. Debriefing police officers involved in critical incidents, being informal consultants, and providing referrals for officers in need of mental health treatment also foster a close working alliance (Zealberg et al. 1992).

In recent years, major disasters such as Hurricanes Hugo and Andrew, the California earthquakes, and flooding in the Midwest have dramatically illustrated the advantages of having clinicians trained and equipped for work in the field. Places that are familiar become unrecognizable due to lack of lighting, signs, communication, or other means of obtaining orientation and direction. Food, ice, batteries, and generators are scarce and water is often undrinkable. Local emergency rooms become rapidly overcrowded because of the large number of accidental injuries in the community (i.e., chain saw accidents, cuts from broken glass or nails, fractures caused by falls, and traffic-related injuries). Mobile services can provide sustenance, support, and direct treatment for disaster victims and relief personnel throughout all phases of disaster relief (Kinston and Rosser 1974; Zealberg and Puckett 1992).

Finally, the presence of mental health clinicians in the field sends a strong message about the mental health system's responsibility for psychiatric patients. By accepting responsibility for the difficult task of emergency intervention, mobile crisis teams become highly visible ambassadors for the public mental health system. A high-profile mobile crisis team can also take advantage of every encounter with the media to help diminish the stigma associated with mental illness, to teach about the needs of mentally ill persons, and to inform the public about local mental health resources (Zealberg et al. 1993). Field-based services can also provide excellent training experiences for health care professionals; trainees are challenged and stimulated to think in new ways and to apply all their problem-solving skills to real-life situations (Santos et al., in press; Zealberg et al. 1990).

## Profile of One City's Program

The Mobile Crisis Service in Charleston, South Carolina, is staffed by psychiatrists, residents, nurses, and master's-level clinicians. The service area is a mixture of urban and rural, has a population of approximately 325,000, and is about 35% African-American. Between 200 and 225 patients are seen per month, about half in health care facilities of various kinds and the remainder in the community (i.e., private homes, shelters, hotels, malls, bridges, police cars). Referrals include self, family, friends, landlords, health professionals, police/court, or community agencies. Calls are carefully screened by clinicians to estimate the level of any potential danger before making a mobile visit. The field team always consists of at least two individuals. Team physicians and nurses are capable of administering medications in the field and they carry an array of psychopharmacological agents to each emergency. When necessary, the team will visit patients several times until a crisis is resolved. If appointments arranged for patients are not kept, the team often follows up with a mobile response. The mobile team and police together have resolved dozens of potentially dangerous situations. Being on the streets and "in the trenches" with police affords mobile crisis clinicians extra professional validity in the eyes of law enforcement officials, the kind of rapport that simply cannot be created in hospital- or clinic-based programs. Clinical DSM-IV (American Psychiatric Association 1994) disorders of targeted clients are schizophrenia (20%), bipolar disorder (15%), major depression (20%), substance abuse or dependence (50%), and a large percentage of dual diagnoses. Roughly 35% have a history of suicidal ideation or attempts. Approximately 25% have a medically significant problem requiring evaluation and treatment at the time of crisis.

Yearly recurring costs for the team are approximately $479,392. Table 14–1 outlines a typical year's budget. The total number of emergency patients served in FY 1992–1993 was 2,389; thus, the cost per emergency patient served was approximately $200.66 The program is supported by the state mental health authority. Only $35,783 (7.5% of cost) in fees were generated during FY 1993, primarily through Medicaid. Revenue generation therefore is proportionately less than for other Medicaid-supported programs because a large number of clients served are not enrolled at the time of service. Many of the persons served are not, and do not become, ongoing clients of the mental health center. For such persons, it is often difficult to determine their eligibility for or to obtain their cooperation in obtaining

**Table 14–1.**   Charleston mobile psychiatric EMS expenses FY 1992–1993

| | |
|---|---|
| Personnel and fringe | $436,502 |
| Office supplies and medications | 20,100 |
| Lease of office space | 15,855 |
| Travel | 4,252 |
| Discretionary patient fund (e.g., taxi, food) | 500 |
| Utilities | 1,383 |
| Gasoline | 800 |
| **Total** | **$479,392** |

payment by insurers. Also, in South Carolina and most other states, mobile crisis units bill on the basis of fees established based on the overall costs of the mental health center. Third-party payment, at least through Medicaid, could likely be enhanced by establishing an aggregate fee for a unit of mobile crisis program services based on the actual cost of using the program and the volume of use. It could also likely be enhanced through additional efforts to determine clients' eligibility for insurance payment during or following the crisis episode. Even if a mobile crisis program generates far less revenue than it costs to operate, it might be considered a "loss leader" for a mental health center and the public mental health system at large when potential savings in other sectors of the system are considered along with the positive relations it facilitates with the larger human service system.

## National Characteristics of
## Mobile Psychiatric EMS

Stroul (1991) reports on 69 mobile crisis programs within 26 states and one Canadian community that differ in their constituent parts, policies, and protocols, but have many common elements (see Table 14–2). These programs vary in mission, scope, and approach, but in general they exist in communities of 90,000 people or more, serve persons of all ages, and provide services in varied settings: on the streets, in homeless shelters, in jails, at home, and in residential care facilities. Most programs are licensed, and all have 24-hour telephone capability. Programs typically provide 24-hour walk-in service, but the locations vary from hospital emergency rooms and mental health centers to specifically designated mobile crisis walk-in centers. Most programs have 24-hour mobile response capability, and most perform prehospital screening. Team composition varies, ranging from mental health professionals with master's level degrees and above to volunteer staff trained specifically for their roles in the mobile crisis program. Patient populations include those with

**Table 14–2.**  States and cities with mobile crisis units

| | | |
|---|---|---|
| **California** | **Massachusetts** | **North Dakota** |
| El Cajon | Fall River | Bismarck |
| Long Beach | Holyoke | **Ohio** |
| Merced | Milford | Canton |
| Redwood City | Plymouth | Cincinnati |
| **Colorado** | **Michigan** | Lorain |
| Boulder | Battle Creek | Ravenna |
| Colorado Springs | Cadillac | Toledo |
| **Connecticut** | Detroit | **Pennsylvania** |
| Bridgeport | Grand Rapids | Harrisburg |
| | Holland | Philadelphia |
| **Delaware** | Ionia | **Rhode Island** |
| Milford | Lansing | Pawtucket |
| Wilmington | Sault Ste. Marie | Providence |
| **District of Columbia** | Traverse City | Warwick |
| Washington | **Minnesota** | Woonsocket |
| **Florida** | Minneapolis | **South Carolina** |
| Delray Beach | **Nebraska** | Charleston |
| Jacksonville | Lincoln | **Utah** |
| **Illinois** | **New Hampshire** | Salt Lake City |
| Chicago | Lebanon | **Virginia** |
| Dixon | Salem | Alexandria |
| East Saint Louis | **New Jersey** | Arlington |
| Elgin | Passaic | Lynchburg |
| McHenry | **New York** | Manassas |
| Melrose Park | Poughkeepsie | Williamsburg |
| Metropolis | Valhalla | **Washington** |
| Peoria | **North Carolina** | Bremerton |
| Wheaton | Chapel Hill | **West Virginia** |
| Wood River | Greensboro | Petersburg |
| **Indiana** | High Point | **Wisconsin** |
| Indianapolis | Thomasville | Madison |
| **Kentucky** | | Racine |
| Ashland | | |

Adapted from Stroul (1991).

long-term mental illness, major affective disorders, acute suicidality or homicidality, individuals responding to acute situational stressors, and those with substance abuse disorders, who are often dually diagnosed.

## Discussion

In the United States, financial incentives primarily support hospital care, not basic health care, and the emphasis is on quality of hospital care rather than access to care (Keisler 1992). Because it is predicted that one in three Americans will develop a major psychiatric syndrome sometime during their lives (Regier et al. 1984), access to quality mental health services must be closely examined in this era of cost containment. The past 20 years have witnessed the gradual growth of mobile crisis response teams for psychiatric emergencies in the United States as well as in Europe, Canada, Australia, and New Zealand (Reynolds et al. 1990; Tufnell et al. 1985). Some programs, such as the program in Amsterdam that started in the 1930s, significantly predate U.S. programs.

There are a multitude of potential benefits from mobile emergency services: benefits to individuals, families, neighborhoods, the public at large in the community, and agencies that serve the community. The outreach response may allow early initiation of treatment, crisis resolution, strengthening of the family and support system, and appropriate linkage to aftercare. Mobile services are an effective means of demonstrating the system's assumption of responsibility for the welfare of mentally ill persons beyond the usual "9–5" mode of operation.

Mobile teams have the potential to reduce costs indirectly. Law enforcement personnel are often first responders in crisis calls, and thus are frequently required to accompany psychiatric patients taken to emergency departments. The presence of the mobile team can allow police officers to return to duty more quickly. Other potential savings can be realized through reduced court costs and hospital use because many patients can be treated without hospitalization following crisis intervention, evaluation, and initiation of treatment. Although these cost concepts seem intuitively valid, little systematic analysis has been done and, to date, results are mixed. One study of catchment areas with and without mobile crisis programs (Fisher et al. 1990) demonstrated that the presence of a mobile crisis program showed no significant effect on either first or total admission rates. However, no attempt was made to quantify the integration of mobile crisis units into community service systems, or to define the extent of mobile capacity and use, factors that can clearly affect the number of hospitalizations.

West et al. (1980) noted that their mobile crisis unit played an equivocal role in reducing admissions, and that facilitation of hospitalization in the face of inadequate family and community supports became an unexpected role of their mobile crisis program. Reynolds et al. (1990), however, found that inpatient admissions were halved during a 3-month study period. A key component of the crisis team's role was continued in-home treatment and follow-up after the initial contact. These data suggest that a mobile crisis unit may be most effective as an integral division of a comprehensive, outreach-oriented community mental health service system. Most importantly, however, the costs of providing a responsive mobile psychiatric EMS are offset by gains in good will, credibility, and in-kind responsiveness by other community agencies to the needs of persons with mental illnesses.

As society struggles with health care reform, managed care, and cost control, it is interesting to speculate on the future evolution of mobile emergency psychiatry. In this final decade of the twentieth century, the mental health community could begin to put into practical use technological advances that are well suited to growth and development of more comprehensive and cost-effective delivery of health care. As the entertainment media ponders the marriage of computer, video, and network television programming into a "supersystem," it is likely that more and more clients will have access to interactional computers and modems in their homes. As has been shown (Selmi et al. 1990), computer interactive displays with diagnostic assessment tools can elicit reliable information. This technology could be effective in initial assessment and planning for follow-up outreach to selected clients. For instance, one can imagine a program comparable to a telecommunications system for the blind and deaf, in which high-risk patients could access equipment to facilitate daily assessments with outreach workers. Likewise, mobile video telecommunication systems could enable clinicians, case managers, physicians, and other workers to collaborate effectively in assessment without each person being physically present on each call. Rural areas could hook up their mobile programs to more centralized facilities for consultation, supervision, and practical advice.

One of the more frustrating aspects of mobile crisis work involves patients whose presenting symptoms include medical as well as psychiatric diagnoses. In most programs it is then necessary to arrange for transport to a health care facility for evaluation before appropriate psychiatric therapy can be implemented. At other times, the diagnostic component is relatively straightforward, but medical screening for treatment implementation is a limiting factor. The future holds multiple possibilities for addressing these concerns. The progress of microchip technology could result in completely portable mobile diagnostic units available to crisis outreach teams for laboratory evaluation, ECGs, and diagnostic imaging.

Increased collaboration between local EMS/ambulance services and mobile crisis outreach teams might serve to limit future police involvement in the transportation of acutely ill persons. Psychiatrically trained personnel might be included on ambulance services. Where paramedic services are available, linkage with emergency psychiatrists via radio, telephone, and videotelephone may improve crisis stabilization through administration of medication in emergency settings, and may broaden the concept of humane mobile outreach to acutely ill patients. As we evolve more systems in which transport can be facilitated without the use of police cruisers, handcuffs, leg irons, and other hard restraints, we move further toward the recognition that psychiatrically impaired individuals are truly medically ill with treatable health problems, and further away from the stance that medically oriented services should avoid psychiatrically ill patients.

# References

American Psychiatric Association: Diagnostic and Statistical Manual of Mental Disorders, 4th Edition. Washington, DC, American Psychiatric Association, 1994

Andreoli AV, Muehlebach A, Gognalons M, et al: Crisis intervention response and long-term outcome: a pilot study. Compr Psychiatry 33:388–396, 1992

Bard M, Berkowitz B: Training police as specialists in family crisis intervention: a community psychology action program. Community Ment Health J 3:315–317, 1967

Bengelsdorf H, Alden DC: A mobile crisis unit in the psychiatric emergency room. Hosp Community Psychiatry 38:662–665, 1987

Blansjaar BA, Bruna T: DSM III in outreach emergency psychiatry. Int J Soc Psychiatry 36:308–314, 1990

Bonovitz JC, Bonovitz JS: Diversion of the mentally ill into the clinical justice system: the police intervention perspective. Am J Psychiatry 138:973–976, 1981

Chiu TL, Primeau C: A psychiatric mobile crisis unit in New York City: description and assessment, with implications for mental health care in the 1990s. Int J Soc Psychiatry 37:251–258, 1991

Factor RM, Stein LI, Diamond RJ: A model community psychiatry curriculum for psychiatric residents. Community Ment Health J 24:310–327, 1988

Fisher WH, Geller JL, Wirth-Cauchon J: Empirically assessing the impact of mobile crisis capacity on State Hospital admissions. Community Ment Health J 26:245–253, 1990

Gillig P, Dumaine M, Hillard JR: Whom do mobile crisis services serve? Hosp Community Psychiatry 41:804–805, 1990

Goldberg HL: Home treatment. Psychiatric Annals 3:59–61, 1973

Keisler CA: U.S. mental health policy: doomed to fail. Am Psychol 47:107–108, 1992

Kinston W, Rosser K: Disaster: effects on mental and physical state. J Psychosom Res 19:437–456, 1974

Lamb HR (ed): The Homeless Mentally Ill: A Task Force Report of the American Psychiatric Association. Washington, DC, American Psychiatric Association, 1984

Matthews AR, Jr: Observations on police policy and procedures for emergency detention of the mentally ill. Journal of Criminal Law, Criminology, and Police Science 61:283–295, 1970

Mechanic D, Aiken LH: Improving the care of patients with chronic mental illness. N Engl J Med 317:1634–1638, 1987

Meisler N: State mental health agency responsibility for outreach, in Psychiatric Outreach to the Mentally Ill, Vol 52. Edited by Cohen NL. San Francisco, CA, Jossey-Bass, 1991, pp 81–92

New York City Mental Health Department: Crisis in Mental Health: Issues Affecting HHC's Psychiatric Inpatient and Emergency Room Services: Summary Data. New York, New York City Health and Hospitals Corporation, Offices of Mental Hygiene Services and Strategic Planning, January 1989

Regier DA, Myers JK, Kramer M, et al: The NIMH epidemiologic catchment area program. Arch Gen Psychiatry 41:934–941, 1984

Reynolds I, Jones JE, Berry DW, et al: A crisis team for the mentally ill: the effect on patients, relatives, and admissions. Med J Aust 152:646–652, 1990

Selmi PM, Klein MH, Griest JH, et al: Computer-administered cognitive-behavioral therapy for depression. Am J Psychiatry 147:51–56, 1990

Stroul BA: Profiles of Psychiatric Crisis Response Systems. Rockville, MD, National Institute of Mental Health, 1991

Tufnell G, Bouras N, Watson JP, et al: Home assessment and treatment in a community psychiatric service. Acta Psychiatr Scand 72:20–28, 1985

West DA, Litwok E, Oberlander K, et al: Emergency psychiatric home visiting: report of four years experience. J Clin Psychiatry 41:113–118, 1980

Zealberg JJ, Puckett J: Function of mobile crisis intervention teams after Hurricane Hugo, in Responding to Disaster: A Guide for Mental Health Professionals. Edited by Austin L. Washington, DC, American Psychiatric Press, 1992, pp 185–199

Zealberg JJ, Santos AB, Hiers TG, et al: From the benches to the trenches: training residents to provide emergency outreach services—a public/academic project. Academic Psychiatry 14:211–217, 1990

Zealberg JJ, Christie SD, Puckett J, et al: A mobile crisis program: collaboration between emergency psychiatric services and policies. Hosp Community Psychiatry 43:612–615, 1992

Zealberg JJ, Santos AB, Fisher RK: Benefits of mobile crisis programs. Hosp Community Psychiatry 44:16–17, 1993

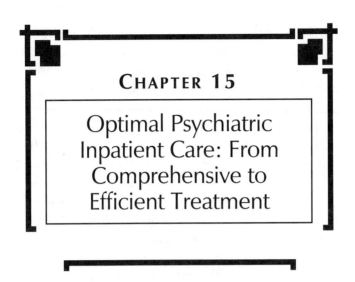

# CHAPTER 15

## Optimal Psychiatric Inpatient Care: From Comprehensive to Efficient Treatment

**Stephen McLeod-Bryant, M.D., George W. Arana, M.D., Laura J. Rames, M.D., and Alberto B. Santos, M.D.**

In the planning and development of a new psychiatric service, we decided at the outset to address four major problems that faced us specifically but had also been described by others nationally. First, the cost of inpatient treatments was becoming increasingly prohibitive. Second, the longer patients stayed in these inpatient facilities, the more difficult it was to reintegrate them into their homes and communities. Third, there was a lack of evidence that inpatient psychiatric treatment yielded any sustained benefit for the patient beyond discharge from the hospital. Fourth, there was no generally accepted model employed by inpatient services to develop improved services.

We established in our approach two hypotheses about the use of inpatient psychiatric services. First, the hospital bed is for containment of dangerous behavior. Second, the goal of hospitalization is the extinction of this dangerous behavior, with as rapid a return of the patient to his or her community as possible.

Adopting these hypotheses as the core mission of the service allowed us to focus on the primary issues of behavior, containment, extinction, and rapid discharge. Secondary factors, such as development of an operational model and staffing needs, followed from consideration of these primary issues.

Our approach led to an acute inpatient service with an average length of stay of 10 days. Outcomes were favorable in the areas of recidivism and safety to patients and community, as well as reduction of dangerousness, at a reduced cost per patient. Reintegration of these patients into the community has been facilitated by their brief stays in the hospital and by the structures we employ in focusing on community reintegration. Finally, we have shown that long stays are most often not necessary for these populations, and we have developed a new services model based on our results that supports our original hypotheses.

We describe in this chapter the forces that led to the need to change our models and assumptions regarding inpatient psychiatric treatments. We outline the operating assumptions used in the development of our service. We describe in detail the way in which this service was operated, and we outline staffing assignments and use. In addition, we discuss the problems inherent in the development of such a unit and the education necessary to our staff and students in order to achieve a successful outcome. Finally, we speculate on ways we can further improve and refine this model so that we can address the issues that will face us in the future.

## Need to Change Model for Inpatient Treatment

In an article about strategies for coping with prospective payment, Fogel and Slaby (1985) noted: "At the same time that organized psychiatry continues to lobby against applying the current DRG system to psychiatric units and health care researchers continue to gather data, the individual psychiatric unit or psychiatry service cannot merely wait and hope for the best" (p. 763). At this writing, some 8 years later, the literature gives little or no data or models guiding reform in professional thinking about inpatient psychiatric care. Over the past 20 years, average lengths of stay for psychiatric hospital patients have been reduced from 1 year to under 2 weeks as a result of external pressure. Yet, remarkably little change in the thinking of mental health professionals and in their training programs about the nature of inpatient care has been documented (Marks 1992).

In most U.S. communities, the role of the psychiatric hospital is dominant in the care of patients. The term *aftercare* in effect relegates anything other than hospital care to a secondary position, placing a premium on comprehensive inpatient care rendered by a multidisciplinary staff. Environments in which managed care is practiced within model HMOs have already undergone "health reform" and offer us a view of what may transpire as federal health reform is debated, legislated, and subsequently implemented (see Table 15–1). In the following two sections we describe a highly efficient psychiatric inpatient service, which is part of a comprehensive, community-based system of care; and we present service-use data to evaluate the efficiency of the program and highlight its specific efficiency-oriented strategies for potential replication in other sites. The service provides a model for cost-effective community-based inpatient care in local general hospitals.

**Table 15–1.** Trends in psychiatric hospital services reform

| Characteristics | Traditional | Reform |
|---|---|---|
| Role | Primary | Consultant |
| Staff | Multidisciplinary | Limited |
| Focus | Comprehensive | Limited |
| Values | "Leave no stone unturned" | Comfort and efficiency |
| Site | Centralized | Localized |
| Sponsor | State | Community hospital |

# Description of Service

## Background

In 1983, the South Carolina mental health authority adopted a plan that included the decentralization of hospital services. Funds were made available to any locale that could develop local programs to reduce admission to the central facilities. Charleston was 120 miles away from the state's central facilities in Columbia. It was often financially burdensome for a family member or an interested party to transport the patient to Columbia, and it was also clinically suboptimal, with risk to patients and professionals incurred with such a cumbersome procedure. The only practical alternative was for a sheriff's officer to transport the patient, requiring the psychiatrist to obtain an involuntary emergency commitment order. Indigent patients who were often willing to be admitted locally had the option been available, would refuse to go to the centralized hospital, therefore requiring transportation under emergency commitment orders. In 1985 a psychiatric unit was opened at the county general hospital through state, county, and university support (Santos et al. 1994). Given the limited number of beds (in 1982 nearly 1,000 Charleston-area patients were admitted to centralized hospitals in Columbia), we developed a set of strategies (Ellsworth et al. 1972; English et al. 1986; Faulkner et al. 1989) to streamline the clinical, functional, and administrative processes (Table 15–2).

## Clinical Operations

With a critical role of reducing admissions to the centralized hospitals, operations are designed for maximum bed use. This goal is discussed openly with patients and disseminated broadly to provide referral sources with realistic expectations about goals of hospitalization. Principal interventions are rapid stabilization using crisis management and somatic therapies and rapid mobilization of aftercare resources (Maxmen et al. 1974). Before admission, requisite medical and surgical consultations are arranged and medical services are planned, including accepting

**Table 15–2.** Program characteristics

Unit mission
- Attention to service and outcome
- Premium on efficiency

Bed control
- Admissions and discharges are coordinated by one person for maximum bed use
- Expectations for hospitalization and arrangements for aftercare are clarified prior to admission

Clinical focus
- Rapid stabilization through crisis intervention and aggressive pharmacotherapy
- Indicated medical and surgical evaluations are obtained prior to admission
- Evaluation and interventions are begun at the time of admission
- Aggressive accessing of support network and resources
- Common knowledge among staff is maximized
- Resolution of the specific behavior or condition that required inpatient care

Personnel, job descriptions, staff identity
- Group identity as consultants to outpatient providers
- Individual job descriptions instead of traditional roles of disciplines
- "Multiservices" rather than "multidisciplinary" team
- The number of disciplines involved in decision making is streamlined

Unit activities
- Staff meetings are limited
- Interactions in staff meetings are highly structured
- Nonproductive patient stimulation is limited

patients requiring close medical monitoring and intravenous lines. Psychiatric treatments are not delayed by administrative or educational processes. The support and provider network is assertively consulted for information and engaged in discharge planning. Information about each case—working diagnoses, reasons for hospitalization, medication dosages and levels, pending laboratory studies, staff assignments, projected discharge date, legal issues, and aftercare arrangements—is tracked on a large blackboard. The blackboard provides a common and practical source of information for all staff, reducing the time spent consulting charts and limiting inefficiencies that may result from staff miscommunications (see Figure 15–1). For each admission, staff identify the indication for hospitalization (Table 15–3) and note it on the blackboard (e.g., suicide or homicide risk, combativeness, dangerousness based on nonfocused agitation, profound psychomotor retardation and inability to care for oneself, severe psychotic thinking, and confused sensorium). Resolution of the specific behavior or condition that precipitated hospitalization serves as a marker of discharge readiness (Colson et al. 1986; Grazier 1992; Robinson and Avallone 1990; Stein and Test 1980).

## Roles and Processes

Staff roles are psychiatrists (and residents), head nurse and nurses' aides, aftercare coordinators, and clerks. A psychiatrist takes all calls for referrals and is responsible for decisions about admission, course, and discharge. The referring clinician is asked to articulate realistic expectations and goals for the hospitalization. The aftercare coordinators are charged with promoting continuity of care and decreasing recidivism.

The unit avoids duplication of clinical efforts by using job descriptions that outline specific services the incumbent is expected to perform (Goodban et al. 1987; Marcos 1988; Munich 1986). The job descriptions are consistent with the services provided by medical, social service, and nursing disciplines for accreditation of health care organizations, as required by the Joint Commission on Accreditation of Healthcare Organizations (JCAHO) (Joint Commission 1994). The staff professional identity, therefore, is that of consultant to outpatient providers, being vigilant in guarding against competitive attitudes toward outpa-

| Admit date | Patient name | Physician | Aftercare coordinator | Need for hospital[a] | Diag- nosis | Medica- tion | Tests pending[b] | D/C date[c] | f/u[d] |
|---|---|---|---|---|---|---|---|---|---|
|  |  |  |  |  |  |  |  |  |  |
|  |  |  |  |  |  |  |  |  |  |
|  |  |  |  |  |  |  |  |  |  |
|  |  |  |  |  |  |  |  |  |  |
|  |  |  |  |  |  |  |  |  |  |
|  |  |  |  |  |  |  |  |  |  |
|  |  |  |  |  |  |  |  |  |  |

**Figure 15–1.** Blackboard display for case information.

*Notes.* [a]Lists indications for hospital-based care. [b]Notes any studies or evaluations pending to complete the current treatment plan, (e.g., Head CT, EEG, Psychological testing). [c]Lists a projected discharge date. [d]Lists scheduled follow-up appointments and aftercare arrangements.

**Table 15–3.** Indications for hospital-based care

1. Suicidal risk
2. Homicidal risk
3. Combativeness
4. Danger assumed on the basis of nonfocused agitation
5. Danger assumed on the basis of psychomotor retardation, lack of self-care, and social withdrawal
6. Irrational thinking
7. Confused sensorium
8. Anxiety
9. Neurovegetative signs of depression (to discriminate suicidality with or without major affective disorder).
10. Other _____

tient providers (Adler 1973; Gordon and Beresin 1983).

We limit staff time spent in meetings by allowing only one staff meeting each day. The daily meeting is structured so that a limited number of persons address a predetermined set of variables for each patient (see Table 15–4). For example, a nurse may report on the patient's compliance with treatment, the aftercare coordinator may present new information about the patient's aftercare arrangements, and the physician may give an update on resolution of the patient's target symptoms. The expected structure is displayed on a blackboard in the meeting room for easy reference. Focus is thus maintained on the patient's response to interventions and on coordinating effective aftercare. The presentation of irrelevant historical material is discouraged.

Patients are not engaged in lengthy or provocative individual or group therapeutic activities that are unrelated to crisis management or stabilization (Blake et al. 1990). For expression of community concerns, everyone is invited to meet for a short gathering each day after breakfast. Nonproductive stimulation (i.e., television) is minimized, and formal "activity therapy" is not provided. Other activities are provided that are consonant with the goals of acute stabilization as mandated by JCAHO (Joint Commission 1994). Leaves or passes occur very infrequently.

**Table 15–4.**  Structured team rounds

| Staff | Variable to report |
|---|---|
| Nursing | Ward activity |
| | Compliance |
| | Prn medication use |
| | Sleep |
| | Appetite |
| Aftercare coordinators | Individual and family psychosocial assessment (residential, financial, and social resources) |
| | History of outpatient compliance |
| | Aftercare arrangements (clinical, housing, social supports) |
| Physicians | Target symptoms→medications |
| | Side effects |
| | Resolution of reason for hospitalization |

## Evaluation

To assess the impact of the unit on patterns of care, we collected demographic, clinical, and fiscal data for each patient admitted during the period between April 15, 1985 and February 28, 1987 (Santos et al. 1988). The needs for hospitalization clustered predominantly around unmanageable, agitated psychotic states and high risk of suicide. The average length of stay was 10 days. At discharge, 80% of the patients returned directly to their previous residence. The unit's occupancy rate remained above 90%, and recidivism to the unit was under 5%. Admissions to the unit during the study period totaled 802. Previously, the overwhelming majority of these patients would have been committed involuntarily to central state facilities. In fact, 715 of the 802 admissions, or 89%, met state criteria for emergency commitment (i.e., imminent danger to self or others or inability to care for self). However, given the option of treatment locally, 532 of the 715 patients (74%) admitted themselves voluntarily. Only 183 of the 715 committable patients (26%) required emergency involuntary commitment orders to be hospitalized locally.

At the time of the study in South Carolina, a probate court hearing was held within 21 days (usually within 14) following an emergency commitment order. However, a facility could request dismissal of an emergency commitment order from the court on the grounds that the patient no longer met criteria for commitment, thereby avoiding the need to remain in the hospital awaiting a hearing. Such a request had to be made before the fifth hospital day. When the dismissal or early release was granted, the patient could be discharged but could also elect to remain in the hospital on a voluntary basis.

A request for dismissal of the commitment order and early release was made for 104 of the 183 committed patients and was granted for 101 (55%) of the total group of committed patients. Therefore, only 82 of the 715 Charleston patients (11%) who met commitment criteria actually required a probate court hearing because of the option of local voluntary admission and the requests for court dismissal of involuntary status.

During the study period, 544 patients were committed to the state's centralized facilities in Columbia under emergency involuntary orders for lack of an available bed in the local unit. According to DMH, the average length of stay in those facilities for this overflow control group was 33.6 days. In contrast, the average length of stay of the 802 patients hospitalized in the local psychiatric unit was 10 days. The difference represented a theoretical reduction in use of 12,555 patient bed-days for the 532 voluntary admissions to the local unit who met commitment criteria. At the Medicare fee of $150 a day, this represented a cost savings for the study period of $1,883,280.

Only 183 of 715 patients who met commitment criteria actually required involuntary admission to the local unit. Of those patients, 101 were granted early release, thereby avoiding the need to remain in the hospital awaiting a hearing. Given the difference in average length of stay between the central state and local facilities, this early-release option represented a reduction of approximately 2,384 patient bed-days. At $150 per patient bed-day, additional savings totaled $357,600.

The total cost savings made possible by the reduction in bed-days on the unit when compared with central state facilities are estimated at $2,240,880 for approximately 2 years of operation, or more than $1 million a year. Of course, it is not reasonable to assume that when an admission is prevented, the hospital savings per patient are equal to the bed-day costs per patient in the hospital, because the fixed costs of the hospital continue whether or not a few hospitalizations a day are prevented. Substantial savings occur only when a hospital can close an entire ward with its fixed costs (mostly personnel), or when the provider is required to pay for patient hospital bed-days, as in a capitated or managed-care system. In summary, the high-acuity inpatient service was specifically developed to provide high-efficiency care to public sector patients who had previously been transported 120 miles to the state's central hospital facilities (Rames et al. 1993; Santos and MacLeod-Bryant 1991). Length of stay and frequency of probate court civil commitment intervention were significantly lower in the local unit than for patients hospitalized in central facilities (Rames et al. 1993; Santos and MacLeod-Bryant 1991; Santos et al. 1988). These bed-days were actually used by other patients needing care. In fact, far more patients were served, and the funds were disbursed locally, to the benefit of the local community, its taxpayers, and its patients.

Interestingly, the staff of the centralized hospital facility (G. Werber Bryan Psychiatric Hospital) visited the unit in Charleston to learn more about our local strategies. They were able to implement the probate court early-release option with the cooperation of most, but not all, of the judges. The results were highly significant: requests for early release rose from an average of around 3 per month prior to implementation to 125–150 per month. This resulted in a reduction in monthly average length of stay from 35–45 days to 13–14 days per patient (Rames et al. 1993).

## Obstacles to Implementation

Although coordination of clinical, legal, and social support services is best achieved in a patient's own community, and although such coordination results in more rapid stabilization and return to normal living in familiar surroundings within a supportive network of available professionals (National Center for State Courts 1986), staff required considerable direction to maintain clinical focus on resolution of a patient's specific behavior or condition and to adhere to the agenda for staff meetings. Staff who had previously been employed in traditional, psychiatric inpatient settings had particular difficulty adjusting to this focus, but staff who had previously worked in medical or surgical wards did not experience this difficulty. As desired outcomes were obtained, staff began to experience rewards from the system. An important consideration in the overall success of such a unit is the comprehensiveness of the system of care for public sector patients in the community. When our unit first began operating, there was significant resistance from outpatient providers to our focus on increased efficiency and the more limited goal of extinguishing the reason for hospitalization, rather than the "cure" of an illness. However, through active dialogue with outpatient providers, including provider-invited participation at staff meetings and sharing of information regarding the current state of the art in the acute treatment of severe and persistent mental illness, we were able to identify opportunities for the development of outpatient services (mobile crisis services, day hospital, and rural outreach services) that better meet the needs of patients than staying in the hospital (Santos et al. 1994).

At least three countries (Great Britain, Australia, and Italy) have legislated the treatment of psychiatric inpatients to units in general hospitals. In Italy, for example, the end to long-term psychiatric hospitalization was legislated in 1978 with the establishment of units in general hospitals not to exceed 15 beds (Lesage and Tansella 1993). In the United States, the specific role of the psychiatric hospital and the general hospital psychiatric unit in the spectrum of mental health services will continue to be a focus of debate. Because a significant portion of mental health providers, administrators, and shareholders have been influenced by and/or have a stake in the hospital treatment model, any transition to a system that challenges the traditional values is likely to be met with considerable resistance. Such professional resistance to change combined with profit-based concerns of lobbying groups will likely delay reforms in practice patterns, despite increased public interest and scientific attention (Brook 1989; Eisenberg 1989).

# References

Adler G: Hospital treatment of borderline patients. Am J Psychiatry 130:32–36, 1973

Blake DO, Owens MD, Keane TM: Increasing group attendance on a psychiatric unit: an alternating treatments design comparison. J Behav Ther Exp Psychiatry 21:15–20, 1990

Brook RH: Health services research: is it good for you and me? Academic Medicine 64:124–130,1989

Colson DB, Allen JG, Coyne L, et al: Profiles of difficult psychiatric hospital patients. Hosp Community Psychiatry 37:720–724, 1986

Eisenberg JM: Clinical economics: a guide to the economic analysis of clinical practices. JAMA 262:2879–2886, 1989

Ellsworth RB, Dickman HR, Maroney RJ: Characteristics of productive and unproductive unit systems in VA psychiatric hospitals. Hosp Community Psychiatry 123:261–267, 1972

English JT, Sharfstein SS, Scherl DJ, et al: Diagnosis-related groups and general hospital psychiatry: the APA study. Am J Psychiatry 143:131–139, 1986

Faulkner LR, McFarland HH, Bloom JD: An empirical study of emergency commitment. Am J Psychiatry 146:182–186, 1989

Fogel BS, Slaby AE: Beyond gamesmanship: strategies for coping with prospective payment. Hosp Community Psychiatry 36:760–763, 1985

Goodban NA, Lieberman PB, Levine MA, et al: Conceptual and methodological issues in the comparison of inpatient psychiatric facilities. Am J Psychiatry 144:1437–1443, 1987

Gordon C, Beresin E: Conflicting treatment models for the inpatient management of borderline patients. Am J Psychiatry 140:979–983, 1983

Grazier KL: A resource-use model for long-term psychiatric facilities. Med Care 30:872–877, 1992

Joint Commission for Accreditation of Healthcare Organizations (JCAHO): JCAHO Accreditation Manual for Hospitals. Oakbrook Terrace, IL, JCAHO, 1994

Lesage AD, Tansella M: Comprehensive community care without long stay beds in mental hospitals: trends from an Italian good practice area. Can J Psychiatry 38:187–194, 1993

Marcos LR: Dysfunction in public psychiatric bureaucracies. Am J Psychiatry 145:331–334, 1988

Marks I: Innovations in mental health care delivery. Br J Psychiatry 160:589–597, 1992

Maxmen JS, Tucker GJ, LeBow MD: Rational Hospital Psychiatry: The Reactive Environment. New York, Brunner/Mazel, 1974

Munich RL: The role of the unit chief: an integrated perspective. Psychiatry 49:325–336, 1986

National Center for State Courts: guidelines for involuntary civil commitment. Mental and Physical Disability Law Reporter 10:409–514, 1986

Rames LJ, McLeod-Bryant S, Alston SG, et al: Trends in public psychiatric inpatient care in a general hospital. Journal of the South Carolina Medical Association 89:475–479, 1993

Robinson AM, Avallone J: Occupational therapy in acute inpatient psychiatry: an activities health approach. American Journal of Occupational Therapy 44:809–814, 1990

Santos AB, McLeod-Bryant S: Strategies for operational efficiency in a general hospital inpatient unit. Hosp Community Psychiatry 42:66–69, 1991

Santos AB, Thrasher JW Jr, Ballenger JC: Decentralized services for public hospital patients: a cost analysis. Hosp Community Psychiatry 39:827–829, 1988

Santos AB, Ballenger JC, Bevilacqua JJ, et al: A community-based public-academic liaison program. Am J Psychiatry 151:1181–1187, 1994

Stein L, Test M: Alternative to mental hospital treatment, I: conceptual model, treatment program, and clinical evaluation. Arch Gen Psychiatry 37:392–397, 1980

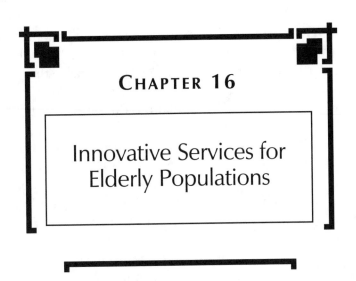

# CHAPTER 16

## Innovative Services for Elderly Populations

Melisa D. Rowland, M.D., Barbara J. Burns, Ph.D.,
Gretchen E. Schafft, Ph.D., Frances L. Randolph, D.P.H.,
and Cecile B. McAninch, Ph.D.

Mental illnesses, the emotional consequences of physical disabilities, and the impact of the environment on an aging person's well-being, all pose significant public health problems. In this chapter, we use the term *neuropsychiatric* (Fogel et al. 1990) to refer to the cognitive, emotional, and behavioral problems in geriatric psychiatry (delirium, dementia, depression, schizophrenia, paranoia, anxiety, phobias, alcohol and prescription drug abuse, and maladaptive emotional adjustment to life stressors). Because the neuropsychiatric disorders affect 12%–25% of the general geriatric population (Regier et al. 1988), it is important to better understand this population in terms of who needs treatment, who is obtaining treatment, and whether the treatment provided is cost-effective.

About two-thirds (69.2%) of elderly neuropsychiatric clients live in the community, whereas the remainder (30.8%) are institutionalized (Burns and Taube 1990). The 1-month prevalence rate for neuropsychiatric illness in the elderly living in the community is 12.3% (Regier et al. 1988). It is estimated that 7.8% of persons over 65 need mental health care; yet 62.6% of these cases (5.7% of the total geriatric population) do not receive treatment (Shapiro et al. 1985). Outpatient services currently available consist primarily of community mental health centers and office-based counseling by psychiatrists and psychologists; however, persons over 65 consistently use outpatient mental health resources to a much lesser extent than their younger adult counterparts (Butler and Lewis 1982; Goldstrom et al. 1987; Light et al. 1986).

Inpatient services, on the other hand, have shifted the primary locus of care from the state hospitals to the community as a direct consequence of policy changes, with 94% of this population residing in community nursing homes (Burns and Taube 1990; 1985 National Nursing Home Survey 1991). Although 47% of all nursing home residents suffer from dementia and an additional 17% have other neuropsychiatric disorders (Burns et al. 1993), few provisions are made for mental health services in nursing homes, and only 4.5% of residents receive treatment for neuropsychiatric disorders (only half of these see a mental health professional). Although the need for treatment is clear and evidence of effective psychosocial interventions for elderly clients exists (Bienfeld and Wheeler 1989; Pinkston et al. 1988; Tourigny-Rivard and Drury 1987), current treatments consist almost entirely of psychotropic medication, which is often prescribed inappropriately (Beardsley et al. 1989; Buck 1988; Burns and Kamerow 1988; Ray et al. 1980). Obviously, the current prevalent service system does not adequately address the complex needs of this population. Below we overview a series of innovative approaches to appropriate care for these individuals designed to surmount obstacles to more rational care. We emphasize a synthesis of empirical support for principles of service effectiveness.

In the general field of aging (not mental health) before the late 1970s, long-term care was synonymous with nursing home placement. In 1977 the National Nursing Home Survey and a 1979 General Accounting Office (GAO) report (General Accounting Office 1979) demonstrated that Medicaid was financing most of the nursing home care in the country and was providing incentives to use nursing homes instead of community-based services. Subsequently, a number of community demonstration projects providing long-term alternative care using Medicaid and Medicare waivers were funded by the federal government with the goal of reducing institutionalization and controlling the rising costs of long-term care. These projects include social and health maintenance organizations, the On Lok program, life-care communities, and The Channeling Demonstration (Robinson 1990). Although only the Channeling Demonstration was tested using a randomized controlled design, and mental health services were variable within these projects, they serve as examples of alternatives to traditional services. A brief description of each program and its evaluation is provided below.

## Social and Health Maintenance Organizations (S/HMO)

Like HMOs, an S/HMO is a managed system of health and long-term care in which a single provider is responsible for all health services in return for a fixed premium. Four demonstration sites were established in 1985 with funding from private foundations and the Health Care Financing Administration. A total of 10,626 elderly individuals were enrolled using Medicare eligibility requirements. S/HMO members receive a full range of medical and long-term care services, including respite, day care, transportation, homemaker, personal aide, and nursing home care. Case management is used to assess, identify, and refer clients in need of specific services (Greenberg et al. 1988). Evaluation of this program from a neuropsychiatric standpoint reveals that finding psychiatrists to treat clients in the S/HMO was difficult, and few formal mental health services were used. In addition, no current system existed to identify clients in need of mental health treatment and no in-home services existed to assist with behavioral management, potentially resulting in use of nursing home placement where it might be avoided if appropriate interventions were available. This suggests that although none of the four sites exceeded their capitation estimates, a more comprehensive model with emphasis on the efficacy of assessment and treatment of neuropsychiatric conditions is warranted (Robinson 1990).

## The On Lok Program

On Lok was developed in 1971 to provide comprehensive health care services for San Francisco's geriatric clients at risk of being institutionalized. Like the S/HMOs, the responsibility for service delivery rests within the On Lok organization, with staff providing or contracting for all medical and support services. Since 1971, On Lok has grown. It currently operates three adult day centers and a 54-unit housing facility, and has been replicated in four sites across the country. The multidisciplinary team is an important component of this treatment model and is comprised of physicians, social workers, nurse practitioners, therapists, paraprofessionals, and support staff with each member having an extensive knowledge of each client's condition. Mental health services are provided, with some on-site treatment available in at least one location (Kane et al. 1992; Robinson 1990). Studies that have been conducted on service-use patterns indicate that On Lok clients use one-third as many hospital days and one-fifth as many nursing home days as comparison groups and have a significant reduction in total expenditures for health care (Zawadski and Ansak 1983). Although this is encouraging, mental health use has not been systematically studied in On Lok clients, which demonstrates again the need for a closer look at this important aspect of health care.

## Life-Care Communities

This model consists of two types of life-care communities (LCC); the continuing-care retirement communities (CCRC), and the life-care-at-home (LCAH) communities. Both of these are housing-based programs that provide residents with health and social services. The primary difference between the two is that the CCRC is campus based; members live in a central location, and the LCAH provides in-home services to clients. Both involve a contract between the life-care community and the resident, an entrance fee, and a monthly service fee. CCRC fees range from $50,000 to $100,000 initially and cost $400 to $1,500 a month. LCAH is less expensive; it costs $5,000 to $10,000 initially, with a monthly fee of approximately $200. In both types of communities these fees cover only long-term care services and do not provide for acute care, which are covered by Medicare policies. Services provided may include nursing home care, home health services, personal care, homemaker services, respite care, meals, day care, recreational activities, transportation, and an in-home monitoring system. LCAH plans do provide nursing home care, whereas many CCRCs do not guarantee complete nursing home benefits (Pies 1984; Tell et al. 1987). No empirical evaluations of the benefits of this setting for people with neuropsychiatric illness have been undertaken to date. Given that the life-care communities are becoming increasingly popular among middle- and upper-middle-class elderly citizens, further research concerning the need for and provision of services to this population is indicated (Robinson 1990).

## The Channeling Demonstration

The National Long-Term Care Demonstration or Channeling Demonstration was funded by the U.S. Department of Health and Human Services (HHS) in 1980. It was developed to test the efficacy of case management in improving the quality of life and reducing the costs of long-term care for impaired elderly individuals at risk of being institutionalized. Designed to broker services with the goal of keeping patients in the community, case managers assessed clients, developed care plans, implemented the plans through service arrangement, and monitored service provision (Carcagno and Kemper 1988). Evaluation using a randomized controlled design revealed that case management was 6%–18% more expensive for the provider but reduced client costs by 7% and improved the quality of life for clients and caregivers. Despite the fact that this study required clients to have a cognitive or behavioral impairment, no systematic evaluation of mental health needs or service provision was undertaken (Kemper 1988).

In each of the long-term care models described above, there is little or no evaluation of the neuropsychiatric status of the client, and no evaluation of the efficacy of services provided for these problems. Given the significant need and the existence of effective services, a systematic evaluation is indicated.

In the field of geriatric mental health, the Community Support Program (CSP) was established by NIMH in 1977 out of a concern for access to treatment and coordination of services. As a pilot program, it was designed to assist states and communities in providing services for adults with seriously disabling mental health problems. Subsequently the concept of a community support system (CSS) was established as a basis for planning and organizing services for this population. The CSS concept identifies the array of services needed to assist persons with disabling mental health problems to function at optimal levels within the community. CSS is not only a network of service components but also represents a philosophy regarding the delivery of services. The 11 service components that constitute a community support system and the operational philosophies encouraged by the CSP are outlined in Tables 16–1 and 16–2 (Schafft and Randolph, in press; Stroul 1988). Within the field of geriatric psychiatry, CSP represents a transition from traditional facility-based, long-term care to a community-based model with a primary concern for the access to and coordination of services. In an effort to develop effective approaches to providing community services for elderly clients, NIMH initiated a program through CSP in 1985 to fund demonstration grants. Subsequently, grants were awarded to 16 state mental health authorities to develop and provide a range of community-based services targeted to prevent or delay institutionalization. These 16 projects brought

**Table 16–1.** Service components of a community support system

- Client identification and outreach
- Mental health treatment
- Crisis response services
- Health and dental care
- Housing
- Income support and entitlements
- Peer support
- Family and community support
- Rehabilitation services
- Protection and advocacy
- Case management

**Table 16–2.** Philosophies encouraged by the community support program

- Services should be consumer centered.
- Services should empower clients.
- Services should be racially and culturally appropriate.
- Services should be flexible.
- Services should focus on strengths.
- Services should incorporate natural supports.
- Services should meet special needs.
- Service systems should be accountable.
- Services should be coordinated.

mental health services to a wide variety of neuropsychiatrically ill elderly clients throughout the country. A summary of the programs is provided in Table 16–3 (Schafft and Randolph, in press).

Most of the programs served elderly individuals who had schizophrenia or affective disorders and many included populations with Alzheimer's and related diseases (ADRD) as well as anxiety, substance abuse, and adjustment disorders. The populations treated ranged from 50 to 105 years of age and included culturally diverse individuals. Residents of nursing homes and the homeless were targeted as well as both urban and rural popu-

**Table 16–3.** Summary of 16 demonstration projects for elderly patients

| Project | Program model | Geo-graphic setting | Service setting | Services provided by program |
|---|---|---|---|---|
| Colorado: The Elderly Empowerment Program | Outreach, networking, and training | Urban | In vivo (SROs, public housing) | Outreach, case mgmt., counseling, improvement groups, empowerment training |
| Florida: Geriatric MH Support Team | Training | Mixed | In vivo and day treatment center | Outreach, assessment, case mgmt., crisis intervention, counseling, respite care, day Tx |
| Georgia: The Respite Care Project | Training and respite care | Urban | In vivo and day care center | Assessment, respite care, emergency care companionship, personal care, support groups, peer counseling |
| Iowa: Rural Geriatric Mental Health Outreach Project | Outreach, supportive therapy, training | Rural | In vivo, MH center | Outreach, assessment, case mgmt., social supports |

| MH characteristics of clients | Number of clients | Staff charac- teristics | Training provided to | Training products |
|---|---|---|---|---|
| Psychiatric Dx, dual Dx | 81 | Geriatric specialists, MH staff, students | Board and care staff, SRO hotel staff, service providers, natural helpers, volunteers | Training modules, audiotapes, and curricul- um on em- powerment |
| Psychiatric Dx or MH problems, including Alzheimer's disease | 190 | PD, SWs, psychiatric nurse, prog. mgrs. | Staff from foster care homes, adult community living facil- ities, and family members | Training curricula |
| ADRD | 132 | PD, CM, registry mgr., nurse consultant | Respite care staff | None |
| DSM-III-R Dx of MI, ADRD | 365 | 1 psychia- trist, 3 gero- psychiatric nurses, 2 SWs | Community gatekeepers (e.g., mail carriers, store clerks, police), care providers, elderly per- sons and families, peer coun- selors | Two-part manual for training gatekeepers |

*(continued)*

**Table 16–3.** Summary of 16 demonstration projects for elderly patients *(continued)*

| Project | Program model | Geo-graphic setting | Service setting | Services provided by program |
|---|---|---|---|---|
| Louisiana: Black Elderly Crisis Counseling Intervention Program | Crisis intervention and training | Rural | In vivo, MH center | Assessment, crisis intervention, home visits, telephone counseling, family support groups |
| Maine: Comprehensive Community Based Care for Elderly Persons With Severe Long-Term Disabling Mental Illness | Interagency collaboration | Rural | In vivo | Assessment, case mgmt., MH Tx |
| Maryland: Psychogeriatric Assessment, Treatment and Training in City Housing (PATCH) | Assessment, Tx, and training | Urban | In vivo (Section 8 public housing) | Medical and MH assessment, referral, case mgmt., counseling, medication mgmt. |
| Minnesota: Elderly Mentally Ill CSP Demonstration Project | Multiorganizational coordination | Rural | In vivo and MH center | Assessment, referrals, residential placement, respite, crisis intervention, day Tx |

| MH characteristics of clients | Number of clients | Staff characteristics | Training provided to | Training products |
|---|---|---|---|---|
| Symptoms of mental and emotional distress | 227 | Project service coordinator, secretary, research assistants, 10 social work students, 3 CMs | Project assistants, care providers | In-home crisis intervention training guide for graduate schools of social work |
| Symptoms of emotional and mental problems | 85 | CM, specialist in aging, 8 psychiatric nurses | Agency staff | None |
| Psychiatric Dx, dementia, and no Dx | 184 | PD, 2 nurse clinicians, 2 psychiatrists, 1 secretary | Public housing staff | None |
| Diagnosed with MI | 300 per year | PD, 2 MH specialists, 1 CM, clerical support | Consultation with board and care homes, senior centers | None |

(continued)

**Table 16–3.** Summary of 16 demonstration projects for elderly patients *(continued)*

| Project | Program model | Geographic setting | Service setting | Services provided by program |
|---|---|---|---|---|
| New Hampshire: North Country Alzheimer's Partnership | Case mgmt. | Rural | In vivo, telephone consultations | Assessment, case mgmt., respite, caregiver support groups |
| New Mexico: Mental Health Service to Native American Elders | Case mgmt. and education | Rural | In vivo and senior center | Case mgmt., counseling, transportation, recreational and educational activities |
| New York: Project Rescue: A Model Program for Homeless Mentally Ill | Outreach and shelter | Urban | Shelter and on the streets | Assessment, financial and other entitlement assistance, clothing, showers, support groups, nutrition, health care |
| North Carolina: Senior Adult Growth and Enrichment Program | Case mgmt. and consultation | Rural | In vivo, rest homes, family care homes | Outreach, assessment, case mgmt., therapy, psychosocial activities, consultation, and education |
| Ohio: Chums & Choices: A Support Network for Severely Mentally Ill Persons | Companionship | Suburban | In vivo, community hospital, senior centers | Socialization activities, home visits |

| MH characteristics of clients | Number of clients | Staff charac- teristics | Training provided to | Training products |
|---|---|---|---|---|
| Diagnosed with ADRD | 161 | PD, SW, LPN, secre- tary, intake worker, CM | Family mem- bers, staff of nursing homes, and home health agencies | None |
| Native Americans with depression | < 30 | Outreach worker, consulting counselor, psychologist | None | None |
| Homeless, elderly with MI | Unknown | SW, out- reach workers, volunteers, secretary | None | None |
| MI and dementia | 154 | 5 SWs, physicians, administra- tors, support staff, volun- teers | Student interns | None |
| Dx of schizo- phrenia | 144 | Prog. dir., community relations dir., 1.5 FTE volunteer directors | Volunteers, community service per- sonnel | Training manual |

*(continued)*

**Table 16–3.**  Summary of 16 demonstration projects for elderly patients *(continued)*

| Project | Program model | Geo-graphic setting | Service setting | Services provided by program |
|---|---|---|---|---|
| Virginia: Project Reach | Enrichment activities | Urban | In vivo | Assessment, socialization, peer counseling, support groups |
| Washington: Community Services to Mentally Ill Isolated Elderly | Outreach and case mgmt. | Urban | In vivo (public housing) | Outreach, re-ferrals, case mgmt., brief counseling, shopping, chores, advocacy |
| Wisconsin: Mobile Outreach to Seniors Team (MOST) | Case mgmt. and educa-tional inter-ventions | Mixed | In vivo | Assessment, counseling, crisis inter-vention, peer support groups, medication monitoring |

| MH characteristics of clients | Number of clients | Staff charac- teristics | Training provided to | Training products |
|---|---|---|---|---|
| Dx of MI | 117 | PD, psychia- tric nurse, MH clinician, consulting psychiatrist | Volunteers | Volunteer training curriculum |
| Elderly with symptoms of MI, including dual Dx | 349 | Clinical spec- ialist, prog. mgr., 3 CMs, students, volunteer substance abuse coun- selor | Public housing staff, students | None |
| Symptoms of MI, including dementia | 601 | SW, psychia- trist, 2.6 FTE nurses, administra- tion and clerical staff, evaluator, students | Graduate stu- dents, pro- fessors, peer counselors, gatekeepers, staff of service agency | None |

*Note.* ADRD, Alzheimer's disease and related disorders; CM, case manager; dir., director; Dx, diagnosis; FTE, full-time equivalent; LPN, licensed practical nurse; mgmt., management; mgr., manager; MH, mental health; MI, mental illness; PD, project director; prog., program; SRO, single-room-occupancy [building]; SW, social worker; Tx, treatment.

lations. Several treatment models were used, with case management, outreach, and training approaches used most frequently. Although evaluation designs were incorporated into each of the projects, with attention given to outcome measures that would be meaningful in planning future treatment models, few of the studies used randomized controls and many experienced difficulty adequately addressing the need for evaluation. Results from two of the projects that were appropriately evaluated are briefly described below.

## Iowa

An independent study of the effectiveness of Iowa's Rural Geriatric Mental Health Outreach Project was conducted by the Center for Health Services Research at the University of Iowa. Findings indicate that this project reached elderly clients with a wide variety of mental health problems who may not have been identified by a more traditional service system at a cost that was substantially less ($622 per patient year) than that of local mental health providers. An evaluation of the effectiveness of services provided was conducted with 30 clients by analyzing scores on pre- and posttreatment evaluations. These indicated significant improvements in depression and other psychiatric symptoms (Buckwalter et al. 1991).

## Wisconsin

The effectiveness of the Mobile Outreach for Seniors Team (MOST) was measured by comparing clinical ratings of severity of impairment at intake with ratings at termination. Of the 77 clients sampled, 61% improved, 38% maintained, and 1% declined in level of functioning. Improvement was consistent across diagnoses and correlated with more MOST contacts. This sample of clients also experienced fewer and briefer hospitalizations. Surveys of consumers, volunteers, and staff found the community support model used in the delivery of MOST services to be both highly acceptable and effective (P. Anderson, personal communication, September 1993).

Overall, these studies served to emphasize the importance of recognizing and treating the multiple emotional, cognitive, physical, and socioeconomic needs of elderly clients. Projects that are home-based, provide auxiliary services (transportation, respite care), and use a multidisciplinary team approach seem to best address the multiple needs of elderly neuropsychiatrically ill individuals.

## Conclusions

A large population of neuropsychiatrically ill elderly persons are currently being underserved despite the existence of an appropriate service technology. New and innovative models of care that strive to treat the individual in a more comprehensive manner have been developed and are being increasingly implemented. Promising models implemented tend to approximate the basic CSP elements (see Tables 16–1 and 16–2). Although these approaches appear to represent progress, care must be taken to rigorously evaluate them to ensure their effectiveness in terms of both cost and outcomes.

Appendix 16–1 lists addresses and contact persons for the programs discussed.

## References

Beardsley RS, Larson DB, Burns BJ, et al: Prescribing of psychotropics in elderly nursing home patients. J Am Geriatr Soc 37:327–330, 1989

Bienfeld D, Wheeler BJ: Psychiatric services to nursing homes: a liaison model. Hosp Community Psychiatry 40:793–794, 1989

Buck JA. Psychotropic drug practice in nursing homes. J Am Geriatr Soc 36:409–418, 1988

Buckwalter KC, Smith M, Zevenbergen P, et al: Mental health services of the rural elderly outreach program. Gerontologist 31:408–412, 1991

Burns BJ, Kamerow DB: Psychotropic drug prescriptions for nursing home residents. J Fam Pract 26:155–160, 1988

Burns BJ, Taube CA: Mental health services in general medical care and in nursing homes, in Mental Health Policy for Older Americans: Protecting Minds at Risk. Edited by Fogel BS, Furino A, Gottlieb GL. Washington, DC, American Psychiatric Press, 1990, pp 63–84

Burns BJ, Wagner HR, Taube JE, et al: Mental health service use by the elderly in nursing homes. Am J Public Health 83:331–337, 1993

Butler RN, Lewis MI: Aging and Mental Health. St. Louis, MO, Mosby, 1982

Carcagno G, Kemper P: An overview of the channeling demonstration and its evaluation. Health Services Research 23:1–22, 1988

Fogel BS, Gottlieb GL, Furino A: Minds at risk, in Mental Health Policy for Older Americans: Protecting Minds at Risk. Edited by Fogel BS, Furino A, Gottlieb GL. Washington, DC, American Psychiatric Press, p. 1–21, 1990

General Accounting Office: Entering a Nursing Home—Costly Implications for Medicaid and the Elderly. Washington DC, General Accounting Office, November 1979

Goldstrom ID, Burns BJ, Larson DB, et al: Mental health service use by elderly adults in a primary care setting. J Gerontol 42:147–153, 1987

Greenberg J, Leutz W, Greenlick M, et al: The social HMO demonstration: early experience. Health Affairs 7:66–79, 1988

Kane RL, Illston LH, Miller NA: Qualitative analysis of the Program of All-Inclusive Care for the Elderly (PACE). Gerontologist 32:771–780, 1992

Kemper P: Overview of the findings: the evaluation of the national long-term care demonstration. Health Services Research 23:161–174, 1988

Light E, Liebowitz BD, Bailey F: CMHCS and elderly services: an analysis of direct and indirect services and service delivery sites. Community Ment Health J 22:294–302, 1986

Pies H: Life care communities for the aged—an overview, in Long-Term Care Financing and Delivery Systems: Exploring Some Alternatives (Conference Proceedings: Health Care Financing Administration, Publication No. 03174). Washington, DC, US Government Printing Office, June 1984

Pinkston EM, Linsk NL, Young RN: Home-based behavioral family treatment of the impaired elderly. Behavior Therapy 19:331–344, 1988

Ray WA, Federspiel CF, Schaffner W: A study of antipsychotic drug use in nursing homes: epidemiologic evidence suggesting misuse. Am J Public Health 70:485–491, 1980

Regier DA, Boyd JH, Burke JC, et al. One-month prevalence of psychiatric disorders in the US: based on five epidemiological catchment area sites. Arch Gen Psychiatry 45:977–986, 1988

Robinson GK: The psychiatric component of long-term care models, in Mental Health Policy for Older Americans: Protecting Minds at Risk. Edited by Fogel BS, Furino A, Gottlieb GL. Washington, DC, American Psychiatric Press, 1990, pp 157–177

Schafft GE, Randolph FL: Innovative Community-Based Services for Older Adults With Mental Illness, Center for Mental Health Services, Substance Abuse Mental Health Services Administration, Public Health Service, Department of Health and Human Services, November 1994

Shapiro S, Skinner EA, Kramer M, et al: Measuring need for mental health services in a general population. Medical Care 23:1033–1043, 1985

Strahan G: 1985 National Nursing Home Survey. US Dept. of Health and Human Services, Public Health Service, CDC. National Center for Health Statistics, DHHS Publication # PHS 91-1766. Hyattsville, MD, February 1991

Stroul BA: Community support systems for persons with long-term mental illness: questions and answers. National Institute of Mental Health Community Support Program, Rockville, MD, 1988

Tell E, Cohen M, Wellock S: Life care at home: a new model for financing and delivery of long-term care. Inquiry 24:253–265, 1987

Tourigny-Rivard MF, Drury M: The effects of monthly psychiatric consultation in a nursing home. Gerontologist 27:363–366, 1987

Zawadski RT, Ansak ML: Consolidating community-based long-term care: early returns from the On Lok demonstration. Gerontologist 23:365–369, 1983

# Appendix 16–1.   Elderly Program Contacts

**The Elderly Empowerment Program**
Ruth Parsons
Associate Professor
Associate Dean
Graduate School of Social Work
University of Denver
University Park
Denver, Colorado 80112
(303) 871-2886

Enid O. Cox, DSW
Associate Professor
Graduate School of Social Work
Director, Institute of Geron-
tology
University of Denver
University Park
Denver, Colorado 80112
(303)871-2886

**Geriatric Mental Health Support Team**
Ray Hinsley
Director, Overlay Services
11401 A Belcher Road South
Largo, Florida 34643
(813)541-7441

**The Respite Care Project**
Harriet L. Cohen, LCSW
Executive Director
Atlanta Area Chapter of
Atlanta Association
3120 Raymond Drive
Atlanta, Georgia 30340
(404)451-1300

**Rural Geriatric Mental Health Outreach Project**
William Dobbs
Mental Health Specialist
Department of Human Services
Division of Mental Health,
Mental Retardation, and
Developmental Disabilities
Hoover State Office Building
Des Moines, Iowa 50319
(515)281-6873

**Black Elderly Crisis Counseling Intervention Program**
Delores Jones (state)
Geriatrics Coordinator
Division of Mental Health
PO Box 4049, Bin No. #12
Baton Rouge, Louisiana 70821
(504)342-2587

Shirley Mitchell (program)
Project Director
BECCI—Basic Elderly Crisis
Counseling Intervention
719 Elysian Fields
New Orleans, Louisiana 70117
(504)942-8315

Arthemease Melancon (alter-
nate)
Program Coordinator
BECCI
719 Elysian Fields
New Orleans, Louisiana 70117
(504)942-8315

**Comprehensive Community-Based Care for Elderly Persons with Severe Long-Term Disabling Mental Illness**
Joyce S. Harmon
Coordinator of Geriatric
   Services
Department of Mental Health
   and Mental Retardation
Bureau of Mental Health
State House, Station #40
Augusta, Maine 04333
(207)289-4230

**Psychogeriatric Assessment, Treatment, and Training in City Housing (PATCH)**
Alison Carter
Federal Program Administrator
Mental Hygiene Administration
201 West Preston Street 4th
   Floor
Baltimore, Maryland 21201
(301)225-6633

**Elderly Mentally Ill CSP Demonstration Project**
Sharon Autio
Mental Health Specialist for
   Older Adults and Nursing
   Home Reform
444 Layfette Road
St. Paul, Minnesota 55155-3828
(612)297-3510

**North Country Alzheimer's Partnership**
Mary Maggioncalda (state)
Program Specialist
Division of Elderly and Adult
   Services
115 Pleasant Street
Concord, New Hampshire 03301
(603)271-4410

Susan Kearns (program)
Director, North Country Elderly
   Programs
253 High Street
Berlin, New Hampshire 03570
(603)752-3336

**Mental Health Services to Native American Elders**
George Wallace, Program
   Manager
Division of Mental Health
Department of Mental Health
1190 St. Francis Drive
Santa Fe, New Mexico 87592-
   0968
(505)827-2611

**Project Rescue: A Model for Homeless Mentally Ill**
Arlene DeRise, Program
   Director
Bowery Residence Committee
   (BRC) Human
Services Corporation
Homeless Seniors Service
30 Delancey Street
New York, New York 10002
(212)353-0955

**Senior Adult Growth and Enrichment Program**
Gayle Goodburn, Program
  Director of SAGE
1946 Martin Street
Burlington, North Carolina
  27215
(919)222-6430

**Chums and Choices: A Support Network for Severely Mentally Ill Persons**
Risa Grimes-Chaffin
Executive Director
CHUMS Inc.
2611 Wayne Avenue #61
Dayton, Ohio 45420
(513)258-6285

**PROJECT REACH**
Jacobs Singer (Program
  Contact)
Geriatric Coordinator
Richmond Community Mental
  Health Center
900 East Broad Street
4th Floor, Room 406
Richmond, Virginia 23219
(804)780-6890

Sundra Rollins (State Contact)
Director, Geriatric Services
Department of Mental Health,
  Mental Retardation, and
  Substance Abuse Services
PO Box 1797
Richmond, Virginia 23214
(804)786-8044

**Community Connections: Services to Mentally Ill Isolated Elderly**
Jane E. Relin, MSW
Program Manager
Community Connections
Community Home Health Care
200 West Thomas, Suite 200
Seattle, Washington 98119-4216
(206)282-5048

**Mobile Outreach to Seniors Team (MOST)**
Patricia Anderson, MSSW
Coordinator of MOST Program
Center of Dane County
625 West Washington Avenue
Madison, Wisconsin 53703
(608)251-7893

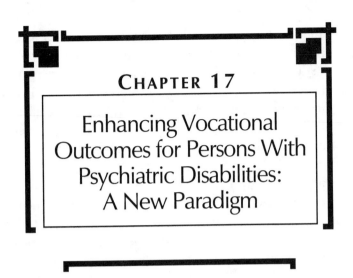

# CHAPTER 17

## Enhancing Vocational Outcomes for Persons With Psychiatric Disabilities: A New Paradigm

**Carol T. Mowbray, Ph.D., Steven Leff, Ph.D.,
Ralph Warren, Jr., Ph.D., Nancy M. McCrohan, Ph.D.,
and Deborah Bybee, Ph.D.**

**W**ork in some sphere—be it paid employment, family work, or church or community volunteerism—plays a significant role in the lives of most adults. Work gives us social recognition, a way to structure our time, contacts with similar others, and a sense of purpose and meaning. However, up until 20 years ago, work was not considered a viable option for most individuals with psychiatric disabilities (National Institute on Disability and Rehabilitation Research 1992). There were multiple reasons for that predicament. First, many persons with severe mental illness experience their initial episodes in adolescence or young adulthood, thereby eliminating opportunities for educational preparation and the acquisition of work skills and experiences, which are part of a normal developmental sequence. Second, the episodic nature of psychiatric disabilities has often meant interrupted work histories for those who did obtain jobs. Loss of a job due to a return of symptomatology usually reduces the probability of getting future employment. Third, for a variety of reasons, persons with a psychiatric disability experience less success in traditional vocational rehabilitation programs. Finally, functional deficits associated with severe mental illness can create workplace problems, such as inconsistent performance and interpersonal difficulties (MacDonald-Wilson et al. 1991; Rogers et al. 1991).

The absolute significance of psychiatric disability in precluding vocational activity is still a matter of debate. Even recent writings have echoed strong negative opinions, as illustrated by the following: "Impairment in work functioning is a diagnostic feature of schizophrenia and a deficit that may persist without improvement for years" (Lysaker et al. 1993, p. 278).

In contrast, numerous studies now support the conclusion that neither diagnosis nor severity of psychiatric impairment rule out positive vocational outcomes for individuals with psychiatric disability, provided adequate services and supports are available (Rogers et al. 1991). Research has also provided evidence of the ability of these individuals to function successfully in the community in other domains, provided adequate services and supports are available (Russert and Frey 1991).

As a result of such research findings and other social and political factors, a fresh spirit of hope and recovery affirms the belief that through a rehabilitative approach, those with mental illness should be able to assume productive and meaningful roles of their choosing in normal settings (Anthony and Blanch 1987; Lawn and Meyerson 1993). Anthony and Blanch (1987) describe a new set of assumptions, which now characterize occupational approaches for persons with psychiatric disabilities: regardless of the severity or type of disability, if they choose to do so, all persons can do meaningful, productive work in normal settings, when provided with the necessary supports; vocational failures are not due to the disability itself, but to the wrong job, the wrong setting, or inadequate/inappropriate supports. The authors' purpose in this chapter is to provide an overview of current vocational approaches for persons with psychiatric disabilities, to delineate barriers to employment and suggest improvements to rehabilitative approaches that are vocationally focused, and to describe what we know about their work histories and work orientation.

## Current Vocational Models

Although there is increasing recognition of the importance of vocational rehabilitation and a variety of recent program innovations, vocational services, for the most part, remain independent of mental health services. Brown and Basel (1988) view the mental health and vocational rehabilitation systems as "more different than alike" (p. 23). They note that the vocational rehabilitation system operates according to clear federal guidelines and shows much less variation across states than does the mental health system. Vocational rehabilitation counselors typically work with consumers under highly structured and time limited conditions. The mental health system, on the other hand, provides a set of services that may vary in their combination, intensity, and duration. Staff in mental health programs are often not skilled in vocational rehabilitation, and vocational rehabilitation counselors similarly lack specific skills needed to aid persons with severe psychiatric disabilities.

Two of the earliest vocational models developed for persons with severe mental illness were the Fairweather Lodge and Fountain House programs. The Fairweather Lodge model establishes small groups of persons with psychiatric disabilities who live together in a common residence and work together in a common business. The basic assumption of this psychosocial approach is that a properly functioning group process in a community lodge will promote the social and vocational rehabilitation of individual members (Fairweather et al. 1969). During the period of time that the deinstitutionalization movement has reduced the number of persons with psychiatric disabilities who have long-term inpatient episodes, the Lodge model has evolved to meet the needs of persons who have more experiences with community living (Marrone 1993).

In the Fountain House/Clubhouse model, work is an essential context for the interaction among members, the development of friendships within the clubhouse, and the attainment of an individual member's sense of effectiveness and self-esteem (Jackson 1992). The clubhouse model sets up various work units in the clubhouse, which are directly related to maintaining its ongoing functioning. Typical work units are clerical, housekeeping, kitchen, and public relations (Marrone 1993). Most clubhouses do not assign members to a specific work unit for a specific period of time. The clubhouse model emphasizes the voluntary nature of participation in work. It also balances practical work needs of the community with personal growth needs of individual members. Clubhouses do not provide specific skills training, however (Anthony and Jansen 1984).

The Fountain House/Clubhouse model recognized the need for members to learn specific vocational skills and created short-term training placements (transitional employment) with businesses (Beard et al. 1982). These placements were developed to create a bridge from the Clubhouse work units to employment in the community. Now, several decades after the initiation of the clubhouse model, questions have been raised about the capability of this model to enable consumers to sustain independent competitive employment in the community. The question of the efficacy of vocational services in the clubhouse model has mainly appeared in comparative discussions of transitional employment (TE) and supported employment (Bond 1992). Although initially available only in clubhouses, TE programs developed within the clubhouse model, but these programs are now also housed in a variety of mental health program models and are, in some cases, stand-alone programs. Marrone (1993) characterizes the main features of TE programs as follows: a consumer is placed in a specific job placement for a time-limited period (usually 6 months); employers pay consumer-workers directly; the program rather than the individual consumer develops job placements; and programs hire and conduct the initial training of individual consumer-workers. Most TE jobs are entry-level service jobs (e.g., clerical, food service, etc.) and require limited training.

According to Bond (1992), "Supported employment represents a paradigm shift in vocational thinking" (p 244). The supported employment (SE) approach to vocational rehabilitation originally developed within services for persons with developmental disabilities and mental retardation in the early and mid-1980s. Anthony and Blanch (1987) identify four primary service settings in which SE programs are located: psychosocial rehabilitation centers, community mental health centers, sheltered workshops, and career placement agencies.

Anthony and Blanch (1987) and Bond (1987) report that TE and SE models share many of the same characteristics. Both approaches provide consumers with community-based work placements and the staff are involved with job coaching. Aside from the defining distinction of the duration of work placement, TE and SE programs also differ in their typical goals and job levels (Anthony and Blanch 1987). TE programs focus on developing basic work skills, establishing a work history, and enhancing self-esteem and a sense of efficacy in new social roles. SE programs instead emphasize the goal of an immediate and hopefully permanent placement in independent competitive employment at any job level (not just entry level). SE programs also appear to be more flexible with respect to consumers' wishes about the way support services relate to an employer. In some cases consumers may not want an employer to be informed about their disability.

As programs have evolved, TE may appear to be less distinct from SE. In some vocational programs, TE placements have been structured to lead directly to SE. As a result, TE and SE eventually may be best distinguished in terms of conceptual frameworks and historical rationales rather than unique modes of implementation in existing programs (Anthony and Blanch 1987).

## Work Histories and Work Orientation

The heterogeneity of functioning among persons with a severe mental illness is now well documented (Braucht and Kirby 1986;

Hazel et al. 1991). Studies have established the fact that a wide range of functioning, skills, disabilities, and independence levels are represented among the psychiatrically disabled. However, despite the diversity displayed in many domains, employment levels appear to be uniformly poor. Thus, Anthony and Blanch (1987) summarized research on competitive employment rates for those with psychiatric illness and reported a consistent figure of 20%–25% for all persons discharged from psychiatric hospitals and 15% or lower for those with severe disabilities. More recent studies show little change from these figures; in statewide studies conducted in New York, Michigan, and Indiana, 3%, 7%, and 17%, respectively, were competitively employed (Bond and Boyer 1988; Donahue et al. 1990; Herman et al. 1988). Another 4%–6% were employed in sheltered or supported work, and 3%–5% were employed in school or training.

It is usually assumed that if they work, those with psychiatric disabilities work at low-paying, low-status jobs with frequent turnover, and some data support this. For example, Cook (1991) found that for a large sample of psychiatric clients receiving vocational rehabilitation services, the median Hollingshead rating of their last job was in the unskilled range; typical jobs included janitor, fast-food service, supermarket stock person, or bagger. However, other data collected on work histories suggest more diversity. For example, Sommer et al. (1984) state that according to family members of individuals with severe mental illness, for 83% of these individuals their current jobs were not in keeping with their education. Other studies also suggest that the work backgrounds of psychiatric consumers may be underestimated. Data reported from Thresholds National Research and Training Center indicate that more than 80% of clients receiving services have prior work experience. A majority have worked at least a year at a single job (Cook 1991; Cook and Roussel 1987). Michigan statewide data support this: 88% of a statewide sample labeled seriously mentally ill have been competitively employed at some time. Given the acknowledged heterogeneity of the population of individuals with severe mental illness (Hazel et al. 1991; Goldman and

Manderscheid 1987), it would not be surprising if their work experiences were equally diverse.

Collecting information only about clients' current or last jobs may be more reflective of their recent symptomatology than of their overall vocational potential and skill levels. Our research on the vocational backgrounds and orientation of persons with serious mental illness in Michigan supports this. We interviewed a sample of clients with severe mental illness who receive case management services from two large agencies in Kent County, which serve a combined total of over 1,000 persons. Our sample of 279 participants was similar in many ways to other samples of seriously mentally ill clients: 60% were male; 80% were white and non-Hispanic; 74% were high school graduates; the average age was 37 years; 68% had a diagnosis of schizophrenia; and nearly all were taking prescribed psychotropic medications (see McCrohan et al. 1994).

Although a higher percentage of our sample was working than in other studies (40%, including competitive and sheltered/supported employment), wages for their current or last jobs were low (median $4.15) and so was job status. As shown in Table 17–1, the modal occupational category (classified according to the Department of Labor's Dictionary of Occupational Titles) was the service industry (51%), which includes food service, janitorial work, personal services (like nurse's aide), and general labor. Another large category (31%) was benchwork, consisting mostly of light assembly in sheltered workshops. Clerical and sales work each made up less than 5% of current or last job categories. Despite the low level of current or last jobs, for most individuals, work aspirations were high: among those not currently working, more than 75% said they wanted to work; 71% of all participants saw themselves working in 1 year and 67% in 5 years.

Besides gathering information about current or last jobs, we also asked participants a series of questions about their best and worst jobs, desired jobs, and the jobs they saw themselves doing in 1 and 5 years from now (also in Table 17–1). Although the worst job classifications appeared quite similar to their current or last jobs, the best job classification was quite different—with

**Table 17–1.**  Classification of past, current, and future vocation of seriously mentally ill clients

| Occupational category | Current/last job (%) ($N = 274$) | Best job (%) ($N = 246$) | Worst job (%) ($N = 211$) | Job in 1 yr (%) ($N = 164$) | Job in 5 yrs (%) ($N = 150$) |
|---|---|---|---|---|---|
| Service | 51.1 | 45.1 | 48.8 | 44.5 | 33.3 |
| Benchwork | 31.0 | 17.5 | 32.7 | 24.4 | 22.7 |
| Profess/tech/managerial | 1.8 | 3.3 | 1.9 | 12.2 | 23.3 |
| Clerical | 4.7 | 15.0 | 2.4 | 6.7 | 7.3 |
| Sales | 4.7 | 5.3 | 4.7 | 4.9 | 4.7 |
| Structural | 1.5 | 4.9 | 1.4 | 3.7 | 4.0 |
| Machine trades | 1.8 | 3.7 | 0.5 | 1.8 | 2.7 |
| Agriculture/fish/forestry | 0.0 | 0.8 | 2.8 | 0.0 | 0.0 |
| Processing | 0.7 | 0.4 | 2.4 | 0.0 | 0.0 |
| Miscellaneous | 2.6 | 4.1 | 2.4 | 1.8 | 2.0 |

*Note.*  Categories based on the Department of Labor *Dictionary of Occupational Titles* 1991. Numbers from McCrohan et al. (1994).

more diversity and more prestige. Somewhat fewer were in service categories (45%) and markedly fewer were in benchwork (18%). The number in clerical occupations tripled, as did structural classifications (e.g., construction work). For best jobs, about 33% were in skilled or white-collar categories, compared with about 15% of current or last jobs.

The participants' future job aspirations showed even more diversity. At 5 years, only 33% saw themselves working in service occupations—less than 25% in benchwork—whereas more than 40% saw themselves in skilled or white-collar occupational categories. Future jobs were more prestigious (as rated on the Hollingshead classification scheme), averaging in the skilled manual category. However, contrary to stereotypes about the inability of psychiatric consumers to set realistic goals, the progression from current or last job to future job did not appear extreme; rather, there was a gradual progression. Indeed, statistical analysis established a significant linear trend from the least to the most prestigious job classification for respondents; on average, the trend was as follows: from worst, to current or last, to best job, to 1-year job aspiration, and finally to 5-year job aspiration (see McCrohan et al. 1994).

Thus, the detailed data on work histories and plans from the Kent County study indicated more heterogeneity and prestige in past (i.e., best) than in current jobs. It also indicated a high level of orientation to working in the future and that most participants have aspirations for better positions. However, expectations seemed reality-based in that a linear progression was found, with participants' future job expectations gradually moving into more prestigious categories. The data paint a much more positive picture of work orientation than has been the case in other studies. Contrary to mythology, it appears that when most psychiatric consumers are asked about work goals, they can be fairly specific and are able to articulate goals for higher level positions that seem appropriate, rather than representing quantum leaps from their present or past occupations. As a cautionary note, however, it should still be acknowledged that many of the participants in this study do have significant problems with their employment potential. Even for their best jobs, half had worked at them for 1 year or less and left their best jobs 10 or more years ago; about 60% of these best jobs were still in service or benchwork classifications.

## Barriers to Employment

Planning interventions to increase the likely employment of persons with psychiatric disabilities requires information on the vocational potential of these clients, as well as on the barriers that prevent them from resuming prior occupational pursuits. Many of the barriers cited in the literature are internal to the client, a direct result of his or her mental illness; that is, symptomatology that includes anxiety, social withdrawal, or problems in memory and concentration (Bolton 1988; National Institute on Disability and Rehabilitation Research 1992; Russert and Frey 1991). Other internal barriers may be better interpreted as secondary to having experienced a severe and persistent mental illness. For example, loss of self-esteem due to stigma and repeated job loss can increase the perceived risk of failure and can lower current motivation to find or maintain work (Bingham 1988). The early onset of mental illness usually restricts the developmental experiences necessary to exploring different vocational options, so adults with mental illness may need to try out a variety of work roles before they find any that motivate job retention (Bingham 1988; National Institute on Disability and Rehabilitation Research 1992). Given the increasingly specialized employment market, many individuals, with or without disabilities, need advanced education and/or training before they are able to work in any occupation of interest (Moxley et al. 1993). Limited work experiences and occupational failures can also contribute to poor work habits, distorted vocational aspirations, and poor job-finding skills (National Institute on Disability and Rehabilitation Research 1992). On the other hand, some of the work barriers identified as internal to the person with mental illness seem to reflect deficits that may be situation-specific, for example, those deficits observed in a treatment program or hospital setting but not necessarily endemic to the person's functioning in a work environment, such as dependency, social naivete, hostility, and aggression (Bolton 1988).

The literature on occupational rehabilitation for psychiatric disabilities has begun to recognize the external barriers that individuals face. For example, stigma and employers' fears of mental illness often produce restricted work opportunities in unskilled settings with low wages, noisome work conditions, low prestige, and no career opportunities (Link et al. 1986; National Institute on Disability and Rehabilitation Research 1992; Russert and Frey 1991). The checkered work histories and/or limited work experiences and education of persons with psychiatric disabilities compound difficulties with employer-based discrimination. Other realities include disincentives to work created by welfare and by Social Security Administration definitions of disabilities; for example, part-time work may pay little more than these entitlement programs, yet provide no stable source of medical coverage, and may risk the individual's eligibility for future financial support. Employment support and training through the vocational rehabilitation system have also been found to provide limited opportunities or assistance to persons with psychiatric disabilities (National Institute on Disability and Rehabilitation Research 1992).

Our research on the vocational orientation of the sample of persons with severe mental illness from Kent County, Michigan, included questions about perceived barriers to employment (McCrohan et al. 1994). When asked why they were not employed, the largest number of responses related to mental or physical health (45.2%), for example, a recent hospitalization, particular health problem, or limitations imposed by psychotropic drugs. About another fifth (17.0%) reflected internal barriers such as having no desire to work, being indecisive about applying for jobs, or preferring to not have the structure of a job. The remaining responses reflected a combination of internal and external factors: external barriers (19.5%) included the poor job market and lack of transportation; references to past jobs were also given as barriers to employment (18.2%) and included a variety of responses with the common theme of why past jobs did not work out; responses concerning money or benefits (9.4%) included concerns over losing entitlements or benefits and fears about not earning enough money to live on; and competing activities (8.2%) identified as barriers to employment included caring for family members, going to day treatment, and school-work. Thus, participants themselves recognized the limitations imposed by their own mental and physical impairments, fears, and anxieties. However, nearly 40% of the barriers cited reflected other reasons.

Barriers to employment can also be implied from participants' listing of reasons for why a job was their worst job (McCrohan et al. 1994). The two most often cited reasons (at about 30% each) were, first, the type of task or work material, referring to the intrinsic aspects of tasks or tools used, such as the amount or difficulty of work, the job pace, and the unpleasantness of tasks; and, second, the environment or working conditions, such as heat and cold, fumes or smells, dangerous conditions, hours, and freedom of movement. In contrast, the reasons most often cited for a job being the best job were people (38.8%) and money (29.0%). Stress, or other reasons more directly reflecting concerns over mental or emotional functioning, were rarely mentioned as reasons for best or worst job choices.

Thus, in contrasting the literature review with our data based on self-reports of persons with psychiatric disabilities, we see that the former may reflect much more of an emphasis than may be warranted on internal deficits contributing to employment problems. Although problems directly reflecting symptomatology and functioning levels are real and should be acknowledged, there are substantial external barriers as well, which interventions focused only on "fixing" the person cannot address. Most of the barriers identified seem to reflect a complex set of interactions between the person and the environment. For example, mental illness may initially limit experiences necessary for healthy development, such as educational and occupational explorations and achievements. These limitations then contribute to poor work histories, restricted work skills, and past job and educational failures. This background then necessarily relates directly to lowered confidence and ability to seek and obtain work and to a lessened probability of being hired. The latter, of course, is exacerbated in the community realm by employer stigma and a poor job market, and in the human services realm by disincentives to employment created by entitlements, vocational rehabilitation policies and practices, and the negative, deficit-oriented attitudes of mental health workers.

We can conclude that getting persons with psychiatric disabilities employed is a complex, ongoing, and probably long-term endeavor (Bond and Boyer 1988). It involves significant amounts of mental health intervention with individuals themselves, such as counseling to address attitudes about past failures, needs for job change due to symptomatology, and medication adjustments to accommodate work schedules. It also may involve providing prevocational adjustment, skill training, and/or advanced education to many. It also involves assisting individuals to access such services, given that they are not readily available to persons with psychiatric disabilities. Other systems must also be negotiated on these individuals' behalf, such as social services and entitlement programs. Finally, the community must also be addressed: employers and others must be educated about their false beliefs concerning persons with mental illness and about discriminatory employment practices, which are now outlawed under the Americans with Disabilities Act.

It is not surprising that traditional ways of offering vocational training and of obtaining jobs for people with psychiatric disabilities have shown only limited success (MacDonald-Wilson et al. 1991). Vocational approaches linked only to mental health or to rehabilitation services could understandably be overwhelmed when confronted with the plethora of individually based needs and systems-level problems that require a response. We now discuss how and why a new approach to meeting these challenges is evolving and describe services now in place that exemplify this model.

# Emergence of Hybrid Programs for Vocational Case Management

There has been a tendency for discrete mental health services for persons with serious and persistent mental illness to evolve into hybrid programs that combine two or more services. (See H. S. Leff, R. Warren Jr., S. Raffe, P. Weinstock, and L. Toms-Barker, "New Developments in Vocational Services for Persons With Psychiatric Disabilities: Services Combining Elements of Case Management and Vocational Rehabilitation," Boston, MA, HSRI, unpublished manuscript, 1994; Trochim et al., in press.) In general, this reflects two facts: first, persons with serious and persistent mental illness need multiple services addressing the different domains to improve their quality of life; and second, linking and coordinating of services has proven extremely difficult in the human services (Baker and Itaglia 1992). The first fact influences providers to seek diverse services for their clients. The second moves them to "one-stop" solutions to problems concerning availability of and accessibility to an array of services. In the area of employment services, this general trend has led, among other things, to hybrid programs that combine vocational services with case management (H. S. Leff, R. Warren Jr., S. Raffe, et al., unpublished manuscript, 1994). Cook et al. (1992), Cook and Razzano (1992), and Trochim et al. (in press) all describe hybrid models that combine TE programs with SE programs.

More specifically, the emergence of hybrid case-management and SE programs can be viewed as resulting from the pressures exerted by three influences: community-support-systems theory and practice; psychosocial rehabilitation theory, research, and practice; and the consumer movement in mental health. Although these three influences can be distinguished, they share key philosophical assumptions, goals, and approaches to service delivery. Taken together, these three influences have contributed to important programmatic changes in the mental health system over the past three decades.

## Community-Support-Systems Theory and Practice

The deinstitutionalization of persons with serious and persistent mental illness, which occurred during the 1950s, 1960s, and 1970s, led to the recognition that community-based mental health services were not available or were inadequate to meet the needs of persons with severe psychiatric disabilities. One positive aspect of institutional care was that it provided a variety of services (e.g., housing and rehabilitation) under one roof (Baker and Intagliata 1992). With the release into community-based care of persons who had been institutionalized, the lack of coordinated treatment, rehabilitative, and support services for persons with psychiatric disabilities became glaringly apparent (Government Accounting Office 1976; Stroul 1989). Community-support-systems (CSS) theory and practice grew out of the recognition of these needs, particularly concerning supportive and rehabilitative services. The CSS paradigm has been guided by a distinctive set of core principles and values. In this paradigm, services should be coordinated; should be accountable, incorporating consumer and family input into the quality assurance process; should be consumer-oriented, and should actively involve clients in planning and delivering services and in setting policy; should be provided in the least restrictive setting and should promote natural supports; should be modified to meet special subgroup needs and should be ethnically, culturally, and racially appropriate (Stroul 1989).

The basic components of the CSS include client identification and outreach; mental health treatment; health and dental services; crisis response services; housing; income supports and entitlements; peer supports; family and community support; rehabilitation services; protection and advocacy; case management; and systems integration (Anthony and Blanch 1989; Stroul 1989). CSS theory and practice began with the realization that mental health systems would have to obtain or provide a variety of services and that these services would have to be sought and coordinated by persons who eventually became known as case managers (Baker and Intagliata 1992). Over time, CSS proponents became more pessimistic about obtaining and coordinating services delivered by diverse providers, especially traditional vocational rehabilitation services. CSS practitioners also learned that in open and complex community environments, service provision and coordination required assertive outreach to consumers (Thompson et al. 1990). As a result, CSS practitioners developed program models of case management, including individual staff- and team-oriented approaches, that would actually provide the variety of services needed by persons with serious and persistent mental illness. Some of these case management models explicitly integrated rehabilitation activities, including vocational services, into the case management process (Russert and Frey 1991).

## Psychosocial Rehabilitation Theory, Research, and Practice

At the same time that community support systems were being developed as a result of federal and state initiatives, psychiatric and psychosocial rehabilitation theory and practice were evolving. Anthony (1980), at the Boston University (BU) Center for Psychiatric Rehabilitation, developed a rehabilitation model that was influenced by client-centered therapy and skills training and that was based on a series of empirical studies in the 1960s and 1970s. Some of the major findings from these studies were that persons with psychiatric disabilities are able to learn skills and that this learning is positively related to more general rehabilitation outcomes; that symptoms and psychiatric diagnoses are poor predictors of rehabilitation outcomes; and that functional assessments for one environment are poor predictors of how a person will function in a different environment. These findings also provided an important impetus for the development of case management and related services that were part of the community support paradigm. These empirical findings also led many psychiatric rehabilitation programs to incorporate formal functional assessments. The BU Psychiatric Rehabilitation Center developed a specific technology for conducting functional assessments and a companion vocational rehabilitation model,

Choose-Get-Keep, which emphasizes client choice (Danley and Rogers 1989). In the Choose-Get-Keep model, clients first enter a structured phase of exploring career interests and options, then engage in job-seeking activities. Finally, after a job is obtained, rehabilitative services are provided to ensure that appropriate vocational and social skills and supports are put in place to aid clients in maintaining their jobs. Programs such as Fairweather Lodge and Fountainhouse, initiated during the early to middle period of deinstitutionalization, were the earliest exemplars of psychosocial rehabilitation principles, such as community integration and normalization. They created vocational and social services independent of traditional treatment-oriented mental health programs. As previously described, their program evolution led to a need to create community-based employment options through TE programs. Subsequently, difficulties in expanding congregate work (sheltered workshop) opportunities, and the time-limited nature of TE led to the development of SE programs (Trochim et al., in press).

## The Consumer Movement

During the 1960s and 1970s, the civil rights and social justice movements and a broad-based focus on consumerism, which affected legal decisions and business conduct, set the stage for a consumer movement in mental health systems (Campbell 1991). From the 1970s to the present, a variety of self-help and empowerment-oriented organizations for the psychiatric consumer have been established. Some of the self-help efforts of persons with psychiatric disabilities were aided by relationships with independent living centers, which had typically served persons with physical disabilities (Deegan 1992). At present, there are several national organizations and hundreds of local consumer groups that are involved in advocacy and education, drop-in and social centers, information clearinghouses, and other activities (Campbell 1991). In 1991, the National Institute of Mental Health funded 14 consumer-operated service demonstration projects. One example of a consumer-operated service demonstration in Michigan is Project Stay, which mobilized consumer volunteers to provide assistance in obtaining social service benefits; medical, legal, and transportation assistance; and other instrumental supports. An evaluation of this program found that it was successful in providing such support services and that it had become an ongoing part of the local community mental health system (Mowbray et al. 1988). Early in their development, CSS and psychosocial rehabilitation theory recognized an expanded role for consumers. More recently, the concepts of consumer empowerment and consumer-operated services have emerged from the consumer movement. Overall, the consumer movement has led to a focus on the opportunity for work in integrated settings (an often expressed desire of consumers), to flexible and accessible (supportive) services that can respond to consumer preferences as to the manner of service delivery, and, in some cases, the consumer movement has led to the employment of consumers in peer-support roles. These foci of consumer concerns and advocacy dovetail with the characteristics of hybrid case-management and SE programs described below.

### Description of Hybrid Program

In 1978, the Rehabilitation Services Administration and the National Institute of Mental Health entered into a cooperative agreement to improve vocational services to persons with serious and persistent mental illness (Katz 1991). Furthering this, the 1986 amendment of the Rehabilitation Act of 1973 authorized grants to states to develop SE services for persons whose competitive employment has been limited by a severe disability. Persons with serious and persistent mental illness were specifically identified as a target group.

Recent research on vocational interventions for persons with mental illness have, directly or indirectly, given impetus to program innovations that integrate SE with other mental health services. Bond's (1987, 1992) reviews of recent research suggest that vocational programs lead to improvements in paid employment (e.g., increased average earnings and length of paid employment), for all types of employment, including sheltered work and TE, but that these vocational programs do not result in improved rates of competitive work. Additional research findings suggest that sheltered settings lead to an "institutional dependency" (Bond 1987). Patients in hospital work programs and consumers in community-based sheltered workshops and prevocational programs may benefit from vocational experiences and associated monetary compensation, but still not move toward competitive employment placements. Some surveys and a controlled study of psychosocial rehabilitation programs also suggest that when consumers are not given suitable opportunities and challenges they do not move toward independent competitive employment.

In contrast, the findings of previous research support the potential of hybrid models combining case management and employment services. Reviews by Bond (1987, 1992) suggest it may be useful to tailor interventions to individual consumer needs and interests rather than to structure the intervention on a particular vocational model. There is also evidence to suggest that ongoing follow-along supports of the type provided by case managers may be required to sustain any gains made in temporary training placements. Also, because many consumers appear to have more success the longer they are involved with a vocational program, it appears that the long-term flexible supports present in the SE model may be a significant feature of successful interventions.

Some of the most recent developments in mental health and vocational rehabilitation services have been to create hybrid combinations of case management and vocational services. Under a grant from the National Institute on Disability and Rehabilitation Research (NIDRR), Berkeley Planning Associates and the Human Services Research Institute identified and described six such model hybrid programs (H. S. Leff, R. Warren Jr., S. Raffe, et al., unpublished manuscript, 1994). A brief description of the ways these programs integrate vocational services with case management follows in the next paragraph.

The Community Companions Program, located in San Jose, California, stresses competitive employment as a desired outcome. Although it separates case management and SE, employment outcomes are seen as the responsibility of case managers as well as employment specialists. Community Support Services at West Central Services, located in Lebanon, New Hampshire, has adopted a continuous-treatment-team approach for their case management services. Case managers participate in job development and skills training for specific consumers. A vocational specialist is also considered a member of a continuous treatment team. This specialist is dedicated to general job development activities and to liaison and coordination with the local Department of Vocational Rehabilitation Office. The Building Bridges Program, located in Decatur, Illinois, is an example of a program that has created the role of a life skills coach. This person provides training, which includes socialization skills, ADL skills, and other life skills along with job skills required at a specific work site. The life skills coach coordinates support services on and off a specific work site as needed. In addition, the life skills coach may provide some basic mental health case management functions, such as linkage with needed services (for example, health care and housing) and advocacy for individual consumers. The Hospital Transition Program, located in Eugene, Oregon, has rehabilitation counselors who coordinate all services. They also provide some skills training but there are other specialists who provide skills training and job coaching. The Center for Mental Health, located in Anderson, Indiana, provides separate case management and SE programs that are integrated through regular staff meetings and case conferences, which include the individual consumer. There is also a single vocational follow-along case manager who provides ongoing support to consumers after their initial involvement with SE. Project WINS (Work Incentives and Needs Study), located in Grand Rapids, Michigan, was designed to promote the integration of case management and vocational services in two ways. First, the program requires that vocational specialists be assigned to and work closely with teams. Second, it employs consumers as peer support specialists to function in part as peer job coaches and case manager extenders. Program characteristics of Project WINS detailed below provide a context for comparing hybrid programs.

**Service focus.**   Some services studied could be classified as primarily case management and others as vocational services. However, some merged the two functions in a manner that made the distinction arbitrary. For example, the Center for Mental Health created a case manager position within its vocational service, whereas the West Central Community Support Program assigned job development and job coaching duties to its case managers.

**Team approach.**   Although all the services we investigated borrowed from the PACT team model of case management, they clearly differed in the extent to which they organized themselves as teams. Several of the services relied primarily upon individual case managers, each with their own caseload. Others totally functioned as teams.

**Vocational staff functions.**   The services studied also differed in the functions they assigned to vocational staff. Some programs had vocational specialists perform both job coaching and job development tasks. Other programs viewed the two tasks as requiring different skills and personalities and assigned different persons to the two functions.

**Use of more traditional services.**   Another way in which the programs differed was in their use of day treatment, clubhouse, and traditional vocational services such as workshops. Some programs continued to use these services, combining them with more normalizing and integrated services. Others turned totally to placing individuals in highly individualized, community-based work settings.

Despite these programmatic differences, there are several common themes that emerge strongly in each of these programs (H. S. Leff, unpublished data, 1994). First, they adopt an assertive approach to service delivery. Case managers do outreach work to engage clients who are in need of services but who, for a variety of reasons, are not receiving them or are not engaged with the system. They make an effort to motivate clients to engage in vocational rehabilitation. Second, these programs make positive vocational outcomes a key indicator of achieving community integration and normalization. Third, these programs adopt an individual approach (doing whatever it takes to find and sustain persons in employment). Persons with psychiatric disabilities have a diverse set of employment histories, coping abilities, interests, and talents. These programs tailor vocational interventions accordingly. Fourth, consumer empowerment is frequently an explicit dimension of these programs. Finally, these programs are committed to follow-along services. The term *follow-along services* refers to the ongoing monitoring of functioning and support activities provided to consumers after they have secured stability in an employment placement. Such ongoing monitoring and support have become a characteristic feature of most case management programs, and many SE programs are similarly incorporating a wider range of ongoing supports. Project WINS is an example of these common themes. As such, its principles, operating characteristics, and impact are further described below.

### Detailed Description of Project WINS

Project WINS (Kent County, Michigan) was a 3-year research demonstration project, funded by the Substance Abuse/Mental Health Administration's CSP Program. During this period of external funding, it operated to enhance vocational opportunities to eligible clients and included process and outcome evaluation components.[1] Kent County, Michigan, has a full-management community mental health (CMH) board and provides a comprehensive array of services for persons with serious and persistent mental illness. Through two agencies, all such clients are provided with case management using a team approach (ACT as well as a less intensive model). There are also two large, traditional vocational agencies, but only a minority of persons served are

---

[1] Once demonstration funding was discontinued, Project WINS was no longer able to operate as described in this narrative because of serious funding limitations at state and local levels in Michigan. However, components of WINS's services, as well as its goals and guiding principles, were retained.

mentally ill. Three major principles guided the conceptualization and implementation of Project WINS.

1. *Toward zero exclusion.* In reaction to what is often labeled creaming in traditional vocational services, WINS set out to increase vocational opportunities for all case-managed clients, with eligibility based primarily on clients' self-selection.

2. *Client self-determination.* From the point of entry, clients were seen to be in total control of the services they received from WINS and how they were delivered; every effort was made to communicate this to clients, to clearly present choices, and to encourage decision making.

3. *Choose-Get-Keep model.* WINS was designed to follow the BU Rehabilitation and Training Center model, with interventions specifically tailored to meet client needs, whatever their employment stage. Vocational opportunities provided were individualized, not following a specific program model, like the clubhouse. The goal was to procure jobs of choice in independent settings in the community, although more traditional VR placements could be offered as appropriate. The community jobs could be transitional or permanent, depending on the client's needs and desires. The amount of support and assistance was also individualized.

The major component of Project WINS's operations were the services provided by five vocational specialists (VS) assigned to seven case management teams across the two participating agencies. Each VS provided direct services to a rotating caseload of about 20 clients each from their assigned team(s). They attended team meetings and worked with case management staff to address vocational goals of WINS clients. They also provided case consultation and overall information about vocational issues to their teams. VSs' education varied from less than a B.A. to master's level. They were hired from positions in either rehabilitation or community mental health, but had to demonstrate significant experience in working with the other system. Clients could also elect to receive services from peer support specialists (PSSs), who were themselves consumers from the case management teams served. The PSSs worked with a VS as a case manager extender and also served as a role model for assigned clients. The PSSs provided services to individuals as negotiated in the WINS intervention plan for that client; for instance, helping clients to prepare resumes, set up bank accounts, acquire clothing for interviews or work, or learn the bus system. PSSs were also responsible for developing and acting as facilitators for job support groups, producing a newsletter, and carrying out other informational activities for WINS. At any one time, between four and seven PSSs were employed at WINS. Each PSS usually worked with 4–5 clients, but this could range from 1–10 (see Mowbray et al. 1996).

Eligibility was based primarily on clients' self-selection, which excluded those who defined themselves as uninterested or unable to work at that time, such as those who opted to be full-time parents or homemakers, or who labeled themselves retired. Clients with a level of medical or substance abuse disability or acute psychiatric symptomatology proscribing labor force participation were also not included. Ineligible clients could be reconsidered at any time. WINS received referrals of eligible clients from each case management team. An ongoing waiting list was kept by the project. Each VS was responsible for prioritizing the referrals by further discussing with the treatment team each individual's needs and work motivation. WINS's first contacts with priority referrals occurred either through the case manager or by the VS directly. An initial interview had the goal of obtaining a basic understanding of the client's vocational background and present needs. An overview of available services was given to facilitate understanding of vocational options and to encourage choice making according to individual interests and abilities. Those services included vocational training programs through vocational rehabilitation (VR) or community education, educational pursuits (GED, community college, or university), volunteer activity, VR placements, and part-time or full-time independent, competitive employment. WINS staff presented the vocational options in a manner that fostered self-determined choices so that clients themselves could decide their vocational endeavors.

The major categories of service provision to individual clients involved plan development, assessment, job preparation and choice, getting a job, and job maintenance.

**Plan development.** Plan development began after the initial interview, once clients made a choice to work with WINS. Vocational intervention plans were formulated in conjunction with the clients' stated interests and were written with clients in non-clinical terms. Each jointly written plan contained four parts: the vocational history, the problem statement summarizing the kind of help needed, a goal statement, and intervention activities. The latter were described in terms of what the staff would do and what the client would do. The relationship between the client and WINS was viewed as a partnership, with joint responsibilities involved.

**Assessment.** Assessment was an extended activity in WINS. It occurred concurrently with plan development, but also continued throughout service provision. Initial assessment was comprehensive, covering education, work history, and career preferences gathered over a period of time by either the VS or PSS. For clients who required a more formal assessment, the project developed an on-site assessment method of monitoring observable work behaviors and interactions, administered by a PSS. Once the initial plan was developed, WINS staff continued assessment activities throughout service provision—monitoring clients' follow-through, assessing their level of motivation, and trying to understand their perceptions of vocational activities. Having the VS sit in on case management team meetings was critical for ongoing assessment to gain awareness of clinical issues that could affect employment, such as prescribed medications and side effects, treatment compliance, substance abuse patterns, and anxiety levels. This is a distinct advantage of a hybrid model that integrates vocational services with case management.

**Job preparation and choice.**     Some WINS clients required preparation before they entered the phase of actively searching for jobs. The intervention plan specified what assistance was needed to develop or rehabilitate necessary skills and how it was to be obtained. Traditional VR services might be accessed for some clients. Assistance could also involve providing reinforcers needed to encourage work-related behaviors. Some specific tasks in the plan might be delegated to a PSS, such as learning about public transportation, helping to set up the environment or the client's schedule to better manage time and improve punctuality, or providing support in a wide variety of living and working skills. Some clients with limited job experiences received additional direction and assistance initially with job choice, such as going through want ads, obtaining information about interesting occupations, and completing vocational worksheets to identify interests, abilities, and vocational choices. For all clients, choice was a continually evolving process; as new knowledge and experiences were gained, new choices were presented.

**Getting a job.**     This phase used hands-on approaches, in keeping with the in vivo team treatment model. Staff spent a lot of time processing past work experiences with clients to maximize what could be learned about preferences and abilities. Once a strategy was selected about the type of job and/or training desired, clients had the option of getting direct assistance in obtaining it or encouragement and background support, as well as of determining how much they wanted divulged about themselves or their work histories. Advocating for clients—whether with VR, individual employers, or training institutions—was always based on clients' individual needs, emphasizing strengths and abilities. In character with the project's commitment to client-driven services, any client advocacy activities were determined by the client. Peer support specialists were used actively in the Get phase, for example, in searching want ads, participating in mock interviews, preparing resumes, filling out job applications, helping clients to use public transportation to get to interviews, and/or attending interviews. To fulfill the client choice philosophy, WINS staff were active in marketing services to employers in the public and private sectors in order to open up community-based competitive job options. Job development involved two approaches. The first was geared toward marketing with businesses that had multiple employment opportunities appealing to one or more clients. The second approach was development of a particular job for a specific client. In either case, the VS met with the employer to obtain information about specific jobs as well as to present information to the employer regarding the WINS program. This could involve persuading employers why they should hire WINS clients: that is, clients were pre-screened; and WINS offered support services and accessibility. Employers could call the VS if there were problems, and the VS would problem solve on-site. The VSs also used job development and follow-along support as opportunities to continually educate employers and decrease stigma regarding workers with a psychiatric disability.

**Job maintenance.** The active involvement of the VS at clients' case management team meetings was a key ingredient in the Keep phase. The VS presented and received status reports on his or her assigned clients and participated in treatment planning with case managers. This helped to assure that all aspects of the client's treatment were integrated and that medication or mental health interventions were complementary to job requirements. For example, the VS could advise about a particularly stressful time at work, so that a planned medication cutback might be postponed. Support through Project WINS at the job site was based on the client's concerns and perceptions of the work environment and also on the employer's expectations. As much as possible, the VS tried to determine these in advance and specify what on-site assessment and support would be provided through the client's vocational plan. If appropriate and agreeable to all parties, on-site contact was arranged. Such contact was typically facilitated by a PSS.

Either through their VS, a PSS, the case management team, or all three, individual counseling was provided on job maintenance skills: how to get along on the job, how to handle conflict, how to establish a peer group, how to avoid personalizing criticism, and so on. WINS staff gave follow-along support coupled with ongoing evaluation of vocational interests and promotion of insight about work identity. This meant that the intervention plan needed to be periodically revised, involving the clients themselves and WINS staff. In so doing, the project recognized the dynamic nature of vocational activities (clients' needs are constantly changing) as well as the importance of learning from all experiences, including those usually labeled as failures. Added work experiences also helped identify other vocational and/or treatment needs that a revised plan should address; for example, problems with use of substances. In the Keep phase, especially, WINS staff constantly encouraged attendance at the job-support group meetings. Through these contacts or one-on-one assignments, the PSSs were active in providing problem-solving assistance, for example, to deal with transportation to work, lifestyle changes required by work schedules, diet and exercise requirements, and so on. Clients were also encouraged to keep updating their resumes. Clients who were stable in the Keep phase for some time exited from WINS's specialized services back to their case management teams. Periodic exits were necessary so that cases could be opened for new clients who had not received assistance from WINS. Inactive clients could still maintain involvement with the job support group. Requests for reentry to WINS came from clients themselves, or were made when the VS attended regular case management team meetings. Over the course of WINS's demonstration phase, only a handful of clients reentered.

WINS's approach to increasing vocational opportunities not only enhanced integration with ongoing mental health services, it also addressed clients' follow-along needs. In working in a team approach with WINS staff, case managers were sensitized to and made more aware of the vocational issues that their clients faced. Thus, even when clients had exited from WINS's direct service component, advocacy and knowledgeable support for vocational involvement was likely to continue through the ongoing case management assignment.

Project WINS was also designed to effect changes in the local mental health and vocational systems. One change strategy used was hiring several VSs from the VR agencies to enhance agency commitment and to help with continuity of program learnings once the demonstration project was over. Secondly, an advisory committee was set up to meet monthly with representation from all local vocational agencies, the regional office of the State VR service, Social Security, and the two case management agencies. The project director also met routinely with the local vocational agencies in order to advise and assist in developing consumer-oriented programs that had not been previously available. As a result of these collaborative efforts, a number of program design changes and new programs were implemented within the county's MI vocational system. These included a vocational and substance abuse treatment program to specifically address the needs of consumers with a dual diagnosis of mental illness and substance abuse; a drop-in work program (with flexible hours and start times after the workshop program is usually closed) geared to address the needs of consumers who cannot handle the stress of structured work programs, or who have a limited work history; TE programs with work experience in the community; and a TE program that functions jointly with a local psychosocial (clubhouse) program to promote and foster social interaction and community integration. One of these VR programs includes a peer support component that was designed after consultation with the WINS program director.

WINS has been credited with opening up vocational slots in the county's VR system as a result of assuming responsibility for long-term follow-along support of psychiatrically disabled persons in SE positions. VR agencies also indicated that because of WINS, mental health referrals were more complete and expeditious to process because there was only one contact person per case management team. Another benefit of the increased collaboration between MH and VR is a sharing of placement slots in the community (rather than competing over the same pool of employers), thus increasing employment options for all appropriate mental health consumers.

WINS also provided an increased awareness of vocational issues and concerns within the Kent County Community Mental Health (CMH) System. With the onset of the project, Kent County CMH began a vocational planning committee. This group developed a mission statement and a long-term plan with a consumer-centered approach to vocational planning as one of its major tenets.

A summary of the accomplishments of WINS vis-à-vis the vocational activities of clients served is contained in Table 17–2. It presents a snapshot of the vocational status of clients on the caseload, quarterly from December 1991 to December 1992. The vocational achievements are diverse, suitable to the Choice emphasis of Project WINS. The number of clients employed in competitive jobs in the community steadily increased over time, in raw numbers and in percentages (from 40% to over 53%). After about 18 months of operations, about two-thirds of Project

**Table 17–2.**  Description of vocational activities for project WINS clients on the caseload as of quarterly dates

| | Quarterly date | | | | |
|---|---|---|---|---|---|
| **Vocational activity** | **12/91** | **3/92** | **6/92** | **9/92** | **12/92** |
| Employed in community work setting | 24 | 33 | 44 | 59 | 62 |
| Employed in sheltered work setting | 9 | 16 | 16 | 13 | 10 |
| Attending school | 6 | 8 | 5 | 8 | 5 |
| Day treatment/ psychosocial programs | 2 | 3 | 3 | 6 | 8 |
| Volunteer positions | 2 | 1 | 5 | 6 | 5 |
| Looking for work | 17 | 33 | 33 | 21 | 26 |
| Total caseload | 60 | 94 | 106 | 113 | 116 |

WINS's caseload was working in competitive jobs, VR placements, or going to school. The data also show that the number of clients in the Get phase (looking for work) decreased, relatively speaking, from about 28% to 22% of those on the caseload. These sets of figures reflect the success of WINS staff in finding independent jobs matched to clients' choices, and in doing so more efficiently over the duration of the project.

For a sample of WINS's clients involved in the research sample for the project ($N = 106$), service data collected showed that the duration of direct contact with WINS' staff varied from 1 month to 15 months, with a median value of 4 months. The intensity of direct contact per month also varied substantially, from less than 1 hour to 8.5 hours (median value of 1.1 hours). About 35% of this sample received the services of a PSS (probably an underestimate due to service recording problems).

Thus, the service data indicate that WINS achieved some success in getting jobs for clients and that their efficiency in doing so (especially regarding independent employment) increased over the duration of the project. The data indicate that WINS's duration of service to clients was as originally conceptualized. The somewhat lower intensity of services actually delivered may reflect the demand for WINS services, in other words, efforts to maximize coverage of all the clients being referred. It should be noted that the service data presented do not include vocational activities of the case management teams (because this was not recorded per se). A significantly higher amount of vocational activity would be observed if these figures were available because the WINS model focused on working directly with clients, as well as on a case consultation basis with their case managers.

Like the previously reported data on client work history, the service data also show the diversity of the client sample. The length and intensity of vocational services provided was highly variable. Future projects that focus on expanding vocational activities will need to anticipate this diversity in client needs in planning for staff assignments, client turnover, and total service projections. (For further information, see Mowbray et al. 1993).

# Conclusions

Hybrid models, as exemplified by Project WINS, offer the potential to overcome some of the barriers that have traditionally kept individuals with psychiatric disabilities from participating in the labor force. Through integration with case management and mental health services, they can better address individuals' internal barriers directly related to their psychiatric disability (such as medication side effects, symptomatology, etc.) and indirectly related (such as fears and anxieties due to past failure experiences, stigmatization, lack of work experiences, etc.). On an individual level, they can improve external barriers posed, such as access to training programs, VR support, and collateral services like medical treatments. However, despite these advantages, programs like WINS are still far from maximizing the employment potentials of the clients they serve. As noted by the National Institute on Disability and Rehabilitation Research (1992), individual level strategies are not sufficient to produce employment success. Substantial systems-level barriers still exist beyond those that can be addressed and successfully resolved at the individual community level.

Barriers produced by disability-related programs themselves still need to be reckoned with. Substantial attention has focused on disincentives created by SSI and SSDI program structures wherein psychiatric clients' return to work can permanently affect their ability to receive future financial support or access to medical insurance if they reexperience psychiatric problems. Improvements have been made in these regulations. However, additional corrections are still necessary (National Institute on Disability and Rehabilitation Research 1992), because clients still perceive loss of benefits as a barrier (McCrohan et al. 1994).

Perhaps less attention has been paid to several other systemic barriers. The first involves the development of educational and training opportunities, and the second, increased employment opportunities. Vocational opportunities are often conceptually limited, in the minds of service providers, consumers, and the public, to lower-level service occupations ("food and filth") or to blue-collar positions in industry. The experiences of programs working to maintain psychiatric consumers in community jobs, however, indicate the importance of having a wide array of jobs available with good pay, benefits, and career opportunities. That is, job success is optimized when there is a positive match with the consumer's job preferences and abilities (Russert and Frey 1991). Of course, given the great heterogeneity in the population of individuals with psychiatric disabilities, this can only occur if there are a range of jobs available. A wide variety of paid, part-time, volunteer, and full-time positions are needed at multiple levels and in many different settings.

Furthermore, we know that "work is a developmental process" (Russert and Frey 1991, p. 12). A better understanding of the factors relevant to the success of individual clients (such as medication, stress tolerance, and work habits) can only be achieved after the individual has tried out a variety of work experiences. Horizontal as well as vertical movement in jobs should be possible within the same or different occupational classifications. We also know that for all individuals with a vocational orientation, the attainment of higher education and more specialized training is increasingly an issue in obtaining desirable, career-oriented, good-paying jobs with benefits (Moxley et al. 1993). Research on persons with psychiatric disabilities finds that this generalization applies to them as well, in that forward occupational movement relates to number of years of education (Cook et al. 1989). Thus, many individuals need to have continuing access to higher educational opportunities as they refine their occupational choices and as they move to develop skills and abilities to match job requirements. In refining their occupational choices, individuals also need to be continually provided with information about developments in the job market and about which career paths lead to jobs that are likely to be readily available in the future, with career ladders and secure benefits.

These conclusions about what is desirable concerning vocational support and assistance are in stark contrast to what we know is currently available. Persons with psychiatric disabilities have experienced stigma and discrimination in entering higher education and in pursuing degree requirements. Little in the way of support is usually available through academic services or mental health providers; active discouragement of educational goals is often apparent (see Moxley et al. 1993, for a discussion). In the employment arena, employer bias is still noted as well as the difficulties associated with employment development and the limitations shown by current strategies (National Institute on Disability and Rehabilitation Research 1992). Herculean efforts are expended in some cases, even in conjunction with VR agencies. However, creating the appropriate range and number of vocational slots is a lot of work and is sometimes very inefficient when no incentives but goodwill can be leveraged to engage employers. It may be that larger initiatives at federal and state levels are needed to address these systemic deficits—for example, more active anti-stigma campaigns aimed at employers, educators, and mental health providers themselves; or the availability of specific incentive programs for businesses that hire individuals, or for educational institutions that enroll students with psychiatric disabilities.

Although we have continued to make progress in evolving models for increasing the vocational participation of persons with serious mental illness, it is clear that we have far to go. The vocational aspirations of persons with psychiatric disabilities have often been assailed by negative stereotypes, discrimination, and supposed good intentions of providers and caregivers. However, the employment opportunities made available and the supports necessary to sustain them have not even begun to match the vocational aspirations that our clients present. Indeed, better addressing of vocational needs and potentials is probably one of the greatest challenges facing providers of mental health services in this decade.

# References

Anthony WA: The Principles of Psychiatric Rehabilitation. Baltimore, MD, University Park Press, 1980

Anthony WA, Blanch A: Supported employment for persons who are psychiatrically disabled: an historical and conceptual perspective. Psychosocial Rehabilitation Journal 11:5–23, 1987

Anthony WA, Blanch A: Research on community support services: what have we learned? Psychosocial Rehabilitation Journal 12:55–81, 1989

Anthony WA, Jansen MA: Predicting the vocational capacity of the chronically mentally ill: research and policy implications. Am Psychol 39:537–544, 1984

Baker F, Intagliata J: Case management, in Handbook of Psychiatric Rehabilitation. Edited by Liberman RP. New York, Macmillan Publishing Company, 1992, pp 213–244

Beard JH, Propst RN, Malamud TJ: The fountain house model of rehabilitation. Psychosocial Rehabilitation Journal 5:47–53, 1982

Bingham WC: A vocational psychology perspective on rehabilitation, in Vocational Rehabilitation of Persons with Prolonged Psychiatric Disorders. Edited by Ciardiello JA, Bell MD. Baltimore, MD, The Johns Hopkins University Press, 1988, pp 137–149

Bolton B: Vocational assessment of persons with psychiatric disorders, in Vocational Rehabilitation of Persons with Prolonged Psychiatric Disorders. Edited by Ciardiello JA, Bell MD. Baltimore, MD, The Johns Hopkins University Press, 1988, pp 165–180

Bond GR: Supported work as a modification of the transitional employment model for clients with psychiatric disabilities. Psychosocial Rehabilitation Journal 11:55–73, 1987

Bond GR: Vocational rehabilitation, in Handbook of Psychiatric Rehabilitation. Edited by Liberman RP. New York, Macmillan Publishing Company, 1992, pp 244–275

Bond GR, Boyer SL: Rehabilitation programs and outcomes, in Vocational Rehabilitation of Persons with Prolonged Psychiatric Disorders. Edited by Ciardiello JA, Bell MD. Baltimore, MD, The Johns Hopkins University Press, 1988, pp 231–263

Braucht GN, Kirby MW: An empirical typology of the chronically mentally ill. Community Ment Health J 22:3–20, 1986

Brown MA, Basel D: Understanding differences between mental health and vocational rehabilitation: a key to increased cooperation. Psychosocial Rehabilitation Journal 12:23–33, 1988

Campbell JF: The consumer movement and implications for vocational rehabilitation services. Journal of Vocational Rehabilitation 1:67–75, 1991

Cook JA: Independent community living among women and men with severe mental illness. Presented at the University of Chicago, School of Social Service Administration Conference, Mental Health Research: Critical Issues for the 90s and Beyond, Chicago, IL, May 3–4, 1991

Cook JA, Razzano L: Natural vocational supports for persons with severe mental illness: Thresholds Supported Competitive Employment Program. New Directions for Mental Health Services 56:23–41, 1992

Cook JA, Roussel AE: Who works and what works: effects of race, class, age and gender on employment among the psychiatrically disabled. Paper presented at the annual meeting of the American Sociological Association, Chicago, IL, 1987

Cook JA, Solomon ML, Mock LO: What happens after the first job placement: vocational transitioning among severely emotionally disturbed and behavior disordered adolescents, in Programming for Adolescents with Behavioral Disorders, Vol IV. Edited by Broaten S, Rutherford R, Reilly R, et al. Reston, VA, Counsel for Children with Behavioral Disorders, 1989, pp 71–93

Cook JA, Jonikas JA, Solomon ML: Models of vocational rehabilitation for youths and adults with severe mental illness: implications for AMERICA 2000 and ADA. American Rehabilitation 32 (Autumn):6–11, 1992

Danley KS, Rogers ES: A psychiatric rehabilitation approach to vocational rehabilitation, in Psychiatric Rehabilitation Programs: Putting Theory into Practice. Edited by Farkas MD, Anthony WA. Baltimore, MD, The Johns Hopkins University Press, 1989, pp 81–131

Deegan PE: The independent living movement and people with psychiatric disabilities: taking back control over our own lives. Psychosocial Rehabilitation Journal 15:3–20, 1992

Donahue SA, Martin RJ, Shern DL: Adult intensive case management evaluation: second year final report. Albany, NY, New York State Office of Mental Health, 1990

Fairweather GW, Sanders DH, Cressler D, et al: Community Life for the Mentally Ill: An Alternative to Hospitalization. Chicago, IL, Aldine Press, 1969

Government Accounting Office: Comptroller General's Report to the Congress: Returning the Mentally Disabled to the Community: Government Needs To Do More. Washington, DC, U.S. Government Accounting Office, 1976

Hazel K, Herman SE, Mowbray CT: Characteristics of adults with serious mental illness in a public mental health system. Hosp Community Psychiatry 42:518–525, 1991

Herman SE, Amdur R, Hazel K, et al: Clients with Serious Mental Illness: Characteristics and Typology. Lansing, MI, Michigan Department of Mental Health, 1988

Jackson R: How work works. Psychosocial Rehabilitation Journal 16:63–67, 1992

Katz LJ: Interagency collaboration in the rehabilitation of persons with psychiatric disabilities. Journal of Vocational Rehabilitation 1:45–57, 1991

Lawn B, Meyerson AT: A modern perspective on psychiatry in rehabilitation, in Psychiatric Rehabilitation in Practice. Edited by Flexer RW, Solomon PL. Boston, MA, Andover Medical Publishers, 1993, pp 31–44

Link BG, Dohrenwend BP, Skodol AE: Socio-economic status and schizophrenia: noisome occupational characteristics as a risk factor. American Sociological Review 51:242–258, 1986

Lysaker P, Bell M, Milstein R, et al: Work capacity in schizophrenia. Hosp Community Psychiatry 44:278–280, 1993

MacDonald-Wilson KL, Revell WG, Nguyen N, et al: Supported employment outcomes for people with psychiatric disability: a comparative analysis. Journal of Vocational Rehabilitation 1:30–44, 1991

Marrone J: Creating positive vocational outcomes for people with severe mental illness. Psychosocial Rehabilitation Journal 17:43–62, 1993

McCrohan NM, Mowbray CT, Bybee D, et al: Employment histories and expectations of persons with psychiatric disorders. Rehabilitation Counseling Bulletin 38:59–71, 1994

Mowbray CT, Wellwood R, Chamberlain P: Project stay: a consumer-run support service. Psychosocial Rehabilitation Journal 12:33–42, 1988

Mowbray CT, Bybee D, McCrohan N, et al: Project WINS: initial results from an innovative CSP research demonstration project. Paper presented at the NASMHPD Research Institute Conference on State Mental Health Agency Services Research and Program Evaluation, Annapolis, MD, October 2–6, 1993

Mowbray CT, Moxley DP, Thrasher S, et al: Consumers as community support providers: challenges created by role innovation. Community Ment Health J 32:47–67, 1996

Moxley DP, Mowbray CT, Brown KS: Supported education, in Psychiatric Rehabilitation in Practice. Edited by Flexer PW, Solomon P. Boston, MA, Andover Medical Publishers, 1993, pp 137–153

National Institute on Disability and Rehabilitation Research: Consensus Statement 1(3): Strategies to Secure and Maintain Employment for People With Long-Term Mental Illness. Washington, DC, National Institute on Disability and Rehabilitation Research, 1992

Rogers ES, Anthony WA, Toole J, et al: Vocational outcomes following psychosocial rehabilitation: a longitudinal study of three programs. Journal of Vocational Rehabilitation 1:21–29, 1991

Russert MG, Frey JL: The PACT vocational model: a step into the future. Psychosocial Rehabilitation Journal 14:7–17, 1991

Sommer R, Williams P, Williams WA: Self-survey of family organizations. Psychiatr Q 56:276–285, 1984

Stroul BA: Community support systems for persons with long-term mental illness: a conceptual framework. Psychosocial Rehabilitation Journal 12:9–26, 1989

Thompson KS, Griffith EEH, Leaf PJ: A historical review of the Madison model of community care. Hosp Community Psychiatry 41:625–634, 1990

Trochim WK, Cook JA, Setze R: Using concept mapping to develop a conceptual framework of staff's views of a supported employment program for persons with severe mental illness. J Consult Clin Psychol 62:766–775, 1994

U.S. Department of Labor: Dictionary of Occupational Titles, 4th Edition. Washington, DC, U.S. Government Printing Office, 1991

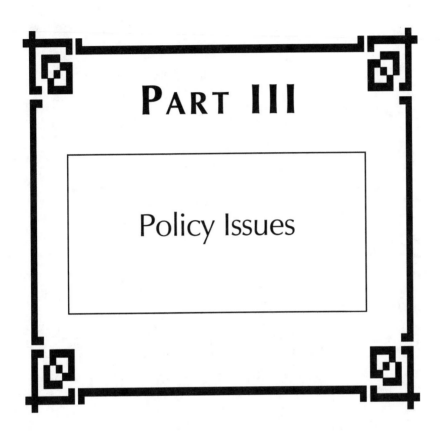

# PART III

## Policy Issues

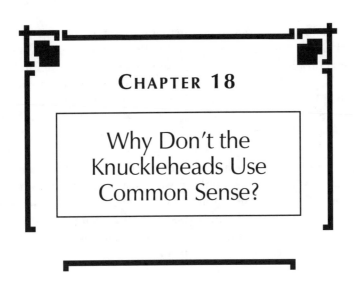

# CHAPTER 18

## Why Don't the Knuckleheads Use Common Sense?

**Gary B. Melton, Ph.D.**

Commonly available services for difficult-to-treat populations—most of the clients of the public mental health, substance abuse, child welfare, special education, and justice systems—defy common sense. Often the response is so minimal or misdirected that it is misleading to say that services are delivered at all. For example, 40% of substantiated cases of child maltreatment result in no service other than the investigation itself (McCurdy and Daro 1994). Unfortunately, when services are available, they often bear little logical relation to clients' needs.

> Seriously emotionally disturbed delinquent youth commonly not only have aroused the ire of the guardians of public order (not to mention neighbors, teachers, and parents), but they frequently have a host of other problems that are likely to be persistent across time and pervasive across situations. These include low educational achievement, distorted perceptions of social interaction, impaired problem-solving skills, troubled

and delinquent friends, conflictual family relationships, poverty, and deteriorating neighborhoods. Indeed, the list of personal problems is often longer: substance abuse, vulnerability to accidental injury, a history of maltreatment, depression, learning disabilities, and so forth. Given such a picture, why should one expect that going to an office to talk for 50 minutes a week (if indeed one can expect such a level of attendance at therapy sessions) is going to make a significant difference in the adjustment of most emotionally disturbed youth in the juvenile justice system? Similarly, when youth are removed from their homes and communities for incarceration or residential treatment, why should one expect a lasting change in their adaptation to those families and communities, once they return? (Melton and Pagliocca 1992, p. 114)

The same points about the mismatch between client and service characteristics—presentation of a multiplicity of serious problems for clients, their families, and their neighborhoods and provision of a narrowly constructed service model—could be made about the populations subject to virtually any public human service system (see, e.g., Dryfoos 1990; Osgood and Wilson 1991; Panel on High-Risk Youth 1993; U.S. Advisory Board on Child Abuse and Neglect 1993). For example, services provided after a child protection investigation (when any services are provided) often are limited to a packaged parent education program, even though there is little reason to believe that such a program by itself will prevent further maltreatment by abusive parents, who typically face enormous social, economic, and psychological problems (Olds and Henderson 1989).

By contrast, the innovative services described in this volume are based largely on common sense, as described below.

- When people have a multiplicity of serious problems, develop a multifaceted service plan.
- To maximize client involvement, go where the clients are, address problems that they find significant in their everyday lives, and do so in a form that minimizes stigma.
- To maximize the service efficacy and efficiency, work on mul-

tiple aspects of an individual's problems in the settings in which problems arise. For example, enhance the school's capacity to serve children with serious emotional disturbances, build the child client's competence in adapting to teachers' expectations and forming and maintaining peer relationships, and build the parents' competence in maneuvering through the school system.

■   To maximize the long-term efficacy and efficiency of services, design services in a manner that enhances client responsibility, that builds skills in obtaining help at times when it is needed, that develops a stable support system, and that assures a decent standard of living in a safe environment.

Given that innovative community- and family-based services rest on a commonsense foundation, why didn't someone think of them earlier? The answer, of course, is that the "innovations" have antecedents in social and mental health services across several decades. Today's client-centered, family-focused, neighborhood-based services, such as family resource centers, bear substantial resemblance to the settlement houses and community action programs of earlier days (Levine and Levine 1992; Levine and Levine, in press). Intensive, integrated-service models have clear roots in some of the best studied—but, until recently, little emulated—programs of 30 years ago (see, e.g., Hobbs 1966; Massimo and Shore 1963; Shore and Massimo 1966, 1969, 1973, 1979; Weinstein 1969).

What may be new is that the current innovations have been designed with an eye to systems of services. Mindful of the bureaucratic, professional, and fiscal pressures toward unduly specialized and rigid services, planners increasingly have attended to establishment of the interagency fiscal and administrative structures necessary to sustain integrated, flexible services. Prime examples are the Community Support Program and the Child and Adolescent Service System (CASSP) Program of the Center for Mental Health Services. Such efforts take on particular significance in light of the continuing and accelerating disruption of natural support networks (see, e.g., Garbarino 1995; Melton

1992; Panel on High-Risk Youth 1993; U.S. Advisory Board on Child Abuse and Neglect 1993)—change that results in a need to make diligent efforts not simply to use but also to construct systems of social support for people with serious, complex problems.

With such a strong and intuitive conceptual base, a history of successful implementation, and a current political foundation, the question remains why innovative services have not become conventional. Why wouldn't policy makers, program administrators, and third-party payers rush to adopt service models that—in contrast to the services that now are widely available—are inexpensive, carefully and positively evaluated, easy to understand, and consistent with long-established values of respect for family integrity and personal privacy and liberty? If an innovation is cheaper but more effective than current practices, why wouldn't it be quickly and widely adopted?

Some may argue that such change is taking place. Service system reform is taking place in remarkably diverse contexts but with a remarkably consistent conceptual foundation. In the area of child and family services alone, movements toward family-focused, integrated, or coordinated service systems have occurred in child welfare, public assistance, job training and employment programs, preschool special education, services for children with chronic health problems, primary and secondary education, and child mental health (Gittler, in press). Model programs for prevention and treatment of child abuse and neglect differ little from model programs with broader goals of family support (Wilson and Melton, in press) and narrower goals of prevention and treatment of parental substance abuse and its effects on the family (Flood 1992).

This recent change in the professional zeitgeist has been accompanied by establishment of thousands of family- and community-based programs in the United States. For example, the number of comprehensive school-based health centers (including school-based mental health services; see, e.g., Adelman and Taylor 1991) grew from single digits in the mid-1970s to about 50 in 1985 to several hundred in 1993 (Robert Wood Johnson

Foundation 1993; "School-Based Clinics," 1993). Similarly, since the development of the intensive home-based treatment model (in social service parlance, family preservation services) in the mid-1970s, such programs for troubled—often maltreating—families have become available in most states, with most of the growth having occurred since 1985 (Barthel 1992). This expansion has been supported by substantial investments on the part of several major foundations and by legislative action in about half the states (Barthel 1992; Smith 1991). Analogous programs in adult services (e.g., day treatment programs for adults with serious mental illnesses) have proliferated at a similar rate.

Such a rate of program expansion is hardly trivial. A franchiser who experienced such proliferation of a service would undoubtedly be ecstatic—and very wealthy! The pioneers of such exemplary services can be justly proud of the number of professionals who have imitated them and, more important, the number of troubled people—tens of thousands—who have received help tailored to their needs.

Considered in context, though, the innovative programs are barely significant. For example, the number of comprehensive school-based centers in the entire country is about the same as the number of schools in one or two metropolitan districts. To my knowledge, not a single community has implemented comprehensive school-based mental health services on a districtwide basis (cf. Knitzer et al. 1990). Such a modest scale of implementation—a school here, a school there—is especially remarkable when one considers that the movement for school-based centers has enjoyed the enthusiastic support of major foundations (e.g., Robert Wood Johnson Foundation 1993), influential professional associations (e.g., Council on Scientific Affairs 1989), and the general public (Elam et al. 1992).

Indeed, the direction of aggregate growth of human service programs has been opposite to the thrust of public policy and professional opinion. The growth of foster care—from about 245,000 foster children in 1985 to about 429,000 in 1991—has been far greater than the addition of family preservation programs, despite a dramatic loss in the number of foster homes, from about 137,000 to about 100,000 during the same period (Evans 1993). The expenditures for foster care have grown at a still faster rate (Gershenson 1992). Similarly, the growth of community-based alternatives in the mental health and justice systems has been dwarfed by increases in the frequency of, and expenditures for, hospitalization in general hospitals (Kiesler and Simpkins 1993), establishment of proprietary psychiatric hospitals (Dorwart and Schlesinger 1988), and incarceration in juvenile (Schwartz and Van Vleet 1992) and adult (Darrington 1994) correctional facilities.

Even when well-designed evaluations have shown innovative prevention and treatment programs to be substantially more effective and much less expensive than conventional services, the general pattern has been that the replication of model programs has been small-scale, occasional, and unsystematic. The replications continue to be perceived as demonstration programs that stand apart in their states and communities from ordinary services.

The experience that my colleagues and I have had in developing family preservation programs for serious juvenile offenders in South Carolina is illustrative. In a series of studies, we have demonstrated home- and neighborhood-based intervention to be markedly more effective and much less expensive than usual juvenile justice services for serious juvenile offenders (see, e.g., Henggeler et al. 1992, 1993; Scherer et al. 1994). These findings have been embraced with enthusiasm by state agency directors in the fields of mental health, juvenile justice, and child welfare and have been noted favorably in both news articles and editorials in South Carolina newspapers (e.g., Allard 1993; "Intervention Works," 1993). The initial federally funded demonstration programs have been sustained with fees for services and state funds, and several replications have occurred with new federal grants and additional state support.

This picture is generally quite positive, but the reality remains that administrators have failed to adopt our innovations on a broad scale. Although the grossly overcrowded conditions in South Carolina's juvenile prisons have been found to be unconstitutional, even the most adamant reformers in the state have looked primarily to less restrictive residential alternatives, despite their expense and their lack of demonstrated efficacy.

When administrators repeatedly assert their support for reform and both common sense and evaluation research clearly favor innovative over conventional services, why aren't the innovative models widely adopted? Aren't administrators able to learn from experience? Do they care only about the opinion polls? Are they so rigid that they are capable only of doing what they've always done?

Of course, some administrators and clinicians *are* unintelligent, cynical, lazy, or rigid. More often, though, the nearly universal failure to adopt innovative service models as standard practice reflects intrinsic but often tractable obstacles to reform. The remainder of this chapter identifies some of these obstacles and suggests some means to overcome them.

## Obstacles to Change

### We Just Didn't Know

The most common explanation that is given for failure to replicate successful programs—certainly the explanation that is most commonly given by administrators and clinicians themselves—is that practitioners have not been informed of them. The state of practice would match the state of the art, so the argument goes, if only the researchers would descend from the ivory tower and disseminate their findings to busy practitioners in a succinct, nontechnical, easily applicable form in an easily accessible forum.

Certainly, there is some truth to this line of argument. The evidence is clear both that practitioners are able to spend only a small portion of their time reading professional journals and that researchers have little incentive to publish in the journals that are widely read by practitioners (see, e.g., Grisso and Melton 1987). Scholars in the human services have much to learn from their peers in agriculture and other technical disciplines, which have been typified by elaborate structures for knowledge diffusion and substantial research on the process (see generally Havelock 1969; Rogers and Shoemaker 1971).

The significance of the problem of knowledge diffusion should not be overestimated, however. As in the South Carolina example, widespread adoption of innovative services seldom occurs when administrators do know the relevant findings, even when their agencies have sponsored the original research and occasional replications.

## We Just Didn't Think

A more serious problem is that many state agencies lack the planning capacity needed to implement and fine-tune new services. In working with one state social service agency, for example, we requested county-level data on reports and investigations of suspected child maltreatment. Apparently no one ever had conducted such an analysis, despite the obvious significance of such data for ongoing system management and the ease with which they could be summarized periodically. (The data in fact showed enormous variation in reporting and substantiation rates; colleagues have proposed research to identify the sources of the variation.)

This problem should be easily alleviated when data actually are being collected and there simply is no one charged with their analysis. The more fundamental problem is that there may be active resistance to scrutiny of services. This response is often not defensive; rather, it reflects a view that "everybody knows" what the situation is and what it ought to be in child and family services and some other domains of human services (cf. Melton 1987). When problems are undiscussable, careful planning becomes a near-impossibility.

## We Were Thinking About Something Else

In some instances, planning does occur, but the primary goals of policy makers are not directly related to the values underlying innovative services. For example, a failure in diversion of clients from institutional placements may rest on the desire to maintain public jobs (cf. Rothman and Rothman 1984). More subtly, development of effective alternatives to inpatient treatment may be impeded by a preoccupation with symbolic issues—for example, focusing on who has the authority to decide about treatment rather than on the need to develop and implement alternative treatments (cf. Parham v. J. R. 1979).

No other factor is as powerful, however, as money in diverting policy makers, program administrators, and clinicians from pursuit of policy goals. Medicaid, private insurance, and Title IV-E of the Social Security Act all reward out-of-home placement, but third-party payers rarely reimburse policyholders for innovative, flexible services. With such reinforcement contingencies, there is little incentive for broad adoption of innovations, even when their effectiveness has been clearly demonstrated.

## We Had to Be Sure

The fiscal issues in human services may mask more fundamental problems. It is easy to say (and is sometimes true) that the primary reason a program has not been implemented is a lack of funds. Often, though, other problems are driving policy.

Politically, a particularly formidable obstacle to adoption of home- and neighborhood-based services is the desire for certainty. I have heard policy makers who rarely use the presence of evaluation research as a factor in their decisions argue for additional replications of research on new service models, even when the relevant research base already is much stronger than for traditional, often institutional, service models.

Two points are important here. First, the service models that are featured in this book often are sufficiently flexible that it is difficult to discern whether they are being delivered—in contrast, for example, to a day of hospitalization. Therefore, administrators charged with maintaining accountability to taxpayers or investors may feel anxious about their ability to fulfill their duty when they must do case-by-case accounting and, even then, they may lack standards against which to judge the quality of care.

Second, adoption of innovations inherently requires some risk taking by relevant administrators, in that conventional practices—even if widely acknowledged to be ineffective, inefficient, and expensive—nonetheless are normative by definition. In a social context in which malpractice is defined in terms of departure from prevailing standards of practice, administrators and clinicians know that they incur a risk of condemnation and perhaps even civil liability if they diverge from conventional treatments. There is safety in numbers, even when most practitioners are pursuing courses of action that appear to defy both common sense and empirical research.

## We Could Have Seen the Forest but for the Trees

Part of the risk lies in the availability heuristic (Tversky and Kahneman 1973). Whether the case involves John Hinckley, Willie Horton, or a figure who becomes known in the local press for an especially heinous act, the public, legislators, and often administrators themselves remember particularly salient events and exaggerate their generalizability. Therefore, even if a new program is demonstrating effectiveness in reducing criminal behavior, the recidivists are the ones who typically are remembered. An aggregate increase in public safety may be lost because of the hue and cry resulting from a single case.

This failure to differentiate individual and aggregate effects has other, more subtle aspects that may present difficult ethical dilemmas. In part because of the difficulties inherent in broad-scale implementation of any innovation, administrators must be willing to accept some casualties while the bugs are being worked out. Some individuals may be worse off because they are "lost" while new service systems are being put into place.

More generally, a dilemma in child and family policy is that policies that may have desirable aggregate effects may have a catastrophic impact on individuals, and vice versa. For example, marriage as an institution is likely to be strengthened by a policy that results in making divorce extremely difficult to obtain, but such a policy would require that society knowingly subject some families to insufferable levels of conflict and even abuse. Similarly, elimination of the current system of child maltreatment reporting and investigation might result in greater safety for children in the aggregate because there would be less confusion of investigation with child protection and perhaps, therefore, more investment in development of a functional safety net for children in their everyday lives. Such a policy would result, though, in knowing tolerance of egregious wrongs against individual children. Although the dilemma is less dramatic, administrators face similar problems when they must weigh whether possible short-term harm to individual clients can be justified by the potential aggregate client benefits.

## We Didn't Know Where to Start

Another impediment to broad implementation of innovative services is that, although the ideas underlying their design often are simple, the implementation is complex. An analogy is instructive. Imagine that research showed that driving on the left side of the road had many advantages over driving on the right side and that the legislature accordingly decreed that, effective immediately, everyone would drive on the left. Undoubtedly, chaos would ensue. The word would need to get out, and people then would have to overcome well-established driving habits. The roads would have to be reengineered, road signs would have to be rewritten and relocated, and every car would need to have its steering mechanism moved. These changes would need to be implemented not only quickly but simultaneously.

This hypothetical example illustrates the complexity of broad-scale reform. Instead of changing a single behavior, service system planners must be concerned with an array of complicated policies and programs. Moreover, they must attempt to synchronize change across systems. With several systems that have essentially the same mission, change in one system alone may simply shift clients from one system to another without achieving any significant reform (see, e.g., Weithorn 1988).

## It's Hard to Teach an Old Dog New Tricks

Such attempts to integrate systems are likely to challenge professional fiefdoms. They do so in three ways. First, flexible service models almost by definition are not discipline-based. Because they blend a variety of interventions in a manner to which traditionally trained clinicians are not accustomed, they potentially threaten each of the major mental health professions.

Second, the new service models often rely on MA-level counselors, paraprofessionals, or volunteers. Given the increasingly impressive outcome research related to new service models, the new models raise questions about the necessity of extensive professional training in order to deliver (if not to design, supervise, and evaluate) mental health services.

Third, even if mental health professionals are open to new roles and nonprofessional colleagues, problems remain in implementing the new service models. Traditional training and practice probably creates negative transfer in learning integrated service models. Such models require experienced clinicians not only to adopt some new strategies but also to unlearn old habits. For example, it is probably easier to develop a home-based practice when one has not had an office-based practice. It is hard to jettison comfortable routines (e.g., scheduled office visits)—a necessity in many of the new service models.

These issues have two implications for policy makers and program administrators. First, they sometimes will encounter resistance by the professional guilds. Because the relevant client populations are found primarily in the public mental health system (if they currently are in the mental health system at all), this political problem generally is not as serious as it first appears. Nonetheless, policy makers and program administrators often will find that they have to spend some time justifying the use of clinicians without terminal degrees.

A second, more serious problem is that the pool of clinicians (whatever their degrees) who are trained and experienced in integrated service models is small. Moreover, expansion of the pool through training of new clinicians who may not have traditionally requisite degrees may require rewriting of Medicaid standards, negotiation with private third-party payers, and redesign of civil service classifications. In short, even if administrators want to adopt new approaches to treatment of difficult-to-treat populations, they may be stymied, at least for the short-term, by a lack of human resources.

## We Needed a New Coach

Another problem in implementing highly flexible, individualized service models is that, by definition, they require creativity in design and implementation of treatment plans. The problem involved in replicating a program that has flexibility as a hallmark is obvious.

In that regard, the most highly regarded demonstration programs typically have the same leader with which they began (see Wilson and Melton, in press), and evaluation studies of treatment innovations typically focus on programs that the researcher himself or herself designed. Questions remain about how well flexible service models can be taught and how well such programs can be replicated by people who do not have the vision and enthusiasm of the program originators.

Although the ideas underlying the new service models are simple, their implementation is complex. There may be a need for development of a corps of highly trained program administrators who have no difficulty seeing relationships among factors, who are skilled in ongoing program evaluation, and who can design and fine-tune programs and treatment plans to manipulate factors preventing healthy adaptation as well as factors promoting such an outcome.

## Small Is Beautiful

A variant of the replication problem is that, with rare exceptions, demonstration programs are small-scale. There is a question whether treatment flexibility can be maintained as programs grow and, by growing, become bureaucratized, with concomitant demands for accountability up and down the hierarchy.

Beyond the special issues in large-scale replication of flexible service models, the tasks involved in building a large-scale program are far different from those involved in implementing the same service model on a small scale. Consider the difference in development of human resources and assurance of program integrity between the two programs. Similarly, imagine the difference between financing a program for 20 clients in one location and the problem of financing a program for 10,000 clients in widely dispersed locations.

## The Budget Was Tight This Year

Although the new service models often are much cheaper on a per-client basis than are their institutional counterparts, a major issue in financing such programs is that they typically require new (rather than redirected) money. Given that institutional programs now consume the lion's share of resources in mental health, corrections, and juvenile justice and that many of the new service models have arisen from a desire to minimize out-of-home placements, institutional budgets are the logical targets for administrators seeking funds for innovative programs.

Although such a strategy is logical, it also typically has five major flaws. First, because many institutional costs are fixed, downscaling (without closing) facilities generally results in few savings.

Second, because many facilities are overcrowded (especially in corrections and juvenile justice), downscaling may result in no savings because the cost of delivering humane care to the number of residents who remain is essentially the same as the amount that had been spent (inadequately) on a much larger number of residents. Accordingly, even the costs that are unfixed (e.g., staff costs where civil service and union rules do not prohibit releasing or transferring staff as the client load decreases) are unlikely to be recovered.

Third, the availability of new, less restrictive programs may result in net widening that increases the boundaries of the client population well beyond the pool of clients who are released or diverted from residential programs.

Fourth, even if the cost of administering an institutional program diminishes, there is no guarantee that the savings will follow the clients. Third-party payers' policies may limit reimbursement to inpatient programs. Even if state-appropriated dollars are freed, mental health program administrators may find themselves competing with highway builders, university presidents, hospital and nursing home administrators, and prison superintendents for the loose cash.

The last point implies the real kicker. A de facto requirement for new dollars in order to implement innovative programs, however effective they may be, is likely to be impossible—or at least very difficult—to meet. In a slow-growth economy, state budgets are likely to continue to be strangled by prison construction, health care, and infrastructure repair and replacement. Accordingly, program developers must be creative not only in leveraging existing potential sources of funding but also in creating new ones (E.g., creative employee benefit menus).

## The Need for Planning

There can be no doubt that broad-scale system reform is difficult, even when proposed reforms comport with common sense. That it is difficult does not mean that policy makers are mean-spirited or stupid. Rather, the level of difficulty suggests the need to build a much stronger planning apparatus than is typical in government agencies, especially at state and county levels.

To develop a fairer, more efficient, and more complex service system for those people who are most in need of help, policy makers must create opportunities to apply new preventive and therapeutic technologies, or at least they must be prepared to take advantage of them as they arise. Health care reform is an example. As shown by a recent General Accounting Office (1993) study of preventive services for children in several industrialized countries with universal health care, well-child care could serve as the base for a host of preventive social and health services of documented efficacy. Such integration also could apply to children and adults who already have serious mental health problems. Mental health planners ought already to be designing such systems in such a way that they could be incorporated into whatever health-care system ultimately emerges.

Systematic planning also can overcome the hurdles in moving from demonstration program to modal practice. An important first step is analyzing the key problems in accomplishing such incorporation of innovations into conventional practice. For example, the author of this chapter is currently helping to construct a planning process for districtwide and ultimately statewide school-based mental health services. Community task forces are systematically addressing programmatic, curricular, community, and fiscal issues that must be resolved.

Another general point is that rational construction of a system of services will be facilitated by an ongoing commitment to research. In that regard, research itself should be seen as an intervention. By its nature, research results in more careful practice, a commitment to innovation, and communication of respect for clients. Asking clients what they think and indicating concern about the quality of services are steps that themselves are important ethically and perhaps therapeutically. Most important for systems change, the establishment of new programs as demonstration projects with rigorous evaluation components permits legislators and administrators to go out on a limb with minimal risk and ultimately results in data that may be persuasive in promoting systemwide innovations.

In short, the irrationality and, to some degree, randomness of the existing service system is typically not the product of ignorance or blind resistance. It is the result in part, though, of a failure to recognize and implement careful planning and systemic research. We can do better to match the state of practice to the state of the art.

# References

Adelman HS, Taylor L: Mental health facets of the school-based health center movement: need and opportunity for research and development. Journal of Mental Health Administration 18:272–283, 1991

Allard J: Going to source: family based programs help youths, DYS finds. The State, Columbia, SC, May 24, 1993, p. 4B

Barthel J: For Children's Sake: The Promise of Family Preservation. New York: Edna McConnell Clark Foundation, 1992

Council on Scientific Affairs: Providing medical services through school-based health programs. JAMA 261:1939–1942, 1989

Darrington D: Testimony on behalf of the National Conference of State Legislatures before the House Judiciary Committee, Intellectual Property and Judicial Administration Subcommittee, February 10, 1994

Dorwart RA, Schlesinger M: Privatization of psychiatric services. Am J Psychiatry 145:543–553, 1988

Dryfoos JG: Adolescents at Risk: Prevalence and Prevention. New York, Oxford University Press, 1990

Elam SM, Rose LC, Gallup AM: The 24th annual Gallup/Phi Delta Kappa poll of the public's attitudes toward the public schools. Phi Delta Kappan 74:41–53, 1992

Evans G: Foster Care Facts and Figures. Houston: National Foster Care Association, 1993

Flood MF: Innovative (and Successful!) Programs: A Presentation for Rural Nebraska Communities on Program Options for Helping Substance Using Pregnant Women and Parents. Unpublished manuscript, University of Nebraska—Lincoln, Center on Children, Families, and the Law, 1992

Garbarino J: Growing up in a socially toxic environment: life for children and families in the 1990s, in the Nebraska Symposium on Motivation: Vol. 42. The Individual, the Family, and Social Good: Personal Fulfillment in Times of Change. Edited by Melton GB. Lincoln, University of Nebraska Press, 1995, pp 1–20

General Accounting Office: Preventive health care for children: experience from selected foreign countries (Report No. GAO/HRD-93-62). Washington, DC, General Accounting Office, 1993

Gershenson C: Statement before the U.S. Advisory Board on Child Abuse and Neglect at a symposium on family foster care, Washington, DC, January 8, 1992

Gittler J: Efforts to reform services for children and families: the lessons to be learned, in Toward a Child-Centered, Neighborhood-Based Child Protection System. Edited by Melton GB. Lincoln, University of Nebraska Press, in press

Grisso T, Melton GB: Getting child development research to legal practitioners: what way to the trenches? in Reforming the Law: Impact of Child Development Research. Edited by Melton GB. New York, Guilford, 1987, pp 146–176

Havelock RG: Planning for innovation through dissemination and utilization of knowledge. Ann Arbor, University of Michigan, Institute for Social Research, Center for Research on Utilization of Knowledge, 1969

Henggeler SW, Melton GB, Smith LA: Family preservation using multisystemic treatment: an effective alternative to incarcerating serious juvenile offenders. J Consult Clin Psychol 60:953–961, 1992

Henggeler SW, Melton GB, Smith LA, et al: Family preservation using multisystemic treatment: long-term follow-up to a clinical trial with serious juvenile offenders. Journal of Child and Family Studies 2:283–293, 1993

Hobbs N: Helping disturbed children: psychological and ecological strategies. Am Psychol 21:1105–1115, 1966

Intervention works best. The State, Columbia, SC, June 21, 1993, p. 6A

Kiesler CA, Simpkins CG: The Unnoticed Majority in Psychiatric Inpatient Care. New York, Plenum, 1993

Knitzer J, Steinberg Z, Fleisch B: At the Schoolhouse Door: An Examination of Programs and Policies for Children with Behavioral and Emotional Problems. New York, Bank Street College of Education, 1990

Levine M, Levine A: Helping Children: A Social History. New York, Oxford University Press, 1992

Levine M, Levine A: The historical context: lessons from the settlement house movement and the war on poverty, in Toward a Child-Centered, Neighborhood-Based Child Protection System. Edited by Melton GB. Lincoln, University of Nebraska Press, in press

Massimo JL, Shore MF: The effectiveness of a vocationally oriented psychotherapy. Am J Orthopsychiatry 33:634–643, 1963

McCurdy K, Daro D: Child maltreatment: a national survey of reports and fatalities. Journal of Interpersonal Violence 9:75–94, 1994

Melton GB: The clashing of symbols: prelude to child and family policy. Am Psychol 42:345–354, 1987

Melton GB: It's time for neighborhood research and action. Child Abuse Negl 16:909–913, 1992

Melton GB, Pagliocca PM: Treatment in the juvenile justice system: directions for policy and practice, in Responding to the Mental Health Needs of Youth in the Juvenile Justice System. Edited by Cocozza JJ. Seattle, WA, National Coalition for the Mentally Ill in the Criminal Justice System, 1992, pp 107–139

Olds DL, Henderson CR: The prevention of maltreatment, in Child Maltreatment: Theory and Research on the Causes and Consequences of Child Abuse and Neglect. Edited by Cichetti D, Carlson V. Cambridge, England, Cambridge University Press, 1989, pp 722–763

Osgood DW, Wilson JK: Covariation among health compromising behaviors in adolescence. Prepared for the Adolescent Health Project of the U.S. Congress, Office of Technology Assessment. Springfield, VA, National Technical Information Service, 1991

Panel on High-Risk Youth, National Research Council: Losing Generations: Adolescents in High-Risk Settings. Washington, DC, National Academy Press, 1993

Robert Wood Johnson Foundation: The answer is at school: bringing health care to our students. Washington, DC, Robert Wood Johnson Foundation, 1993

Rogers EM, Shoemaker JF: Communication of Innovations, 2nd Edition. New York, Free Press, 1971

Rothman, DJ, Rothman SM: The Willowbrook Wars. New York, Harper and Row, 1984

Scherer DG, Brondino MJ, Henggeler SW, et al: Multisystemic family preservation therapy with rural and minority families of serious adolescent offenders: preliminary findings from a controlled clinical trial. Journal of Emotional and Behavioral Disorders 2:192–206, 1994

School-based clinics gaining greater acceptance across U.S. Nation's Health, November 1993, p 7

Schwartz IM, Van Vleet R: Public policy and the incarceration of juveniles: directions for the 1990s, in Juvenile Justice and Public Policy. Edited by Schwartz IM. New York, Lexington Books, 1992, pp 151–164

Shore M, Massimo J: Comprehensive vocationally oriented psychotherapy for adolescent delinquent boys: a follow-up study. Am J Orthopsychiatry 36:609–616, 1966

Shore MF, Massimo J: Five years later: a follow-up study of comprehensive vocationally oriented psychotherapy. Am J Orthopsychiatry 39:769–774, 1969

Shore MF, Massimo J: After ten years: a follow-up study of comprehensive vocationally oriented psychotherapy. Am J Orthopsychiatry 43:128–132, 1973

Shore MF, Massimo J: Fifteen years after treatment: a follow-up study of comprehensive vocationally oriented psychotherapy. Am J Orthopsychiatry 49:240–245, 1979

Smith SL: Family Preservation Services: State Legislative Initiatives. Denver, CO, National Conference of State Legislatures, 1991

Tversky A, Kahneman D: Availability: a heuristic for judging frequency and probability. Cognitive Psychology 5:207–232, 1973

U.S. Advisory Board on Child Abuse and Neglect: Neighbors Helping Neighbors: A New National Strategy for the Protection of Children. Washington, DC, U.S. Government Printing Office, 1993

Weinstein L: Project Re-Ed schools for emotionally disturbed children: effectiveness as viewed by referring agencies, parents, and teachers. Exceptional Children 35:703–711, 1969

Weithorn LA: Mental hospitalization of troublesome youth: an analysis of skyrocketing admission rates. Stanford Law Review 40:773–838, 1988

Wilson K, Melton GB: Exemplary neighborhood-based programs for child protection, in Toward a Child-Centered, Neighborhood-Based Service System. Edited by Melton GB. Lincoln, University of Nebraska Press, in press

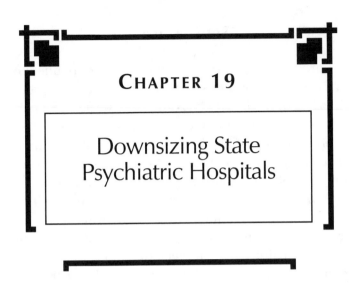

# CHAPTER 19

## Downsizing State Psychiatric Hospitals

**Paul A. Deci, M.D., Elizabeth C. McDonel, Ph.D.,
Jeanette Semke, Ph.D., Trevor R. Hadley, Ph.D.,
Michael Hogan, Ph.D., James K. Dias, Ph.D.,
Bernice A. Pescosolido, Ph.D., and Eric R. Wright, Ph.D.**

Thirty-three state mental health authorities downsized one or more state psychiatric hospitals in 1993, according to the State Mental Health Authority Profiling System of the National Association of State Mental Health Program Directors Research Institute (National Association of State Mental Health Program Directors Research Institute 1994). Relatively little research has been done on the process of downsizing state psychiatric hospitals, on the corresponding process of developing enhanced systems for providing community mental health services, and on the impact of these system changes on their targeted populations. In this chapter, we describe the initiation and ongoing evaluation of hospital downsizing projects in three states and we provide an overview of the political, systems, legal, fiscal, and organizational circumstances that potentially affect the downsizing process.

# South Carolina

South Carolina has a history of being highly dependent on institutional care. Its long-term-care state psychiatric hospitals, South Carolina State Hospital (SCSH) and Crafts-Farrow State Hospital (CFSH), are centrally located in Columbia. They both are outdated physical plants in need of much renovation. The U.S. Department of Justice entered into a consent decree with South Carolina in 1986 mandating that the state rapidly move toward a community-based system of care and that it markedly improve the conditions and treatment at the state hospitals.

South Carolina is only one of six states that has a centralized state mental health system in which the state psychiatric hospitals and community mental health centers (CMHCs) are owned and operated by the state department of mental health. Joseph J. Bevilacqua, Ph.D., former commissioner of mental health in Rhode Island and Virginia, was recruited to be director of the South Carolina Department of Mental Health (SCDMH). The director works for a commission whose members are appointed by the governor and approved by the legislature. South Carolina's state government consists of a strong legislature and a governor with limited powers. Although the centralized system appears to be relatively easy to change, it is complicated by each of the 17 CMHCs' having a local board, which is appointed by local legislators. This results in a situation in which the CMHCs are both state agencies under the direction of the director of mental health and local agencies answerable to local boards with strong legislative connections.

Dr. Bevilacqua set out to develop a consensus of all interested parties for a transition plan to move the institution-dependent system to a community-based system of care. In February 1989, the SCDMH hosted a national (NIMH-funded) conference to explore the process by which other states had made the transition to community-based services. A Transitional Leadership Council was appointed by Dr. Bevilacqua in the spring of 1989 with all the major interest groups represented (i.e., advocacy groups as well as staff from hospitals, the central office, and the CMHCs).

This council established six broad principles or goals to guide the transition process: implement the transition through the use of a joint management council; establish a funding plan using the patient-paying-fee account as bridge funds for the transition; establish a public academic liaison program with the state's colleges and universities to prepare the workforce that would accomplish the transition; establish a working environment supportive to staff pursuing careers in public mental health; establish a regional capability only for those services that cannot be provided close to home; and establish a systemwide client and management information system to monitor and evaluate the accomplishment of goals and objectives (South Carolina Department of Mental Health 1990). Public support was elicited through a series of statewide public forums during the spring and summer of 1990. Over a thousand people attended these town meetings to debate the plan, express their concerns, and help develop strategies for achieving its aims.

In 1991, a joint management and implementation group known as the Transition Council was created. This group surveyed all 665 long-term care adult psychiatric patients in the state's psychiatric hospitals to determine patient functioning and needs and to guide the Council in their efforts. The Council decided after much deliberation to downsize and consolidate the two existing long-term care facilities and to not build replacement hospitals. Priority was placed on enhancing community services while reducing the census and budgets of the state hospitals in the face of shrinking state appropriations and increasing dependence on Medicaid revenue.

Even though a general consensus was developed, there was still resistance and doubt from various parts of the system and anxiety about job security for hospital employees. Labor organizations are very limited in South Carolina so this was not a major concern as it has been in other states. However, in order to move the transition ahead and to address the concerns of employees, the director pledged that no layoffs would occur, although some staff would be transferred to community programs or other facilities.

In order to facilitate the dramatic system changes necessary, the Council in February 1992 issued a request asking the CMHCs for proposals to develop programs that would move a specific number of long-term care psychiatric patients from their catchment areas into their community. Any project was considered as long as it provided appropriate residence, medication monitoring, psychiatric and general medical services, assertive case management and outreach, meaningful daily activity, and employment assistance. All projects had to include an evaluation of service implementation and patient outcomes.

Sixteen Towards Local Care (TLC) project proposals were received from 12 CMHCs. The proposals were reviewed and ranked by a subcommittee of the Council. Based on available SCDMH funds of $2.9 million set aside in FY 1992–1993, eight projects from seven CMHCs were funded in July 1992 according to their ranking. These eight projects proposed to move a total of 145 patients into the community over a 2-year period from July 1992 to July 1994. Two of the projects were targeted at adult patients from SCSH, two at geriatric patients from CFSH, and four were designed for a mix of both groups from both hospitals. Of the eight projects, three used supervised apartments as their primary residential placement, two used the shared private home model of adult foster care (see Chapter 13), one used contracted enhanced proprietary residential care facilities, and the remaining two used a flexible mix of residential options. All of the projects included intensive and assertive case management, with staff-to-patient ratios ranging from 1:4 to 1:10 and 24-hour-a-day staff availability. High priority was placed on continuity of care and caregivers and the individualization of services and placements based on patient strengths, needs, and preferences.

The primary goals of the TLC evaluation were to evaluate the outcomes and costs of the eight TLC programs, to survey consumer perceptions and satisfaction regarding the TLC programs, and to provide timely information to SCDMH policy makers to guide decisions related to the continuing transition to local care. Secondary goals included the education of hospital and staff about successful patient placement in the community and the incorporation of objective assessment instruments into wider hospital and community practice.

The uncontrolled evaluation assesses patients in the eight programs using repeated measures (baseline and at 6-month intervals). There is staggered entry of patients into the programs over time. To be eligible the person must be a long-term psychiatric inpatient at SCSH or CFSH with length of stay on their current admission exceeding 90 days. If the patient's length of stay on his or her current admission is less than 90 days, the patient must have a prior history of long-term hospitalizations and must be at high risk for continued hospitalization. In addition, the patient must be 18 years of age or older, must not require 24-hour skilled nursing services, and must not have severe assaultive or other dangerous behavior not associated with psychosis.

Measures assess demographics, functioning (American Psychiatric Association 1987; Leff et al. 1985; Schneider and Struenig 1983), quality of life (Lehman 1988), symptomatology (Derogatis 1977), alcohol and substance use, medication usage and compliance, information on the use of mental health services (obtained from clinical service tickets and hospital databases), costs, and consumer satisfaction.

As of September 1, 1993, 123 patients had been discharged from SCSH and CFSH into the eight TLC programs. Fifty-five patients were living in supervised apartments, 20 were in residential care facilities, 18 were living independently, 17 were in Homeshare adult foster-care placements, 2 were living with family, and 11 had been returned to the hospital. Preliminary baseline results are presented below on 73 subjects from seven of the projects (information on 50 subjects from one of the projects was not yet available). Of the 73 TLC patients, 62% were male and 38% were female; 53% were white and 47% were black. The average age was 53 years, with a range from 20 to 78 years. The average educational level was 11 years, with a range from 3 to 16 years. The average length of stay during the patient's hospitalization just prior to entry into the TLC program was 2 years, with a range from 1 to 9 years. The average amount of money received by patients in the hospital per month was $295, with a range from $0–$915. Fifty-one percent had never married, 3% were currently married, 11% were divorced, 25% were widowed, and 8% were separated. Primary Axis 1 diagnoses were available on 61 of the 73 subjects. Of these 61 patients, 41 had schizophrenia, 9 had schizoaffective disorder, 4 had bipolar mood disorder, and 7 had organic mental disorders. The mean Global Assessment of Functioning score for the 73 subjects was 55, with a range from 21 to 82, and an instrument range from 1 to 90; 90 represented the highest functioning. The mean Resource Associated Functional Level Scale score was 4, with a range from 2 to 6 and an instrument range from 1 to 7; 7 represented the highest functioning. The mean total Specific Level of Functioning score was 165, with a range from 102 to 209; the scale's highest functioning score was 215, going down to a lowest possible functioning score of 43. The mean SCL30R score was 56, with a range of 30–111 and an instrument range of 30–150; 150 was the most symptomatic score. On the Quality of Life Interview general satisfaction item, the median score was 5 (mostly satisfied) on an instrument scale of 1–7, with 1 being terrible and 7 being delighted. Fifty-two percent of the patients were pleased (delighted, pleased, or mostly satisfied), 21% were mixed, 19% were dissatisfied (terrible, unhappy, or mostly dissatisfied), and 8% didn't know about their general satisfaction.

Both hospital and community staff have been surprised at the success of the programs as measured by client community tenure and functioning. In the 1991 long-term-care inpatient survey, hospital and community staff jointly indicated that 70% of the inpatients would require residential care facilities, nursing homes, or mental retardation facilities for successful discharge. They indicated that only 3% would be able to live independently. The preliminary data from the TLC evaluation have helped change the attitudes and practices of hospital and community staff alike and have changed the most skeptical critics of the transition toward local care into supporters. Plans are being made for further expansion and dissemination of these and similar programs throughout all of South Carolina's community mental health centers along with continued downsizing of the state's long-term-care hospitals. The evaluation will continue as a valued part of the process of downsizing state hospitals and making the transition to a local system of care for people with severe mental illnesses.

# Indiana

In 1992 Indiana's governor announced that Central State Hospital in Indianapolis, the oldest of Indiana's seven state-operated psychiatric hospitals, would close. The Indiana Division of Mental Health (IDMH) had been interested in closing or downsizing parts of its state-run psychiatric hospital system for a number of years and redeploying these resources to improve community-based services for persons with severe mental illness. In addition, the physical plant needed capital improvements estimated at $5 million–$8 million in order to meet code deficiencies. In 1974, and over the subsequent years, several reports generated by planning committees at IDMH or by Indiana's Legislative Services Agency (ILSA) recommended downsizing of inpatient facilities and increasing development of community-based services (e.g., Indiana Department of Mental Health 1988; Indiana Legislative Services Agency 1984, 1990, 1991; Little 1974; Murray 1980).

The political climate became more favorable to serious pursuit of this goal following five well-publicized patient deaths in Central State Hospital occurring between 1990 and 1992. Through the end of the 1993 legislative session, the closure of Central State became the primary focus of attention for Indiana's state legislature's Long-Term Needs of Persons with Developmental Disabilities and Mental Illness Study Committee (which was formed by an act of the 1991 legislative session). The Senate Finance Committee held a public hearing in 1993 to hear testimony about the closure of Central State; this hearing was well-attended and covered extensively by the local media. Leaders of neighborhood organizations and private, nonprofit social service agencies asked for more involvement in planning and implementation of the closure. Labor union (AFSCME) representatives addressed job security of hospital employees as well as the appropriateness of hospital closures.

The principles and proposed funding mechanism for community care of persons with severe and persistent mental illness were spelled out in Indiana House Bill 1702: Mental Health Care Reform. This bill proposed a number of reforms of the public mental health system in Indiana; it was forwarded by IDMH and debated during the 1993 legislative session. This bill initially passed the Indiana House with little resistance and by unanimous vote. However, when the bill was forwarded to the Indiana Senate, a controversial amendment (Senate Bill 57) to transfer authority for closing Central State from the governor to the legislature was added to House Bill 1702. This amendment caused the bill to go to a committee of two Democrats and two Republicans; this committee debated the inclusion of the amendment until the final hours of the legislative session but could not reach a unanimous decision, and so the bill died in committee.

To finance the closure, Indiana state government created a special Community Mental Health Transition Fund of $3.3 million for FY 1993 to develop new community services for approximately 170 persons. This money was an IDMH reallocation of CMHC funds. The preclosure budget for Central State Hospital was approximately $23 million for a census of 409 patients.

To build new community services, IDMH formed planning committees, held focus groups with clinical staff from Indiana's 30 CMHCs, wrote standards for new programs it wanted to fund, and issued requests for proposals from Indiana's CMHCs for new services to support patients discharged from Central State.

Concurrent with the plan for closing Central State Hospital (Indiana Division of Mental Health 1992, 1993a) and the reorganization of IDMH, with its attendant changes and turnover in central office staffing, the Hoosier Assurance Plan was drafted and implementation was begun (Indiana Division of Mental Health 1993a). This plan spelled out many significant and controversial changes in the organization and financing of services in the public mental health system. Most importantly, the plan refocused the priority for persons who are at or below 185% of poverty level in the following clinical populations: adults with serious mental illness, children with serious emotional disorders, and substance abusers.

Indiana's 30 community mental health centers constitute a network of private, nonprofit agencies providing comprehensive outpatient mental health services to all of Indiana's 92 counties. The seven psychiatric inpatient hospitals are public and are centralized as part of Indiana's Division of Mental Health. In 1985, a Justice Department consent decree affected Central State and Logansport hospitals; this decree established staffing patterns in major clinical disciplines and dealt with life-safety code issues. Annual compliance reviews are ongoing.

Since the reorganization, budget cutbacks and transfers of money to other divisions have occurred. Thus, the closure is concurrent with significant and substantial changes in the fiscal operations of IDMH. Also since that time, the CMHCs increased their dependence on Medicaid revenues, especially after the Medicaid Rehabilitation Option was implemented in 1992.

A recent development is the growing concern about potential massive employee layoffs or transfers of employees to other facilities. State personnel policy allows for transfers of more senior Central State Hospital staff to other state facilities within the same county, with the potential displacement of more junior staff. Thus, personnel changes at Central State will have substantial impact on the organizational environments of one other state psychiatric hospital and the IDMH central office. It is reasonable to conclude that the political and services system contexts surrounding the closure are marked by major concurrent systems changes and a degree of media attention that is atypical for mental health issues.

In order to track discharged patients, data are collected monthly through telephone interviews from six CMHCs and case managers from residential settings, supplemented with information from the client and other community sources as necessary. The tracking service answers the following questions for each discharged patient: Where is the client living? What medical and psychiatric services is the client receiving? What CMHC is the outpatient gatekeeper of services? What medications is the client currently receiving? What is the client's global level of functioning? What significant health problems is the client currently experiencing? Has the client spent any days in an inpatient facility or a jail, or been arrested in the last month? Does the client have any special problems for receiving outpatient services?

To examine the impact of Central State closure on the clients, their families, and the community, all clients discharged from Central State Hospital after March 23, 1992 (approximately 300) will be assessed at baseline and 6 months into community life using the following measures. A detailed chart review will be conducted to collect basic demographic and clinical information on all discharged clients. A series of three 30-minute, confidential, face-to-face interviews conducted with the patient in the month prior to being discharged (each client receives compensation for participation) focuses on changes in discharged patients' social networks in transition from inpatient to outpatient treatment settings, and the influence of those social ties on patient symptoms, attitudes, and behaviors. These symptoms, attitudes, and behaviors include opinions and reactions to the decision to close CSH, expectations and fears about life after discharge, overall quality of life, client satisfaction with hospital and social services, use of services, number and types of personal relationships to others in the hospital and in the community (both positive and negative), subjective health status and perceived stress, sexual relationships, sexual risk behaviors, employment, financial resources, self-esteem/mastery, subjectively experienced stigma, devaluation and discrimination experienced from others, medication compliance/side effects/usage, service needs, attitudes and beliefs about mental illness, perceived role of medications in treating mental illness, alcohol and drug use, and safety and victimization rates. To assess networks, client-identified community caregivers will be contacted and invited to participate in a similar confidential, face-to-face interview within a month of the focal client's interview. Domains to be measured include demographics, reactions, and expectations related to the hospital closing, the feelings and responsibilities the family or community caregivers experience because of the focal client's illness, and their perceptions of the client's overall quality of life. Additional domains will be added to the postmeasures, including information about clients' violent behaviors and experience of victimization, and about costs of care.

# Washington

One policy issue addressed by the Washington State Mental Health Reform Act of 1989 (2SSB5400) was the use of inpatient psychiatric services. Policy makers were concerned that a considerable number of individuals with mental illness experience inappropriate psychiatric hospitalizations or unnecessarily long hospital stays due to lack of alternatives in the community for mental health treatment. Several mandates within the Act focused upon stabilizing the state psychiatric hospital census and serving mental health consumers in the least restrictive setting. In implementing the 1989 legislation (to be phased in over 6 years), managers of the Washington State Mental Health Division (MHD) launched a strategic plan to shift greater service resources to high users of psychiatric hospital services. Prior hospital use became a principal basis for targeting public mental health services in Washington State through performance contracts.

In Washington State, "high users," meaning the approximately 38% of individuals who experience a psychiatric hospitalization in a 2-year period, account for 92% of total hospital bed days in that same period. The Washington State Mental Health Division defines high users as those individuals who, in a 2-year period, experience at least one hospitalization of 30 days or more or three or more hospital admissions. All publicly funded hospitalizations that occur in state hospitals, community hospitals, and freestanding private hospitals are included.

Essentially, the Washington State legislature mandated a multicomponent intervention aimed at increasing the capacity of local mental health authorities to provide outpatient alternatives to inpatient psychiatric treatment, at reducing unnecessary psychiatric hospitalizations, and at treating patients requiring short hospital stays within local communities. The intervention decentralized the mental health system, provided new dollars to develop comprehensive community support programs, set in place financial incentives to reduce use of the two state psychiatric hospitals, and created linkages between local mental health authorities and state and community hospitals. In contrast to the initiatives in Indiana and South Carolina that downsized hospitals, the Washington plan did not explicitly call for hospital or ward closures. It did, however, allow for the possibility that ward closures could occur.

Washington State centralized fiscal, clinical, and administrative authority for all public patient care at the level of the local mental health authorities (Frank and Goldman 1989). The State MHD contracts out mental health service to authorities called Regional Support Networks (RSNs), which are composed of counties or groups of counties. Each RSN takes responsibility for all outpatient client services and resources within its region. It is hypothesized that heavy use of psychiatric hospital services will be reduced when one organizational entity has control over the full array of psychiatric services supplied to an individual (Harris and Bergman 1988; Stein 1989; Taube and Goldman 1989). This control enables the local mental health authority to track all mental health treatment experiences for an individual client over time and to select less costly community care over hospital care when it is clinically appropriate.

Each RSN bears the responsibility for identifying individuals most in need and admitting them into ongoing services. Fundamental to the intent of a single point of responsibility for mental health care are procedures for assigning an RSN of residence to each consumer. The RSN determines who is admitted into psychiatric units for acute care, who receives ongoing services in residential or community support programs, and when services are discontinued for consumers no longer in need.

During the first 3.5 years of reform, Washington State MHD gradually consolidated mental health funding from diverse sources into a single block grant. These sources include grants-in-aid, residential funding, involuntary treatment funds, and federal block grants. In Washington State, increase of state allocations to local mental health authorities (RSNs) for community support capacity in Washington State was contingent upon local use of new resources for acute and long-term residential beds, crisis response services, and community support capacity, including case management services. Appropriations to each RSN were tied to commitments to develop capacity in these areas; however, as required in the statute, details of clinical programming were left to the RSNs. The state provided some technical assistance for program development.

Financial policies were also a part of the Washington State mental health reform. By January 1992, the MHD had negotiated goals for reduced use of state hospitals in 1991–1993 RSN biennium contracts. Based upon the assumption that short-term hospitalizations could be shifted from the state hospital to local community hospitals, RSNs by contract are required to provide short stay inpatient treatment within their communities. These goals were tied to receipt of $6.4 million in new state appropriations, which must be used to increase access to local acute care beds, and $9 million to increase capacity and reduce the use of the state hospitals.

Also, in 1992, the legislature enacted language that encouraged agreements between RSNs and state hospitals to reduce census and to transfer resulting savings to the RSNs. RSNs in western Washington did negotiate such an agreement with Western State Hospital, reducing the census by 60 beds and transferring $2.7 million to the RSNs. To date, this agreement has been successfully and smoothly implemented. Examples of how transferred dollars were used include the development of specialized programs for difficult-to-serve clients and the hiring of specialized staff to facilitate the placement of difficult-to-place patients at the state hospital when they are ready for discharge.

Another important goal for system development was to increase continuity of care. By January 1, 1992, RSNs had developed agreements with Washington's two state hospitals regarding admissions and discharges. Agreements stipulate notification procedures for when clients are hospitalized and participation of community staff in discharge planning.

In summary, the initiatives seek to reduce inappropriate use of psychiatric services through two basic mechanisms. The first mechanism involves substitution of psychiatric hospitalization with comprehensive community mental health treatment programming. The system of programs includes several types of crisis response services, increased availability of case management services, and an array of residential services with different levels of structure.

The second mechanism involves strengthening interorganizational relationships within the mental health system and between the mental health system and other systems serving mental health clients. Strengthened interorganizational relationships are expected to result in increased continuity of care, a critical factor in access to care over time and in achieving good connections from one episode of treatment to the next (Bachrach 1981).

Through the mechanisms of substitution and interorganizational relationships, individuals with severe and persistent mental illness are expected to experience increased stability and support in the community. As a result, fewer crises that lead to risk of hospitalization are expected to occur. (Crisis here refers to a situation in which a person is acutely mentally ill or is experiencing serious disruption in cognitive, volitional, psychosocial, or neurophysiological functioning. Also, the responsiveness of the mental health system when an individual with mental illness is experiencing a crisis is also expected to increase. As a result, resolution of crises will more frequently result in community treatment, and discharges from psychiatric hospitalizations will be more timely.

Core elements of the statewide intervention are continuity of care, case management services targeted to high users, crisis response services, and residential services. Each element is reflected in contract terms that are consistent across 1991–1993 state and RSN contracts. Preliminary data from the program evaluation indicate that catchment areas differ in the degree to which hospital diversion interventions are implemented. The study will attempt to answer the degree to which direct service providers (e.g., case managers, crisis staff) take actions in keeping with the HDCA model and examine the steps that local mental health authority and provider agency managers are taking to mobilize resources and organize each component of the HDCA intervention. Measurement of implementation will therefore focus upon actions of direct providers and availability of community treatment alternatives. Examples of objective measures for level of implementation are hours per year of community mental health service received, frequency of contacts between community mental health and hospital staff during a client's psychiatric hospitalization, and number of crisis beds per 100,000 population. Regional socioeconomic conditions will be studied simultaneously with level of implementation. Original data collection using subjective measures will also be used to measure level of implementation of case management, crisis services, residential services, and continuity of care. A service inventory will be used to gather subjective assessments by direct service providers of the extent to which clients needing each service received each service. The interview approach is an adaptation of Grusky and Tierney's (1989) measure of "key service components." Respondents will be asked whether all, most, some, few, or none of those in need of the service in their RSN were receiving it. It is expected that RSN implementation will vary for different services or conditions within each of the four components. For example, in the case of crisis services, an RSN may have a high degree of implementation for 24-hour-per-day crisis phone services, but not for mobile outreach services. Also, it is expected that regional implementation will vary across the four hospital diversion and community alternative components. For example, an RSN may have focused its main effort on crisis service, whereas another may have focused upon residential services.

Other research questions include: Do population characteristics (age, gender, ethnicity, diagnostic category, prior hospital use) of high users change over time? How does hospital use vary for subgroups of high users according to prior hospital use? How does hospital use vary for subgroups of high users according to age, gender, race, and diagnosis? How do regional differences in overall implementation affect hospital use by high users? Do differences in implementation of specific components of the hospital diversion and community alternatives make a difference in hospital use by high users?

# Discussion

Each of the studies outlined in this chapter approaches a major state policy initiative from an analytic perspective. Each involves a multifaceted review of state hospital downsizing in the context of community mental health program development, and each applies thoughtful research methods in an on-line fashion, in which results may be applied to adjust later stages of implementation. Finally, each of the studies has as its principal investigator a research fellow supported by the Public Academic Liaison fellowship program of the National Association of State Mental Health Program Directors Research Institute. This program, funded by the National Institute of Mental Health, intends to help develop the research careers of investigators who focus on services research that involves public mental health systems.

This background alone signals subtle but important changes in the arena of mental health policy and research. The fact that states are studying system change seriously is a sign that we are perhaps moving beyond an era of misplaced certainty about the dynamics and effects of new policies. The focus on data about effects on individuals affected by the policy change is also refreshing, as is the fact that the studies have been launched coterminously with the change efforts themselves, rather than pulled together post hoc to rationalize policy. The leadership role being played by a multidisciplinary group of researchers interested in real time services research also marks a new era, with a focus on knowledge development in areas beyond neuroscience.

Each of the studies is in a relatively early stage, and there are not as yet many findings to discuss. But it is timely to consider some of the questions that the studies raise when viewed from the perspectives of the research literature and of experience. This highly selective review places the studies in a context of ongoing knowledge development and policy problems, and may suggest opportunities for further reflection on the results as they emerge.

## Efficacy of Community Treatment

In general, these studies do not seek to test new and novel treatment approaches to the art and science of community support for persons with serious and persistent mental illnesses. They do not rigorously test new models of care, such as the trailblazing studies of Stein and his colleagues in Madison (e.g., Stein and Test 1980), nor do they evaluate theory-based interventions, such as Hogarty's (1991) fusion of pharmacological, rehabilitative, and psychoeducational family therapy interventions. So in a sense, one might be disappointed that these projects do not promise cutting-edge answers to brand-new questions.

But common sense will show that the major problems affecting services for people with serious mental illness do not stem as much from knowledge gaps as from a failure to apply the knowledge we have. These projects all begin to address the problem of translating policy and clinical knowledge into practice. One notable lack in mental health has been thoughtful and even skeptical review of policy changes and real-world service initiatives. The field has made major research investments in the basic science area, which are likely to have substantial payoffs down the road but little short-term practical impact. At the other end of the spectrum, huge policy shifts (e.g., deinstitutionalization) have been launched with virtually no evaluative component. And the huge gap between policy-neutral basic science and scientific policy shifts has by and large been ignored and unfilled. These studies seek to evaluate policy change by using credible methods and by capitalizing on new methods and instruments—for example, Lehman's (1988) approach to assessing quality of life. Thus, they begin to bridge a gap that for too long has been ignored.

## Inpatient Care and the Role of State Hospitals

In the area of downsizing and potential replacement of state-operated psychiatric hospitals, opinion looms larger than knowledge. On one hand, there is little clinical rationale for much of the care provided in state hospitals. Since Kiesler's (1982) thorough, provocative review of research on alternatives to hospitalization, which found no studies showing superiority of inpatient over alternative care, the literature in favor of community alternatives has continued to pile up. Although evidence to suggest elimination of psychiatric inpatient treatment is inadequate, a reduced role for inpatient care is in line with most clinical research literature.

On the other hand, the proper role of inpatient treatment within community support systems is not established. And just as critically, the dynamics of managing the transition from a state hospital-centered system to community-centered systems are a matter of mental health folklore rather than well-established knowledge. This is remarkable given the apparent policy consensus around downsizing state hospitals in favor of community alternatives. The preponderance of the evidence (Herz et al. 1990) does suggest a limited and focused role for inpatient treatment in mental health, rather than the expansive but unfocused approach of the past. There is certainly little evidence to suggest that long-term hospitalization is a good idea, and there are clear indications that it is actually harmful. Ironically, but logically, long-term hospitalization seems to be most harmful for individuals with long-term illness. For these individuals, long hospital stays are likely to contribute to lost skills and greater difficulty resuming community life, whereas very short stays to resolve crises may be useful. But a review of these issues is well beyond the scope of this commentary. The studies described in this chapter focus more on analyzing movement from hospital to community.

There is no comprehensive analysis of replacing state hospitals with alternative systems. In fact, despite the occasional impression that deinstitutionalization is a fait accompli, there appear to be only two regions of the country that exist more or less without a state hospital: Philadelphia (formerly served by the infamous Byberry Philadelphia State Hospital) and the westernmost four counties of Massachusetts (formerly served by Northampton State Hospital). Although there are many episodes of hospitalization in each region, both regions rely almost totally on private and general hospital inpatient care, except for care of forensic patients treated in out-of-region state facilities.

Trevor Hadley and associates are now engaged in a thorough—if partially retrospective—assessment of "the Philadelphia story," which should provide insights on the issues related to state hospital replacement. The western Massachusetts experience has been reviewed retrospectively by Geller et al. (1990a, 1990b) and M. F. Hogan (unpublished paper, January 1987). Although valuable, all of these efforts are by and large post hoc, and none is comprehensive. Yet patterns of issues—some of them troubling—emerge from these and related reviews.

Anecdotally, it appears that total inpatient costs in these regions—and potentially in other areas that are substituting private for public care—may not be reduced. Total state costs are reduced by substituting Medicaid-reimbursable general hospital services for essentially state-funded institutions. Yet the apparently higher per diem costs of private inpatient care may lead to overall cost increases.

A strong rationale for downsizing state hospitals is that their quality of care has frequently been abominable, and that this legacy of poor quality means that state hospitalization is more stigmatizing than treatment in facilities that are generally seen as positive community resources. Yet this begs the question of whether quality of care in private and/or general hospitals is better, and whether the quality of state hospital care can, or should, be improved. And the superiority of private care is certainly not as settled as proponents of privatization would suggest. For example, reviews of discharge planning in private versus public facilities by the New York State Commission on Quality of Care of the Mentally Disabled (1988) find that practices in private facilities are uneven and in some cases worse than in state facilities.

Several other issues related to the transition from hospital-to community-based systems must be better understood. Analyzing state mental health budget trends over the 1980s in relation to organizational and other factors, Schinnar et al. (1992) found that a declining proportion of state mental health budgets devoted to hospitals was predictive of declining overall mental health resource levels as a proportion of state health and welfare spending. The question of how changes in mental health policy affect the potency of the state agency as a funding source is not insignificant. And the consequences of running state hospitals solely for forensic patients have not been thought through. If it is true that care in general hospitals is less stigmatizing (an untested but not unreasonable assumption), what are the effects on stigma of a separate system dealing solely with "the criminally insane," as the press seems to mislabel forensic patients?

There has also been a paucity of satisfying evidence on the effects of downsizing, state employee reductions, and the move to community care in terms of human resource issues. The issues have been fought out in many states in terms of caricatures of unionized state hospital workers as being self-interested, resistant, overpaid, and underskilled. And community agencies and their employees have been branded as having interests that are proprietary, short-term, and selfish; they have been seen as uninterested in seriously ill people and their needs. A more balanced and data-based view is needed.

Finally, we in the mental health field have tended to view these issues and problems through our own narrow lens. Knowledge from other fields, such as the area of implementation analysis (e.g., Williams and Elmore 1976) has not been applied, with the consequence that we may be setting out to reinvent the wheel in too many areas of mental health. The studies we describe in this chapter are valuable efforts to address many of these issues and problems. They bridge client-level and systems views, link research and evaluative data with practice, and demonstrate a new approach to program development and social change. Although we believe our intentions and interventions are right, these studies remind us of the wisdom of thinking about what we are doing, and learning from our successes and failures.

# Conclusions

Despite the fact that expenditures for state psychiatric hospitals make up the majority of state mental health authority budgets, there has been relatively little research on the closing of state hospital beds and the impact of the development of community alternatives (Geller et al. 1990a, 1990b; Schinnar et al. 1990). That is why these three new research projects are so important. There are a number of reasons for the lack of empirical findings in this area. In general they are related to the time lines for decision making in state government and the time lines required for research. In almost every case the decision to close or downsize a state hospital is made in an intensely political and difficult environment. There are often state employee jobs at stake and considerable controversy about the implementation plan with little time to consider the evaluation. On the other hand research demands a longer time frame both to develop research questions and to wait for results. In these three projects the investigators have managed to integrate their research into the larger context of policy and decision making at the state level and provide regular feedback to decision makers.

Although the empirical literature is not particularly robust, a number of studies of these issues have been published in the literature and a large number of implementation reports have been generated by state mental health authorities. What can we generalize from these reports? First, it is clear that it is clinically, financially, and organizationally feasible to place a large percentage of long-term patients in community alternatives (Bachrach 1986). Second, there does not appear to be a dramatic change in the level of functioning of the discharged patients, although they do seem to function with greater independence than previously thought possible (B. Gordon, unpublished paper, March 1991). Finally, clients express far greater satisfaction with their living situation and overall quality of life.

What has not been demonstrated and then supported by empirical findings? First, it is not clear what the impact of major reductions in the availability of long-stay beds will be on the broader care system. The closing of beds and the discharge to the community of a large number of old long-stay patients may have a number of major effects on the community system. It may mean the exclusion of other special target groups such as the elderly or children. It may mean that once patients are moved and the long-stay beds are closed, the care system will not be able to function without a reasonable number of long-stay beds. Patients in long-stay beds have accumulated over very long periods of time, and without long-stay beds, systems will need to deal not only with the discharged cohort but also with the potential new long-stay patients, sometimes referred to as diversion patients (Schinnar et al. 1992).

These are all areas of research that need further exploration. Currently, states are making major decisions about the future of their long-term care systems with relatively little information, which is a chronic state of life for much of the decision making in state mental health authorities. These three studies have the potential to give policy makers further information about the opportunities and risks inherent in the closing of state psychiatric hospitals (Greenblatt and Glazier 1975).

# References

American Psychiatric Association: Global Assessment of Functioning Scale, in Diagnostic and Statistical Manual of Mental Disorders, 3rd Edition, Revised. Washington, DC, American Psychiatric Association, 1987

Bachrach L: Continuity of care for chronic mental patients: a conceptual analysis. Am J Psychiatry 138:1449–1456, 1981

Bachrach L: The future of the state mental hospital. Hosp Community Psychiatry 37:467–474, 1986

Derogatis LR: The SCL-90R. Baltimore, MD, Clinical Psychometric Research, 1977

Frank R, Goldman H: Financing care of the severely mentally ill: incentives, contracts and public responsibility. Journal of Social Issues 45:131–144, 1989

Geller JL, Fisher WH, Wirth-Cauchon JL, et al: Second-generation deinstitutionalization, I: the impact of Brewster v. Dukakis on state hospital case mix. Am J Psychiatry 147:982–987, 1990a

Geller JL, Fisher WH, Simon LJ, et al:Second-generation deinstitutionalization, II: the impact of Brewster v. Dukakis on correlates of community and hospital utilization. Am J Psychiatry 147:988–993, 1990b

Greenblatt M, Glazier E: The phasing out of mental hospitals in the United States. Am J Psychiatry 132:1135–1140, 1975

Grusky O, Tierney K: Evaluating the effectiveness of countywide mental health care systems. Community Ment Health J 25:3–20, 1989

Harris M, Bergman H: Capitation financing for the chronic mentally ill: a case management approach. Hosp Community Psychiatry 39:68–72, 1988

Herz MI, Keith SH, Docherty JP: Early intervention in schizophrenia, in Handbook of Schizophrenia, Psychosocial Treatment of Schizophrenia, Vol. III. Edited by Herz MI, Keith SH, Docherty JP. New York, Elsevier, 1990, pp 25–45

Hogarty GE, Anderson CM, Reiss DJ, et al: Family psychoeducation, social skills training and maintenance chemotherapy in the aftercare treatment of schizophrenia. Arch Gen Psychiatry 48:340–347, 1991

Indiana Department of Mental Health: Indiana's Response to Public Law 99-660. Indianapolis, Indiana Division of Mental Health, 1988

Indiana Division of Mental Health: Central State Hospital: a report to Governor Evan Bayh. Indianapolis, Indiana Division of Mental Health, 1992

Indiana Division of Mental Health: The Hoosier Assurance Plan: addressing public mental health and chemical addictions needs of Indiana citizens. Indianapolis, Division of Mental Health, 1993a

Indiana Division of Mental Health: Central State Hospital closure plan: commitment to community based care. An update report to Governor Evan Bayh. Indianapolis, Indiana Division of Mental Health, 1993b

Indiana Legislative Services Agency: Performance audit of mental health programs in Indiana. Indianapolis, Indiana Legislative Services Agency, Office of Fiscal and Management Analysis, 1984

Indiana Legislative Services Agency: Mental health needs: evaluation audit, Indiana Legislative Services Agency. Indianapolis, Indiana Legislative Services Agency, Office of Fiscal and Management Analysis, 1990

Indiana Legislative Services Agency: Indiana Legislative Services Agency report on mental health needs and local service delivery. Indianapolis, Indiana Legislative Services Agency, Office of Fiscal and Management Analysis, 1991

Kiesler CA: Mental hospitals and alternative care: noninstitutionaliza-tion as potential public policy for mental patients. Am Psychol 37:349–360, 1982

Leff HS, Graves S, Natkins J, et al: Description and field test of a men-tal health system resource allocation model. Administration in Mental Health 13:43–68, 1985

Lehman AF: A quality of life interview for the chronically mentally ill. Evaluation and Program Planning 11:51–62, 1988

Little AD: Will Indiana choose new directions in mental health and mental retardation services? A summary of findings and recom-mendations from our draft report. Indianapolis, Indiana Division of Mental Health, 1974

Murray BE: Indiana Department of Mental Health plan for the 80s. Indianapolis, Indiana Division of Mental Health, 1980

National Association of State Mental Health Program Directors Re-search Institute: State Mental Health Authority Profiling System. Alexandria, VA, National Association of State Mental Health Pro-gram Directors Research Institute, 1994

New York State Commission on Quality of Care for the Mentally Dis-abled: Admission and discharge practices of psychiatric hospitals: a report to the New York State legislature pursuant to Chapter 50 of the laws of 1987, 1988. Albany, NY, 1988

Schinnar AP, Rothbard AB, Hadley TR, et al: Integration of mental health data on hospital and community services. Administration and Policy in Mental Health 18:91–99, 1990

Schinnar AP, Rothbard AB, Yin D, et al: Public choice and organiza-tional determinants of state mental health expenditure patterns. Administration and Policy in Mental Health 19:235–250, 1992

Schneider LC, Struenig EL: SLOF: a behavioral rating scale for assess-ing the mentally ill. Social Work Research and Abstracts 19:9–21, 1983

South Carolina Department of Mental Health: Toward local care—re-port of the Transition Leadership Council. Columbia, SC, South Carolina Department of Mental Health, 1990

Stein L: Wisconsin's system of mental health financing. New Directions for Mental Health, Paying for Services: Promises and Pitfalls of Capitation 43:29–41, 1989

Stein LT, Test MA: Alternative to mental hospital treatment. Arch Gen Psychiatry 37:392–397, 1980

Taube C, Goldman H: State strategies to restructure state psychiatric hospitals: a selective review. Inquiry 26:146–156, 1989

Williams W, Elmore R (eds): Social Program Implementation. New York, Academic Press, 1976

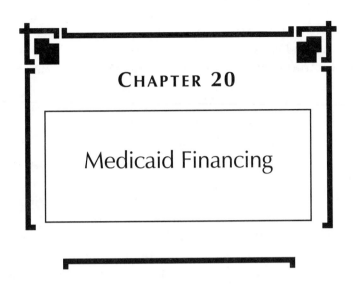

# CHAPTER 20

## Medicaid Financing

**Neil Meisler, M.S.W., and M. Carolyn Gonzales**

Medicaid is a flexible means of increasing financing of community mental health services, of which states have only recently begun to take full advantage. Virtually all components of a comprehensive community mental health system are eligible for federal financial participation through several optional service provisions of Medicaid. In this chapter we provide the reader with an understanding of the ways in which Medicaid can finance community-based treatment for adults with serious mental illness. Medicaid optional services and their restrictions are reviewed, and examples are provided of how several states have used Medicaid to finance community treatment teams.

Title XIX of the Social Security Act, more commonly known as Medicaid, is a medical insurance program for indigent persons, shared and funded by the state and federal government. States' participation in Medicaid is voluntary. The federal contribution toward Medicaid expenditures varies from a low of 50% to a high of approximately 80% in accordance with a formula of economic and performance indicators. Participating states maintain a medical assistance plan, approved by the Health Care Financing Administration (HCFA), which lists Medicaid-eligible groups and services. States must provide Medicaid coverage to recipients of Aid to Families with Dependent Children (AFDC) and Supplemental Security Income (SSI). They must also cover Medicare beneficiaries whose income is below the poverty level, pregnant women whose income is up to 185% of the poverty level, children under 6 whose parents' income is within 133% of the poverty level, and children 6–10 years of age whose parents' income is at or below the poverty level. States may broaden enrollment to include other medically needy persons. Participating states must cover hospital inpatient and outpatient services, nursing facility services (for individuals age 21 and over who are receiving federal income assistance only), and physician services. They must also cover early periodic screening and diagnostic services for children. Moreover, services found necessary through screening and diagnostic services may be covered whether or not they are specifically included in a state's medical assistance plan. States may not limit benefits by diagnosis. They have the option of covering a variety of additional services, including home health services, clinic services, rehabilitative services, and case management services.

When Medicaid was enacted, nearly all state mental health expenditures were for the purpose of maintaining state hospitals, which, at the time, had a national census of more than 500,000 persons. Congress prohibited the payment of Medicaid for patients of state hospitals, other specialty psychiatric hospitals, and psychiatric nursing homes (with the exception, at the state's election, of persons younger than 21 or older than 65 years of age). Congressional intent was that state government would retain sole financial responsibility for the institutional care of indigent persons with mental illness. Because of the prohibition against limiting services based on diagnosis, however, inpatient treatment in general hospital settings and outpatient treatment were covered. During the 1970s and 1980s, state expenditures for outpatient mental health services increased rapidly as part of an attempt to decrease use of state hospitals, the operating costs of which were increasing drastically even as they decreased in size. Few states took full advantage of access to Medicaid to help finance these services. Because there is only vague reference to mental health services in the Medicaid language, awareness among the states of the possibility of obtaining comprehensive coverage for noninstitutional mental health services developed gradually. Another factor that delayed growth in use of Medicaid for mental health services was the reluctance by state budget offices and Medicaid agencies to expand Medicaid coverage to include optional services, out of a fear of uncontrolled increases in expenditures. Additionally, few state mental health authorities had established the necessary infrastructure to comply with Medicaid requirements for utilization control, service documentation, program integrity, and so on. In recent years, however, a majority of states have opted for Medicaid service coverage to finance community mental health services, using the state mental health agencies' appropriations as the match for federal Medicaid expenditures. Thirty-two of 37 states responding to a recent survey reported using one or more of the optional coverage plans for community mental health services (National Association of State Mental Health Program Directors 1992). Today, Medicaid is a significant source of revenue for community mental health services in most states. Federal Medicaid expenditures for community mental health services that are under the control of state mental health agencies grew from $23 million in FY 1981 to $323 million in FY 1990 (National Association of State Mental Health Program Directors 1992).

## Overview of Medicaid Optional Coverage

Although coverage of physician and hospital outpatient services is mandatory, relatively few Medicaid recipients receive mental health services in these settings. General hospitals have not been major providers of outpatient mental health services. State Medicaid agencies have tended to hold the rates paid for a physician's visit for mental health treatment lower than most psychiatrists will accept. Consequently, although physicians and mental health specialists in private practice provide approximately 50% of the total outpatient mental health services rendered (Narrow et al. 1993), relatively few Medicaid recipients receive private outpatient care. Most Medicaid recipients with mental illness depend on the public mental health system for care.

There are four optional provisions under Medicaid that states have used to finance community mental health services in the public sector: clinic services, personal care services, rehabilitative services, and targeted case management services.

## Clinic Services

The Code of Federal Regulations defines clinic services as "preventive, diagnostic, therapeutic, rehabilitative or palliative items or services that are provided to outpatients by a facility that is not part of a hospital but is organized and operated to provide medical care to outpatients and are furnished by or under the direction of a physician." There is specific coverage for mental health and general health clinics and states can opt for either. For mental health clinics, there are detailed requirements and limitations contained in the State Medicaid Manual, the policy manual of the HCFA. Among these are the following.

- Outpatient psychiatric services must be provided at an organized medical facility or distinct part of such a facility, neither of which is providing the patient with room and board and professional services on a continuous 24-hour-a-day basis.
- A physician must directly supervise service provision.
- A plan of care is required for each recipient, containing a written description of the treatment objectives to improve his or her condition to the point where the patient's continued participation in the program is no longer necessary (services representing a departure from the service plan must be explained in detail in regard to how they are

necessary in order to achieve the treatment objectives).

■ An evaluation team must review the plan of care at least every 90 days to determine the recipient's progress toward the treatment objectives, the appropriateness of the services being rendered, and the need for the recipient's continued participation in the program.

These limitations render the clinic option inconsistent with the range of treatment needs of persons with serious mental illness.

## Personal Care Services

Personal care is defined as a range of nonmedical, in-home assistance with self-care, housekeeping, and meal preparation provided to persons who are disabled. Personal care services must be prescribed by a physician and must be provided under the supervision of a registered nurse. State mental health agencies have not tended to use the personal care services option to provide assistance with self-care, housekeeping, and meal preparation to enable a person with severe psychiatric disability to live in his or her own home. The probable reason for this is that such activities are not typically within the scope of services that state mental health agencies finance. However, several states have used the personal care services option to obtain federal financial participation in staffing group homes and other supervised-living situations. They have also used this option to provide activity programs or to otherwise supplement the staffing and care provided in board-and-care facilities. Such use of the personal care option has been controversial in that HCFA's interpretation of congressional intent in covering personal care services is that residential care staffing costs are part of "room and board," which Medicaid does not fund. Moreover, although the person's home can include a congregate, supervised-living facility, he or she must have free choice of services from among all enrolled providers of personal care services. Also, HCFA does not recognize psychosocial activities or supervision as covered personal care services.

## Rehabilitative Services

Title XIX includes, as a state option, "other diagnostic, screening, prevention, and rehabilitation services." Rehabilitation services are defined in the Code of Federal Regulations as "any medical or remedial services recommended by a physician or other licensed practitioner of the healing arts, within the scope of his practice under state law, for maximum reduction of physical or mental disability and restoration of a recipient to his best possible functional level." There are no regulations further defining or restricting the provision of rehabilitative services. The absence of regulatory restriction and the specific reference to reduction of disability and restoration of functional capacity make the rehabilitative services option highly compatible with serving persons with serious mental illness. During the 1980s, emphasis on case management by the federal government became legislated. In 1985, Congress amended Title XIX to include "targeted case management services" as an optional Medicaid-covered service. The legislation defined case management as services that will assist individuals eligible under the medical assistance plan in gaining access to needed medical, social, educational, and other services. Subsequently, HCFA promulgated regulations further defining case management as an activity under which responsibility for locating, coordinating, and monitoring necessary and appropriate services for an individual rests with a specific person or organization. States are permitted to provide case management to all Medicaid-eligible patients or to target them to subgroups of the Medicaid-eligible populations. States are also permitted to limit the availability of case management services to geographic subareas of the state. Both of these provisions are exceptions to the statutory requirements for comparability of services for all Medicaid-eligible persons and for being statewide that apply to all other Medicaid services.

## Targeted Case Management Services

In 1977, the National Institute of Mental Health founded the Community Support Program to promote improvement by states in caring for persons with serious mental illness. It identified case management as an essential component of a community support services system. It defined case management on a system and program level as the presence of a core agency charged with responsibility for providing support services to a community or to identified groups of persons with mental illness; and on the client level as a single person or team responsible for remaining in touch with the client on a continuing basis, regardless of how many agencies get involved (Turner and TenHoor 1978). In 1986 and 1990, Congress enacted legislation requiring states to obtain annual approval from the Department of Health and Human Services for a Comprehensive Mental Health Service Plan as a condition of receipt of the Mental Health Block Grant. The Plan must address the provision of case management services to all persons with prolonged mental illness who use substantial amounts of public funds or services. The NIMH Community Support Program, the Planning Act, and the Medicaid provision for targeted case management services have collectively influenced dramatic growth among the states in the number of case managers and case manager programs. In most states these have been layered onto the existing systems of clinic and day treatment, and psychosocial rehabilitation programs. The range of activities undertaken by case managers in most states include outreach, assistance in obtaining entitlements and services, and support in activities of daily living.

There is some risk, however, in using the targeted case management option to bill for treatment, rehabilitative, or supportive interventions, all of which are covered under other options. HCFA views case management as an outreach and integrative activity, not a therapeutic service. It believes that congressional intent is for targeted case management to be a parallel and separate activity, provided to ensure appropriate access to and use of mental health and other human services. There is no language in either the legislation or the regulatory definition to suggest that targeted case management includes the provision of direct assistance to clients in daily living beyond making appropriate use of services. Neither is there any language to suggest that

Medicaid-covered case management services include provision of any form of therapy or social skills training. Further, during negotiations between some states and HCFA regional offices, direct service by case managers has been a primary reason for denial of the state plan amendment. Clearly, HCFA's intent is to limit billing under case management services to nonclinical interventions of service planning, linkage of clients to entitlements and services, assistance to ensure appropriate use of other Medicaid services, and advocacy for access to service. Claims for Medicaid payment for services provided by case managers that are beyond the functions defined by HCFA as case management would be subject to audit exception. Because HCFA views targeted case management as essentially an administrative service, separation of the function of case management from other mental health services, either through distinctly staffed case management programs within community mental health agencies or through separate agencies that provide case management services only, is most consonant with HCFA's interpretation of congressional intent.

## Medicaid Reimbursement Methodologies

Medicaid allows states flexibility in selecting payment methods. They can elect to fund programs according to their component services or aggregate the various component services within a single program rate. They can base rates upon the average cost of the personnel within a program or they can establish separate rates for each discipline. They can establish statewide rates for a given service based on the average cost across locations, or they can arrive at specific rates for each service and program based on the provider's costs. States can also choose between setting a prospective rate, based on expected costs and volume of services, or setting interim rates with a year-end cost settlement, ensuring that providers are paid neither more nor less than their actual Medicaid-allowable costs.

With the exception of the clinic services option, which ties payment to each specific occasion of service, the options under which mental health services can be covered allow the states to base the rate on the average daily cost of the client's involvement in a program, even though the client may receive services on less than a daily basis. For example, some states pay a monthly fee for targeted case management services, provided that the client receives at least a minimum stipulated amount of case management services within that month.

Most states take at least partial advantage of the opportunity to finance comprehensive community mental health services through Medicaid. The full potential of such financing, however, is only approached by a few states. Not coincidentally, these are the states rated as among the most responsive to the needs of persons with serious mental illness (Torrey et al. 1990). Many state mental health agencies are constrained by a variety of obstacles on the state level, as well as by requirements inherent in Title XIX, which can also present compliance challenges.

There are several factors that limit state mental health agencies from making optimum use of Medicaid. First is the failure by some state mental health agencies to present a vision, a plan, and a strategic set of mental health policies to develop statewide local systems of care that provide assertive outreach, continuity of care, and integrated services for persons with mental illness. In the absence of a coherent strategy, Medicaid and mental health financing in general is likely to lag. A second factor is the constraint of the requirement for state matching. Most state mental health agencies must use their appropriations to finance the matching of Medicaid payments. Most expend in excess of 60% of their budgets on state hospital operations (National Association of State Mental Health Program Directors 1992). The substantial cost of maintaining state hospital services, which many politicians and advocates believe have been excessively reduced in size and number, limits the extent to which state mental health agencies can take advantage of potential Medicaid payments. Many states are, however, in the process of systematically shifting finances from state hospital budgets (where eligibility for Medicaid payment is limited) to general hospital psychiatric inpatient and community support programs where opportunities for federal financial participation through Medicaid are greater (Mauch 1989; McGuire et al. 1990). A third factor is that state mental health agencies are constrained by the low priority that mental illness holds in most state governments relative to other health and social problems. When adjusted for inflation, state expenditures for mental health services have declined nationally, whereas expenditures for other health and welfare services have increased (Hadley et al. 1992). In a number of states, efforts by the state mental health agency to expand service coverage through Medicaid have been rebuffed by the state Medicaid agency or budget office even though the agency would have used its existing appropriation to fund the state match of Medicaid payments. State mental health agencies have been unable to gain the attention and support of their own administrations to make even cost-neutral changes. In other states Medicaid reimbursement has gone to the general fund, or state mental health agencies have had their appropriations reduced in response to increases in federal revenue. A fourth factor is the economic inability of states to take maximum advantage of the liberal eligibility provisions of Medicaid. Many more people could be eligible for Medicaid if states could afford to expand the eligibility criteria for Medicaid coverage. In states that limit Medicaid enrollment to categorical eligibility, state mental health agencies must fund 100% of the cost of care for approximately 50% of clients.

Nearly all states presently cover community mental health services under one or more of these options. In most of them, the state mental health agencies' state appropriations serve as the match of Medicaid payments for the optional services. In this manner, states have attempted to capture federal Medicaid payment while controlling the rate of growth of state expenditures. This has also been accomplished by managing provider enrollment in a manner that allows the state mental health agencies to retain control over total expenditures, program structure, and service mix. Restricting provider enrollment has been controversial in that Title XIX and the Code of Federal Regulations limit states' flexibility in limiting provider enrollment or clients' access to services. However, states have found ways to do so without violating federal laws or regulations.

States need to exercise caution in applying optional Medicaid services coverage to specific services and programs. Title XIX and regulatory language are interpreted quite literally by HCFA, and some states have found themselves subject to audits by the HCFA in which coverage and payments have been retroactively challenged. Comprehensive mental health services can be covered by selectively using the appropriate option for each program component. Following is a brief review of the program components of a typical mental health service system and the applicable optional coverage(s) for each.

## Counseling and Medication Services

Because these are services used both by persons with long-term and episodic mental illness and by those with less serious mental health problems, states should cover them under both the clinic and rehabilitation services options. It is not appropriate to use the rehabilitative services option for service coverage for non-disabling mental illness. On the other hand, the clinic services option has limitations that are not appropriate for persons with long-term service needs. An example is the requirement for re-evaluation to determine medical necessity every 90 days.

## Mobile Crisis Services

Mental health emergency services can be financed as either clinic or rehabilitative services. However, if staff work without continuous, direct supervision of a physician and provide services at the site of the emergency and at other locations away from the mental health facility, such emergency services are more appropriately covered as rehabilitative services.

## Crisis Stabilization Services

Crisis stabilization services provided outside of a hospital inpatient setting can be covered under the clinic services option if they are provided on less than a 24-hour basis at the site of a community mental health center or other ambulatory mental health facility. If such services include overnight care in a nonmedical facility (a facility other than a hospital or nursing facility), they can be covered under the rehabilitation services option. However, costs associated with room and board in such a facility must be excluded from the payment rate.

## Case Management Services

When case management services are provided by staff other than the client's therapist(s), the targeted case management services option is appropriate. Otherwise, the staff effort consumed by case management functions of a program should be incorporated into the cost basis for the rate of the mental health service or program. In this case, case management is not billed as a separate service but as an integral component of another covered service.

## Psychosocial Rehabilitation Services

Services to assist clients who have psychiatric disabilities to cope with and minimize the effects of major mental illness on their cognitive abilities and social functioning are more appropriately covered as rehabilitative services than clinic services. The requirements for 90-day reviews of medical necessity, physician supervision, and facility-based service provision all reduce the appropriateness of the clinic services option for these services. Three activities commonly provided by psychosocial rehabilitation programs are not covered by Medicaid under any option: activities that are primarily recreational, adult or remedial education, and vocational training. Therapeutic interventions to enable a person to get and keep employment are covered by Medicaid. Only such activities as training in a particular job function and supervision of work are not Medicaid-covered services.

## Residential Services

Psychiatric, counseling, and rehabilitative services provided in a client's home, including a group residence, can be covered as optional rehabilitation services. In addition, Medicaid personal care services can be used to cover nonclinical assistance in the self-care and housekeeping domains. States can either cover these as a range of specific services billed individually on each occasion of service, or aggregate them within a daily rate. There are two important caveats. First, the cost of room and board and other components of a residential program that are not Medicaid-reimbursable must be excluded from the basis of the rate. Second, residential programs with more than 16 beds for adults with mental illness are considered by Title XIX as "institutions for mental diseases." Not only are such residential programs ineligible for Medicaid payment, but residents lose their Medicaid eligibility.

## Innovative Community Programs

As suggested by the above overview, Medicaid can be used to finance a broad array of mental health programs, including the more innovative community-based treatment team programs described in other chapters of this volume. Assertive community treatment based on the Training in Community Living (TCL) model described in Chapter 9 is one such treatment program that many states have begun to replicate. Several states have undertaken systematic statewide development of programs based on the TCL approach with Medicaid financing. These states include Wisconsin, Michigan, New Hampshire, Rhode Island, and Delaware. In the remainder of this chapter we describe the different ways in which Wisconsin, Delaware, and Rhode Island have designed Medicaid financing for their TCL programs. Medicaid financing has facilitated statewide TCL program development in all three states. Moreover, they took three quite different approaches to Medicaid financing, which illustrates the flexibility contained in the provisions of Title XIX of the Social Security Act and the regulations of the HCFA. Each state uses a different set of terms to refer to programs that incorporate the TCL approach: continuous treatment teams (CTTs) in Delaware, mobile treatment teams (MTTs) in Rhode Island, and community support programs (CSPs) in Wisconsin.

## Delaware: Bundled Fee for Service

In Delaware, CTT programs are reimbursed by Medicaid as rehabilitative services. Each CTT program has a single unit of service rate determined by its actual Medicaid-allowable costs divided by the expected units of covered services, based on statewide productivity standards. Nonallowable Medicaid costs are paid entirely by the Division of Alcoholism, Drug Abuse and Mental Health through a cost-based contract with the provider. Providers are reimbursed the same unit rate regardless of the staff member (i.e., physician, nurse, social worker, etc.) rendering the service or the particular type of covered service being provided. Payment for group activities is prorated according to the number of client and staff participants in the group. The rate-setting methodology contains an adjustment factor for lower use during new programs' first 3 years of operation, which affords such programs the opportunity to gradually build their caseloads at the rate of approximately four persons per month until they reach full enrollment. After the third year, the rate is based on 100% enrollment.

## Rhode Island: Bundled Per Diem Payment

MTT services for Medicaid-eligible services in Rhode Island are covered through a combination of rehabilitative and targeted case management services. Like Delaware, Rhode Island bundles all Medicaid-covered MTT services into a single fee. Unlike Delaware, however, Rhode Island has established the unit as a per diem. Moreover, providers are paid the daily rate whether or not actual client contact occurs on a given day, provided, however, that the client receives at least 8 face-to-face hours of service in a month. If a provider renders less than 8 hours of service to a client in consecutive months, payment for that client shifts to a fee-for-service basis, using the established rates for targeted case management and conventional outpatient services.

## Wisconsin: Multiple Procedure Codes, Fee for Service

In Wisconsin, certified CSP services are covered by Medicaid as rehabilitative and targeted case management services. Medicaid payment is provided on a fee-for-service basis for a total of 31 separate procedure codes based on a combination of the type of service activity, whether group or individual treatment is rendered, and the qualifications of the staff rendering the service.

# Conclusions

Medicaid offers states a flexible means of obtaining substantial federal financial participation in the provision of community mental health services. Unlike Medicare and private health insurance, Medicaid will finance a broad array of community support programs for persons with serious mental illness. It has been a key factor in the ability of a number of states to shift from an institutional to a community-based public mental health system without abandoning persons with serious mental illness. Although the current political momentum for national health care reform holds promise for providing universal health insurance, including mental health service benefits, for millions of persons who are uninsured it presents a potential threat to the maintenance and expansion of comprehensive community mental health services for persons with serious mental illness. The mental health benefits proposed for inclusion in basic health plans do not approach the comprehensiveness of coverage in many states under Medicaid. It is hoped that the flexibility and comprehensiveness of the Medicaid mental health benefits will be maintained for states to elect. Otherwise, national health care reform could be detrimental to the already uneven national efforts to achieve mental health care reform.

# References

Hadley TR, Culhane DP, Snyder FJ, et al: Expenditure and revenue patterns of state mental health agencies. Administration and Policy in Mental Health 19:213–233, 1992

Mauch D: Rhode Island: an early effort at managed care, in Paying for Services: Promises and Pitfalls of Capitation. Edited by Mechanic D, Aiken LH. San Francisco, CA, Jossey-Bass, 1989, pp 55–64

McGuire TG, Mosakowski WS, Radigan LS: Designing a prospective payment system for inpatient psychiatric services in Medicaid. Administration and Policy in Mental Health 18:43–54, 1990

Narrow WE, Reigier DA, Rae DS, et al: Use of services by persons with mental and addictive disorders: findings from the National Institute of Mental Health Epidemiologic Catchment Area program. Arch Gen Psychiatry 50:95–107, 1993

National Association of State Mental Health Program Directors: Funding Sources and Expenditures of State Mental Health Agencies: Revenue/Expenditure Study Results. Alexandria, VA, National Association of State Mental Health Program Directors, 1990

National Association of State Mental Health Program Directors: Financing Community Mental Health Services Thru Medicaid for Persons with Serious Mental Illness. Alexandria VA, National Association of State Mental Health Program Directors, 1992

Torrey EF, Erdman K, Wolfe SM, et al: Care of the Seriously Mentally Ill: A Rating of State Programs, 3rd Edition. Washington, DC, Public Citizen Health Research Group and National Alliance for the Mentally Ill, 1990

Turner JC, TenHoor WJ: The NIMH community support program: pilot approach to a needed social reform. Schizophr Bull 4:319–348, 1978

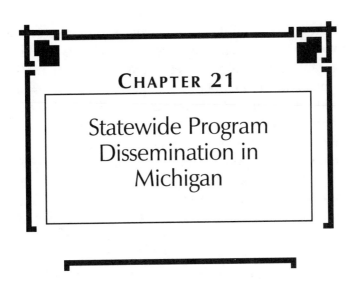

# CHAPTER 21

## Statewide Program Dissemination in Michigan

**Thomas B. Plum, M.S.W.**

In this chapter I provide a retrospective description of administrative processes leading to a successful statewide service program dissemination (issues pertaining to staff training, state funding, reimbursement, community program development, and staff morale). My intention is to help program planners and developers in other states as they continue to create innovative and effective community-based mental health programs for persons with serious mental illness.

When Dr. E. Fuller Torrey, a noted professional advocate for improved mental health services (Torrey 1988, 1992), visited Michigan, he asked, "If your model services work so well, why aren't there more of them?" Since then, the Michigan Department of Community Health has managed to coordinate the establishment of effective services throughout the state, in urban, suburban, and rural areas, for persons with serious mental illness living independently. The service approach is known in the literature as Training in Community Living (TCL); the Program for Assertive Community Treatment (PACT) (Bond 1990, 1991a, b, c; Stein and Test 1974), or, in Michigan, Assertive Community Treatment (ACT). Michigan has created over 110 ACT teams. These teams have had a significant effect on use of services in Michigan. For example, the number of adults in state psychiatric hospitals has decreased from 4,304 in 1985 to 2,219 in 1993. This decline is attributed to sound hospital management and the development of expanded community-based services. Outcome monitoring shows that the community-based program that appears to have had the most effect at reducing unnecessary hospitalization has been ACT. The sections below will highlight the development and implementation of ACT services statewide. The following steps were followed during Michigan's ACT program expansion.

1. *Determining unmet needs (goals of service) and identifying required services to address these needs.* During the mid-1970s, Michigan (along with much of the country) began to expand community-based services for persons with serious mental illness. Day treatment programs, residential placements, medication clinics, and outpatient therapy were the first services developed. Unfortunately, many individuals in need of assistance were either unable or unwilling to participate. For many, clinic-based therapy presented an obstacle to their receiving help. Many would eventually miss therapy appointments, stop taking medication, and drift away from treatment. Renewed psychiatric distress, loss of living arrangements, and a return to the psychiatric hospital would result. The revolving-door syndrome had begun.

2. *Identifying program(s) which can provide needed services and address identified but unmet needs.* The Michigan Department of Mental Health in collaboration with staff from the Kent County (Michigan) Community Mental Health Services Board, planned to establish teams following the PACT model. Consultation was provided by staff from the PACT program in Wisconsin and from the Thresholds program in Chicago. Michigan's ACT programs were designed to faithfully follow the PACT program's principles by encompassing the following elements.

- Services would be provided by a team of mental health professionals and others in the natural community where the clients live, work, and play.
- The teams would provide a wide range of services, such as assuring that basic needs and medical care were available to individuals living independently.
- Treatment would be provided by a team that assumes primary responsibility for as long as is needed (most individuals require long-term treatment).

To provide this service mental health professionals require a broad range of skills and knowledge (Witheridge 1989). The multidisciplinary team involves professionals from at least three separate disciplines. A typical ACT team in Michigan consists of from 5–8 staff (social workers, nurses, psychiatrists, psychologists, and paraprofessionals). The teams have a staff-to-client ratio of 1:10 or less. A staff-to-client ratio of this intensity allows highly flexible and intensive service. It is expected that an ACT team will have the capability to provide multiple contacts a day to an individual client when in crisis.

3. *Establishing demonstration site(s) to evaluate whether the selected program(s) can successfully meet the desired goals and to determine if replication is possible.* Established by the Kent County Mental Health Services board through a National Institute of Mental Health grant managed by the Michigan Department of Mental Health, the first ACT team in Michigan was piloted in 1979. The demonstration project would become a nonprofit organization and was named Harbinger of Grand Rapids Incorporated. Outcome evaluation (Muldar 1982) on the Harbinger program confirmed all expectations. The pilot accomplished the following.

- It significantly reduced the incidence of psychiatric inpatient hospitalization.
- It resulted in notable improvements in the recipient's quality of life.

■ It was a faithful replication of the PACT program.

By comparing pretreatment system expenses to post-treatment system expenses, the cost-effectiveness of ACT was again documented. ACT rendered a significant amount of inpatient hospitalization unnecessary. It also was effective at improving the quality of life for those receiving services and was shown to cost no more than institutionally based services. Other research (Boyer 1992) has identified how ACT teams are a more supportive working environment for providers and how they reduce staff burnout.

4. *Publicizing the results of the evaluation to generate support from stakeholders (e.g., legislature, consumers, advocacy groups, and providers).* In addition to Muldar's work, the Michigan Department of Mental Health collects data regarding hospital use from all ACT clients in Michigan. These data (Plum and Adler 1990) have been used to generate support from various stakeholders (legislature, advocates, administrators, and providers). By using these data, community mental health authorities are able to predict what effect new teams will have on their use of services. For example, outcome data showed the average number of hospital days for ACT clients had dropped by 72% after the first year in treatment and by 91% after the third year. This information has been used to plan the redirection of community mental health resources in order to establish new teams.

5. *Identifying funding sources (e.g., state, local, federal) and developing a fiscal strategy.* Michigan's first 20 ACT teams were funded through expansion funds provided by the state legislature. The Michigan legislature was persuaded by Muldar's research to direct additional resources to the creation of these teams. Local community mental health boards were invited to apply for funding to establish ACT teams with the explicit understanding that a rigorous implementation protocol would be followed, including staff training and state oversight. During the late 1980s, the Michigan Depart-

ment of Mental Health turned to Medicaid for additional resources. Originally Michigan's Medicaid procedures were not well suited for ACT service. Clinic- and discipline-based billing did not reflect the reality of ACT treatment. We overcame this by working with the state manager of Medicaid (the Michigan Department of Social Services) to create a new covered service, called Assertive Community Treatment (see Table 21–1). Under the Psychosocial Rehabilitation Option, ACT service can now be provided without changing the model's basic principles and procedures. For example, ACT can be provided outside of a clinic office by any team staff member. The Medicaid rules were made to fit the model instead of making the model fit Medicaid. Table 21–1 is an excerpt from Michigan's Medical Services Administration Bulletin (Michigan Department of Social Services 1993), which includes Michigan's Medicaid requirements for Assertive Community Treatment. Other states may find this material useful as they craft their own regulations. Additional resources were freed up by ACT's ability to reduce inpatient expenses. Michigan has a community mental health funding strategy (called *full management*), which provides each community mental health board with a budget to purchase both community-based and hospital-based services. If less hospitalization is used, increased resources will be made available to expand community-based services.

6. *Identifying a cadre of experts to provide consultation, training, problem solving, and program monitoring.* To create over 110 ACT teams, the Michigan Department of Mental Health contracted with a nonprofit (Harbinger of Grand Rapids Incorporated) to provide assistance with site visits and training. The enthusiasm of Harbinger's staff has inspired many of us. ACT is best taught by example and Harbinger has been a fine example.

7. *Conducting an evaluation to determine if any of the program's characteristics could be used for other populations with common needs and attributes.* In addition to teams for adults with se-

**Table 21–1.**   Michigan Medicaid requirements for Assertive Community Treatment

---

Assertive Community Treatment (ACT) is an array of services provided by community-based, mobile mental health treatment teams. Teams provide a broad range of essential services for individuals with serious mental illness.

**Program Enrollment.**   ACT is a Medicaid service when provided according to requirements described within this chapter. Medicaid providers intending to bill for ACT and mental health community rehabilitation services must enroll a specific program as an ACT Medicaid provider with the approval of the Department of Mental Health's Division of Licensing, Monitoring and Accreditation. Approval will be subsequent to consultation with the Department of Mental Health's Bureau of Community Mental Health Services, regarding consistency with these standards. Programs meeting these standards and providing a comprehensive, integrated set of medical and psychosocial rehabilitation services, delivered within an interdisciplinary team approach (as defined in this chapter), by qualified staff, may be enrolled as an ACT service provider.

**Elements of ACT.**   The ACT team must ensure that clients enrolled in ACT are provided access to the full continuum of available mental health services. Ideally, each clinical staff person on an ACT team has routine and regular contacts with each client, unless clinically contraindicated. In all cases, each client will receive services, at a minimum, from team members who represent three separate disciplines relevant to the client's needs. An ACT team must have a sufficient number of qualified professional staff (as defined in this chapter) to provide and supervise needed services. Professional staff composition must reflect client need, as identified in the individual service plan. ACT services are provided over a significant time period, with no predetermined discharge point.

**Services.**   ACT teams provide a wide array of services, which are designed to help support mental health service clients as they live independently in the community or during their transition to independent living from a more restrictive setting. Individuals living in specialized community residential settings (i.e., 24-hour supervision with room and board provided) or enrolled in a day program,

*(continued)*

**Table 21–1.** Michigan Medicaid requirements for Assertive Community Treatment *(continued)*

may receive ACT services if the active objective of treatment is to move the client to independent living or to more generic community services. For children and adolescents, ACT services may be provided to sustain the youngster within the family or to assist in the transition from out-of-home placement to the family home.

Services include assistance with addressing basic needs, such as food, housing, and medical care. Other services provided by the team support improved functioning in regard to social, educational, and vocational skills. Clinical consultants, providing other necessary services, may be added to the team. The costs associated with these services should be included in the total team cost for billing purposes.

Although ACT contacts may occasionally occur at the program's office, the majority are provided in other locations, including the client's home, according to individual need and clinical appropriateness.

Services are designed to improve the client's quality of life, to reduce unnecessary residential and hospital treatment, and to reduce other unnecessarily restrictive living situations. All clients enrolled in an ACT program are to receive appropriate assessments and care coordination (such as service plan development, linking and coordination of services, reassessment and follow-up, and service monitoring). ACT contacts provide a range of needed services during face-to-face interactions; these services are provided by an enrolled ACT provider and are based upon an individual service plan. These services may not be billed separately. When the following activities are provided to an individual receiving services from an ACT team, the service shall be billed as an ACT contact.

- Medication monitoring and review
- Medication administration
- Care coordination or case management
- Health services
- Crisis intervention
- Individual, group, child, and family therapy
- Occupational therapy

*(continued)*

**Table 21–1.** Michigan Medicaid requirements for Assertive Community Treatment (*continued*)

**Other Services.**   When the following Medicaid services are required for an ACT client, the activities should be billed separately with the appropriate billing code. The costs associated with these procedures are not included in the ACT contact costs.

- Health assessment
- Occupational therapy evaluation
- Other testing and assessment
- Physical therapy
- Physical therapy evaluation
- Professional treatment monitoring
- Psychiatric evaluation
- Psychological testing
- Quarterly review
- Speech evaluation
- Speech, language, or hearing services
- Treatment planning

Additionally, day program services may also be provided to ACT clients by an approved clinic program.

ACT may not be billed if psychosocial rehabilitation or home-based services are billed.

**Team Meetings.**   Regularly scheduled team meetings must be held a minimum of three times each week (daily meetings are preferable). During meetings the clinical, medical, and social condition of clients are discussed and treatment plan modifications may be initiated. These discussions must include an update on client progress and needs. Staff supervision will occur during these meetings. Documentation of these meetings must be sufficient to identify which individuals were discussed and which staff were present. Clinical decisions must be reflected in the individual service plan.

**Supervision.**   Because the majority of all ACT services are eclectic and supportive in nature, ACT service may be provided by any qualified mental health professional (as defined in the chapter) on the team with staff supervision and consultation occurring during

(*continued*)

**Table 21–1.**   Michigan Medicaid requirements for Assertive Community Treatment (*continued*)

___

routine team meetings, unless the needed service falls beyond an individual team member's scope of practice.

**Professional Treatment Monitoring.**   If a specific service is provided that falls beyond an individual team member's scope of practice (requiring specialized training or professional judgment), another professional who is qualified to supervise the provision of this service must provide professional treatment monitoring, as determined by the interdisciplinary team and documented in the individual service plan. Professional treatment monitoring must occur at intervals determined by the interdisciplinary team, based on client need. Professional treatment monitoring must be documented.

**Quarterly Reviews.**   At quarterly intervals, the physician and other team members must review the treatment plan, revising as necessary. This review provides an analysis of the client's progress over the previous quarter and discusses trends from past months. The quarterly review must be approved and signed by the physician, the professionals(s) who supervise the treatment, and other team members. Reviews are the result of program observations, record reviews, and interviews with staff and clients. The client should participate in the quarterly review process.

**Qualified Staff/Billable Contacts.**   Each face-to-face client contact may be billed (up to the established maximum monthly frequency) as an ACT contact. All ongoing billable services are to be included in the individual service plan. The plan of service is to be developed and authorized by the same interdisciplinary team of professionals providing the ACT service. Billable contacts must be conducted by qualified mental health professionals, as defined in Michigan's Medicaid plan. Provisions must be made for mental health clinics or for professionals who possess, at a minimum, a bachelor's degree in a human service field functioning within the team under the general supervision of qualified mental health professionals or persons without a bachelor's degree in a human service field when providing health services, under professional treatment monitoring provided by a qualified health care professional, when such activities do not require the clinical judgment by a qualified health care professional, or persons with-

*(continued)*

**Table 21–1.**  Michigan Medicaid requirements for Assertive Community Treatment *(continued)*

out a bachelor's degree in a human service field when providing activities of daily living under professional treatment monitoring provided by a qualified mental health professional.

Each billable contact must include a progress note containing the name of the client, date of service, start time and length of the contact, person providing the service, the service provided and how it relates to the treatment plan, and the place of service.

**Billing Instructions.**  To bill for more than one contact per day, the contacts must be separated by half an hour or more, or must be provided by different staff persons and related to different aspects of the treatment plan. An ACT contact cannot be billed solely for the purpose of transportation of the client.

---

rious mental illness, Michigan has established demonstration projects for the elderly with serious mental illness, for children with severe emotional disturbance, for persons with mental illness who also abuse alcohol or drugs, and for persons with mental illness and developmental disability. Our experience has been that all of these populations respond well to ACT treatment.

## Summary

Michigan's public mental health system overcame many obstacles and successfully established an effective and innovative treatment service throughout the state. Outcome surveys, site visits, and statewide training were conducted in order to guarantee positive results and to secure the continued support of various stakeholders. When establishing new program models, it is recommended that mental health administrators, executives, and planners follow steps similar to those described in this chapter. In retrospect, Michigan's success is largely due to the inherent effectiveness of ACT and to our tenacity. We were pleased to find how well received ACT was with consumers, providers, family members, and other advocates. We enthusiastically recommend that states with no ACT teams establish a number of demonstration sites and that states with only a few teams search for ways to create more. Do what we did—know where you are going and take one step at a time.

# References

Bond G: Assertive community treatment for frequent users of psychiatric hospitals in a large city: a controlled study. Am J Community Psychol 18:865–872, 1990

Bond G: Variations in an assertive outreach model. New Dir Ment Health Serv 52:65–80, 1991a

Boyer SL: A comparison of three types of case management on burnout and job satisfaction. Doctoral Dissertation, Purdue University at Indianapolis, 1992

Michigan Department of Social Services: Assertive Community Treatment. Medicaid Bulletin (October), 52–56, 1993

Muldar R: Evaluation of the Harbinger Program (unpublished report). Lansing, Michigan Department of Mental Health, 1982

Plum T, Adler D: ACT Annual Survey. Lansing, Michigan Department of Mental Health, 1990

Stein L, Test M: Gold Award. Hosp Community Psychiatry 25:669–672, 1974

Torrey EF: Care of the Seriously Mentally Ill. Washington, DC, Public Citizen Health Research Group, 1988

Torrey EF: Criminalizing the Seriously Mentally Ill. Washington, DC, Public Citizen Health Research Group, 1992

Witheridge T: The assertive community treatment worker: an emerging role and its implications for professional training. Hosp Community Psychiatry 40:177–183, 1989

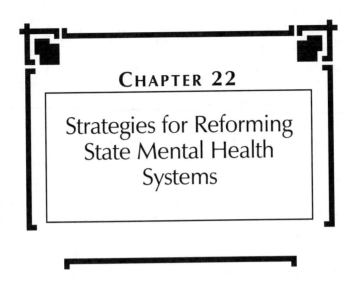

### CHAPTER 22

## Strategies for Reforming State Mental Health Systems

**Joseph J. Bevilacqua, Ph.D., John A. Morris, M.S.W., and J. Donald Bray, M.D.**

*It's one of the happy incidents of the federal system, that a single courageous state may, if its citizens choose, serve as a laboratory, and try novel social and economic experiments without risk to the rest of the country.*

*Justice Louis D. Brandeis*

Since the mid-1930s, the federal government has sought to upgrade human services in the states, with particular focus on health care, the mental disabilities, and basic social services. Washington has used a variety of strategies to achieve its policy goals: regulatory pressure, higher standards for continuing or establishing new participation in federally subsidized programs, and fiscal incentives. However, state participation in these federal initiatives has usually been ambivalent at best. States have always provided the major share of the resources for mental health care, but real improvements in care are of relatively recent vintage (Bevilacqua 1982).

Most state systems of mental health services have certain commonalities, no matter how they are organized, and all have been involved in one way or another in the movement to downsize hospitals and to deinstitutionalize long-term patients (Bachrach 1987). Although continuous system change is arguably both necessary and desirable in the field of public mental health, it is quite possible to radically restructure the formal architecture of an organization without having significant lasting impact on the service product of that agency.

Therefore, public mental health agencies must operate in a larger theater of interests, and successful system revision must formally engage major components external to the agency's operations, even when these external groups are engaged in adversarial dialogue with the public mental health authority. Such adversarial relationships are typical, for example, among private and academic mental health professionals, who often reflect a negative bias in their view of state agencies and public care. Although there is an acknowledgment of the important functions of running prisons, mental hospitals, and helping the poor, there are lingering, stereotypical perceptions of the public system as fraught with patronage, inefficiency, and excessive bureaucracy. The traditional (if unexamined) view is that state government performs important functions but that states are forced to settle for less than optimal standards in health care and social services interventions.

The view of state government as entrenched and unresponsive to the search for excellence has been a significant deterrent to collaborative initiatives for system improvement. All too often, professionals are only comfortable identifying themselves with government and politics when some guild interest is involved (e.g., the rights, prerogatives, and financing of professional practice). It is axiomatic, then, that it would be easier to attract private and academic mental health professionals to advocate for client interests when both guild and client interests are intertwined. Because this confluence of factors has rarely occurred, people with persistent mental illnesses and others served by the public mental health system have received little positive attention.

Until the relationship between the public sector clients and the political process is faced squarely by all stakeholders, including the broadest spectrum of the professional community, satisfactory resolution of the major mental health problems in this country is an unlikely outcome. Historically, the political process has been used to intervene in the economy to circumvent market forces in order to assure the financing of specific communal objectives that would not otherwise be met (Musgrave and Musgrave 1973), or to ensure resource allocation to priority populations (Gil 1976). Because patients who receive services from the public sector are often disenfranchised in many ways, they lack the clout to influence the political process necessary to address their needs. The advocacy of organizations such as the Mental Health Association was often the only avenue for the consumer voice, although the emergence of the Alliance for the Mentally Ill and the burgeoning consumer and ex-patient movement are changing the landscape of the change process.

Current debate about the basic architecture of the health care environment, coupled with the ever-changing face of mental health care, demands significant departures from traditional paradigms of service design. Hanson (1993) reviews the likely outcomes of changes in federal and state relationships under health care reform and concludes that great variability among state approaches is a likely outcome under any plan. In a related article, Peterson (1993) focuses the issue more narrowly: "Institutions matter. Institutions change, and that also matters" (p. 782). He cautions that the current health care debate will be unsuccessful if policy makers assume that the scope of options are limited; the possibility of significant and lasting system change is real at the broadest system level. Changes in the design and payment for specialty services, such as services for mental illnesses, are inevitable and will pose challenges for public and private systems alike.

Sheffler (1993) and his colleagues take the initiative to identify a role for specialized mental health plans under the health care reform, a sort of mental health maintenance organization (MHMO), reflecting the sort of creative strategic approach that will be required of mental health providers in the future.

A final, often ignored factor forcing new approaches to working with difficult clinical populations is the changing needs of such populations and the changing technologies emerging to meet those needs. For example, in a recent monograph on clozapine, Yesavage (1993) devotes several chapters to quality of life issues such as employment and living conditions for patients taking the drug. In previous times, the focus of such a monograph (produced by a pharmaceutical company) would almost certainly have been exclusively on the pharmacological impact on symptom reduction, side effects, clinical trials, and so on. Now the broader dimensions of the patient's life are seen as inextricably tied to the psychoactive agent's effectiveness.

Mental health professionals, especially in the public sector, are demonstrating greater sophistication in identifying and understanding the special needs of discrete subpopulations within the larger community of people with mental illnesses. The unique needs of homeless individuals with mental illnesses and those of people with comorbidity of chemical dependency and mental illness are but two examples.

The interactions between persistent mental illnesses and homelessness have been the subject of considerable attention. Knisely (1993) and others have documented supported housing efforts within mental health systems that are working. Carling (1993) documents the promising evidence that research activities appear to be feeding directly back into the work of service delivery.

The picture is not so encouraging when issues of mental illness and substance abuse are the focus. Durrell (1993), Fox et al. (1992), Drake and Wallach (1989), Kivlahan (1991), Thacker (1989), and others are focusing increasing attention on the complexities of working with persons who have a major mental illness and also a chemical dependency problem. And yet there are major problems integrating the realities of the service and research worlds with that of federal policy and practice. Block grant funds, for example, continue to flow to states in two distinct streams. State policy can allow the streams to continue flowing in separate channels, leaving the dually diagnosed patient on a no-man's-land in between, denied appropriate care.

In the current environment, then, the importance of interconnections and interdependencies among players is highlighted. Attention to the linkages among mental health professionals, universities and their research and teaching faculties, consumers and organized consumer organizations, families and their advocacy voices, and other policy makers is no longer optional for state mental health authorities. Effective system change is unlikely to occur in the absence of conscious, deliberate, and detailed collaborative strategies. In this context, public mental health systems must prepare themselves for an almost entrepreneurial approach to windows of opportunity for change. The capacity to recognize and capitalize on changes in the larger political or public climate is essential.

In this chapter we illustrate these principles as they have been applied in South Carolina to drive change in the mental health service system and in the attitudes of professionals toward the public sector agency and the people who consume its services.

# Background

South Carolina is a small (3.1 million people), relatively poor state (ranking 46th in per capita income), characterized by urban and rural poverty that is particularly evident among ethnic minorities and families with female heads of household. Mental health services are provided through a vertically integrated state system (all hospitals and community mental health centers operate under direct state authority); the State Director reports to a seven-member commission whose members are appointed by the governor and confirmed by the state senate. The Department of Mental Health was not affected by government restructuring that took place in 1993, which eliminated many independent boards and commissions and created for the first time a governor's cabinet.

The state mental health authority has a rich history; South

Carolina was the second state in the country to commission the construction of a public hospital for the care of the mentally ill. It followed Virginia in 1821, and invited the designer of the Washington Monument, native son Robert Mills, to be the architect for its asylum, which still stands in Columbia, the state capital. The South Carolina Department of Mental Health (SCDMH) operates a statewide network of community mental health centers, which have been heavily dependent on centralized inpatient facilities. The system had been relatively isolated from the state's academic institutions as well as private practice clinicians and had a poor record of professional recruitment and retention.

In 1983, the director of the SCMHD was the highly respected psychiatrist William S. Hall, who at his retirement a few years later was the longest-serving commissioner in the country. The system, however, was facing critical scrutiny not only from state legislators and advocates but from the Justice Department as well. An investigation of SCDMH was initiated in 1983 under the Civil Rights of Institutionalized Persons Act (CRIPA), citing intolerable conditions at the South Carolina State Hospital. The census at the hospital in 1983 was 1,244, and its annual operating budget was $ 29.7 million. The community mental health centers in the state operated with great independence, having had their birth in the Community Mental Health Centers Act of 1963 and having maintained a sense of autonomy in spite of their formal affiliation with the state department. There was little sense of common mission with the public psychiatric hospitals, nor shared responsibility for hospitalized patients. In 1983, there were 650 people employed statewide in the community system, with an operational budget of $21.8 million per year.

In 1985, while negotiations about the CRIPA lawsuit with the Justice Department continued, William S. Hall retired. The South Carolina Mental Health Commission conducted a national search, settling on the senior author of this chapter to be the new commissioner. In so doing, the seven-member Commission gave a broad mandate for changing the South Carolina system from a hospital-based system to a community-based system. Although the need for major change in the system was widely acknowledged, there was predictable debate about the degree or exact nature of those changes. The selection of new leadership with a well-articulated commitment to community-based services began the process of defining the mission of the agency.

By 1993, the census at the South Carolina State Hospital had been reduced to 381 (reflecting the first time since the 1870s that the census had been under 400). By January 1996, Crafts-Farrow State Hospital had been consolidated with the SC State Hospital, and the two facilities' combined census was 391. The community system by the mid-1990s employed more than 1,500 staff (two and a half times as many as in 1983), and the FY 1996–1997 budget for community mental health center operations is $115 million (more than quadruple the budget of 1983). Shifts in percentage of total budget allocation between inpatient and community services have been constant.

## Milestones in the Process of Change

### The CRIPA Lawsuit Resolution

The Justice Department had focused on a single facility, the South Carolina State Hospital. The department leadership had a series of alternative strategies to choose from in its response to the court. The first was to expend resources in an expensive and lengthy court battle. The second was to enter into a consent decree to correct the conditions at the hospital site alone (thus accepting the inevitability of large central hospital populations) and engage in major staffing and capital expenditures to more humanely and appropriately house and treat patients at the state hospital. The third was to enter into an agreement with the Justice Department to correct the conditions through a mixed strategy of targeted staffing ratios at the hospital and fire/life safety improvements, coupled with a plan to reduce hospital populations by the mechanism of aggressive community service development.

South Carolina, with the support of then Governor Richard Riley, chose the third course. The governor and new state commissioner worked out a consent decree in 1986 that had the support of the General Assembly and that involved a 4-year strategy of development using $20 million in state appropriations earmarked for the Justice Department consent decree, with the majority of that money targeted for community development. In 1990, on the original target date, the Justice Department released the department from its oversight under CRIPA: "the case is closed and dismissed on the grounds that the defendants have fully and faithfully implemented and maintained all provisions of the agreement"(U.S. v. State of South Carolina 1990, p 2). Obviously, so massive an undertaking involved collaboration among staffs in the hospital, in community mental health centers, and in the central office, as well as among advocates and members of the General Assembly.

## Reaching Consensus Among Stakeholders

Although the consent decree was holding center court for planners and agency management, other voices couldn't be ignored. DMH was operating children's programs and a forensic service that were chronically over census and that acted as lightning rods for community complaint and concern. In one of his Ranking of State Programs from this era, NAMI leader Fuller Torrey, M.D., referred to the presence of a well-staffed and funded university teaching facility (the Hall Institute) on the campus of the beleaguered South Carolina State Hospital as "heaven and hell existing side-by-side" (Torrey and Wolfe 1986, p. 73). The report highlighted another opportunity for action, and in 1986, the department transferred jurisdiction of the two troubled and troubling programs to the Hall Institute. The results of this action have been extremely positive. While these mergers and the consent decree negotiations were taking place, an external consulting firm (D. Goodrich and Associates) was hired to examine the basic structure of the mental health authority. The chief finding was that programs and services were too fragmented, and that the organizational structure was not consistent with the notion of a unified system of care. For example, there was a real gulf between the structure of the centralized hospitals and the community mental health centers.

There was a conscious decision on the part of the agency leadership to counteract the history of press and advocacy criticism by opening the doors of the agency voluntarily to oversight. For example, the agency has strongly supported the activities of one of its traditional critics: the South Carolina Protection and Advocacy (SC P and A) System for the Handicapped, Inc. DMH opens all of its facilities to regular, unannounced reviews by the Team Advocacy Project of SC P and A. The level of commitment to collaboration is reflected in the department's transfer of recurring base funding during a budget reduction to ensure that Team Advocacy representatives could continue to participate statewide in critical incident reviews.

Regular meetings were held not only with SC P and A, but also with representatives from the primary advocacy groups (Mental Health Association in South Carolina, South Carolina Alliance for the Mentally Ill, and the state's primary consumer group, Self-Help Association Regarding Emotion, also known as SHARE), as well as with ad hoc groups of citizens and advocates who had special concerns, such as children's services and services for dually diagnosed and hearing-impaired individuals. These are bread and butter activities that are common across many states, but reflect a change in approach for DMH.

The Public Mental Hospital In a Community-Based System of Care (Shurr et al. 1990) was the title given to an NIMH-sponsored conference that brought together representatives from NIMH and from the University of Illinois Institute of Government and Public Affairs; state mental health directors from Oregon, Ohio, Alabama, New Hampshire, and Vermont; along with a representative from the Dixon Oversight Committee in Washington, DC, and the President of the National Mental Health Association. The conference, jointly sponsored by the department and the NIMH, was envisioned as a way to invite key policy and practice leaders to come to South Carolina and help this state confront the issues of aging, unlicensable hospital buildings, and a community system still struggling for stability. The conference was intended to be an action catalyst, and the facilitators of sessions were expected to provide written feedback to the conference steering committee. Common themes emerged, with a clear consensus in support of greatly increased community development, especially for people with significant mental illnesses. A series of actions were proposed, beginning with a broadly based steering committee composed of "shareholders" who could both plan for change and then sell it statewide. The group further recommended a strategy of community debates on the issues, with the desired outcome being a greater sense of community ownership for the care of people with serious mental illnesses (Morris and Scales 1990).

## Implementation: Creating a Structure for Change

A group known as the Transition Leadership Council was the first in a series of steps designed to follow up on the work of the conference. The State Commissioner convened a group of 22 concerned professionals, advocates, and consumers, and charged them with two major tasks: to conduct a series of public meetings, which came to be known as forums, and to develop an action plan for change that would address the ticking clock of buildings that would need to be replaced or abandoned. The Council membership used a play on the letters of its name to capture its goals: TLC—Toward Local Care. This became the theme of the forums, which were held statewide and attended by over a thousand citizens. Community responses were recorded at each forum and incorporated into the final document of the Transition Leadership Council. The Council, true to its mandate, issued a final report to the members of the Mental Health Commission and the Commissioner, and formally ended its existence (a somewhat unique event in itself). The final report, issued in 1990, included a set of core themes or goals for change.

- People with serious mental illness would receive needed services as close to home as possible through South Carolina's community mental health centers.
- Services that are beyond the capacity of individual community mental health centers would be developed by two or more cen-

ters on a regional basis or provided in a central facility.

- The following groups would be given priority for services: adults with serious mental illness, children and adolescents who are seriously emotionally disturbed, and seriously mentally ill people with special needs, such as alcohol and drug abuse problems, mental retardation, and involvement with the criminal justice system. All services would be designed to be sensitive to the needs of minority clients and their families.
- New funds would be sought to increase the capacity of communities across the state to meet the needs of people with mental illness, including local hospitalization and other community services that have proved ineffective.
- Existing funds would be reallocated as patient care is shifted from central facilities to local communities.
- Mental health professionals who work in South Carolina's public mental health system would be well prepared to provide the range of services needed. All training would be designed to be sensitive to the needs of minority clients and families.

The report identified the following six action steps for change:

1. Establishing a joint management council to implement the transition to local community care
2. Establishing a funding plan using the paying patient fee account as bridge funds for the transition (the paying patient fee account is a special account into which insurance and Medicare payments are deposited; the account's primary purpose is to fund capital projects, but DMH has authorization to use some of the funds for operations)
3. Establishing a public academic liaison with South Carolina colleges and universities to prepare the workforce that will accomplish the transition
4. Establishing a positive working environment that is supportive to staff who are pursuing careers in public mental health
5. Establishing a regional capacity for those services that cannot be provided close to home

6. Establishing a systemwide client and management information system to monitor the transition and evaluate the accomplishments of goals and objectives

Shortly after receipt of the final report of the Transition Leadership Council, the state commissioner implemented the first recommendation and convened the implementation council. This new group chose to continue the TLC theme, but simplified its name to Transition Council. This newest group, which continues to meet, was designed to merge the planning process mandated under P.L. 96-660 (subsequently P.L. 102-321)—the State Comprehensive Mental Health Services Plan Act of 1986—with an action focus on transition. The notion was for this council to have as members, in addition to community and consumer representatives, key DMH officials so that Council recommendations would be assured of implementation. The state commissioner chairs the Council, and all key operational deputies are members. The Council has met monthly since its formation, but has recently opted to go to a bimonthly schedule. The Council operates from an annual action plan, which incorporates the 99-660 system planning activity, but focuses in on issues of community development, and concurrent reductions in dependence on inpatient hospitalization.

The implementation activities were acknowledged to have little hope for creating lasting change if there weren't going to be professionals trained to work in the new environment of more assertive community treatment. Linkages to academia were seen as an essential part of building the workforce needed to affect the total system. During the early stages of the initial council, SCDMH was successful in obtaining an NIMH Human Resource Development Grant (#5T23MH19706). One of the most critical uses of that grant was to fund a Visiting Scholar position, similar to the Galt Scholar program in Virginia (Bevilacqua 1986). J. Donald Bray, M.D., former Commissioner of Mental Health in Oregon, accepted the grant-funded post and devoted 18 months in 1990 and 1991 to full-time, on-site work with DMH. Dr. Bray continues to maintain a relationship with the state as a consultant to the Transition Council and to the Public-Academic Consortium discussed below.

## Reaching Out to Engage the Academics

The confluence of federal and state government interest in public and academic relationships, along with active support from foundations and professional organizations, is creating an important movement in the United States (Bevilacqua 1991; Bloom 1989; Peterson 1991; Talbott and Robinowitz 1986; Talbott et al. 1991). Over the years considerable criticism has been leveled at the preparation of professionals who work with the seriously mentally ill and the paucity of researchers to work and study in public mental health systems (Davis 1986; National Institute of Mental Health 1991). The development of knowledge and its transfer is traditionally seen as the exclusive province of the academic community, and recruitment and retention as the sole concern of the organizations providing services. At the most fundamental level this tunnel vision fails to address the simple economic fact that students want someday to be employed, and public systems want to employ them. When academic training becomes interwoven with the public policy and service mechanisms of a state, fundamental changes in practice can occur.

Most public and academic initiatives have focused primarily on the recruitment and retention of psychiatrists in state hospitals and community programs. Participants typically are state departments of mental health and departments of psychiatry. Although some research has occurred, it does not appear to have been a major goal of most collaborative efforts (Bloom 1989; Boust 1991; Keefer et al. 1991; Neligh et al. 1991; Weintraub et al. 1991; Yank et al. 1991).

Planning for the development of South Carolina's Public-Academic Mental Health Consortium (Bray and Bevilacqua 1993) actually began in January 1990, before the formal creation of the management council described above. All of the colleges and universities in the state that prepare people at the graduate level for work in public mental health were invited to participate in a series of meetings with the state commissioner. Consumer and advocate organizations were also represented along with DMH staff from community programs, state hospitals, and the central office. The planning phase and subsequent work of the consortium have focused exclusively on the state's transition to a community-based mental health system.

The initial step was the development of a vision statement for the consortium describing the plight of children and adults with serious mental illness and defining how a collaborative effort of the member organizations could significantly improve the quality of life of these people. The anticipated positive effects for students, faculty, and mental health workers were also included. Developing this vision statement established a shared focus for the planning group and was essential to achieving the goal of fostering collaborations, which will improve public mental health services in South Carolina by the following means.

- Preparing graduates who possess the knowledge, skills, and attitudes (including expectations of the daily work experience) needed to be effective mental health workers in South Carolina's public mental health system
- Promoting research by faculty and graduate students that is used to improve public mental health services both in South Carolina and nationally
- Providing the educational experiences needed by current workers for continued effectiveness in South Carolina's evolving public mental health system
- Developing a work experience in South Carolina's public mental health system, both in rural and urban areas, that is valued by employees as challenging and satisfying

Concerns were expressed early on that the liaison would not be effective because of its large and heterogeneous membership. Assuring the success of public and academic liaisons with a small number of organizations is difficult enough. Productively involving 27 representatives of participating organizations requires more than a shared vision and a clear understanding of mission and goals. Because of this, the planning group next set about defining how the organization would be structured and how it would function in a detailed set of bylaws. This degree of formality was seen as essential for a collaborative effort of this size and scope. The bylaws are a working document that require amendments as the consortium further defines itself over time.

Another approach to this potential problem was to sharpen the focus of the consortium through a detailed action plan for achieving its four goals. The plan includes specific objectives with clearly defined expected outcomes and finite completion dates. Activities designed to achieve these objectives are assigned to various consortium members and staff. The plan is updated annually. Where possible, initial benchmarks have been established to allow for evaluating progress in achieving the goals (i.e., retention of mental health professionals, recruitment of graduates of South Carolina programs, and levels of extramural funding for research and demonstration activities). Such benchmarks have clear implications for education and continuing education as well as for employee satisfaction and productivity goals.

Once the bylaws and action plan were accepted by the member organizations, the South Carolina Public-Academic Mental Health Consortium was formally established (on November 26, 1990). The member organizations included 13 academic programs from seven colleges and universities that prepare people at the graduate level for work in public mental health. Consumer and advocate organizations as well as the South Carolina Area Health Education Consortium are also members. The SCDMH is represented at the community, state hospital, and central office levels. Additional organizations may join by invitation of the consortium. The consortium's permanent chair is the State Commissioner of Mental Health.

Three levels of outcomes are anticipated for the Public-Academic Consortium. The first level is having academics meaningfully involved in the public mental health system. This will provide each of them with the experience needed to accomplish the second level of outcomes. Second levels include the development of curriculums and placements that are designed to convey the needed knowledge, skills, and attitudes to their students; and the initiation of collaborative research. The third level of outcomes is achieving the goals of the consortium (development of graduates who possess the needed knowledge, skills, and attitudes; facilitating research findings that are used to improve services; and maintaining a high level of effectiveness in a provider pool that values their careers in the public mental health system).

An initial activity of the Public-Academic Consortium was to help its academic members to develop a better understanding of the public mental health system. To accomplish this, a series of focused educational experiences was provided for academic and other consortium members. These were conducted at various sites throughout the state, including state hospitals and community programs, and were designed to give participants an on-site—and often hands-on—exposure to the reality of contemporary clinical practice. Consortium members were assigned to multidisciplinary teams and asked to identify the knowledge, skills, and attitudes needed by each discipline represented in terms of the service environment being visited. The site visits involve a day and a half of time involved in face-to-face interactions with patients, staff, and families. A Literature Syllabus provided team members with a background on the kinds of programs that are essential to an effective community mental health system.

Faculty and students from member academic organizations regularly participate in an administrative seminar at the SCDMH central office designed to provide a broader perspective of the public mental health system and a better understanding of current systemic and governance issues. Participants have discussions with the chairman of the State Mental Health Commission, the commissioner, five deputy commissioners, legal council, and consumer and advocate representatives. They also visit the legislature and have the opportunity to discuss the issues that arise.

Meaningful involvement of academics in public mental health is an indicator that the activities at the consortium have been successful (Bray and Bevilacqua 1993). Some examples follow in the list below.

- A department chair initiated a shared faculty position with a community mental health center based on an idea he had during a focused educational experience.
- One faculty member who completed the administrative seminar in 1990 became a research fellow of the National Association of State Mental Health Program Directors Research Institute and worked on the transition in a variety of ways, such as accomplishing an evaluation of the Transition Council's eight community placement projects.
- A director of a psychiatry training program expanded the clinical training sites from one to eight mental health centers in different parts of the state.
- A college dean is developing a child and adolescent curriculum for the DMH's continuing education program.
- A chief of nursing is working to increase the appropriate utilization of nurses in public mental health through a research project funded by the DMH.
- a faculty member took the lead role in identifying barriers to collaborative research, and has established a consortium office of research (Bray and Bevilacqua 1993).

A series of initiatives are also being taken to improve employee satisfaction and productivity. A broadly representative group of departmental employees has been assembled, joined by a primary consumer and by representatives of the academic and advocacy communities, to aggressively pursue issues of employee morale and support. Special training for all staff at the state's two long-term hospitals has begun to reorient hospital interventions toward a more rehabilitative and community-focused approach. Management has committed to a policy of job-shifting and phased downsizing of hospitals to avoid employee layoffs, reassuring skilled clinicians that their livelihood is not jeopardized by this major systems change. A consultant in public relations works with the department to insure that its message of change is communicated clearly and effectively.

## Other Activities

In addition to the ongoing and targeted activities identified above, DMH has tapped into alternative funding sources for innovative programs. Assertive Community Treatment programs funded by NIMH/Community Support Program grants, family preservation models funded by NIMH/Child and Adolescent Service System Program funds, the Visiting Scholar program funded by NIMH/Human Resource Development Initiatives, and a Robert Wood Johnson capitation project are but a few examples. Late in 1993 the State Department 1) teamed up with the Bazelon Center for Mental Health Law to win a Justice Department grant to improve access to services for the mentally disabled under the Americans with Disabilities Act; 2) received a major demonstration grant from NIMH to create a seamless array of services for children, adolescents, and their families in a major catchment area; and 3) was awarded a second research site by the National Association of State Mental Health Program directors (NASMHPD). These are the fruit of years of focused activities.

DMH has also used its own resources to fuel change strategies, a difficult task in a time of budget constriction. DMH undertook an in-depth survey of 663 long-term psychiatric inpatients to identify clinical, functional, and financial status, and to determine individual preference for where they would like to live, what services they believed they would need, whether they wanted to leave the hospital, and whether they felt ready to leave. Each patient was then assessed by teams of community and hospital personnel, and a consensus plan achieved for each of the patients. Using monies from the Paying Patient Fee Account, DMH subsequently floated a Request for Proposals that would identify specific programming to move 140 of these patients out of the South Carolina State Hospital and Crafts-Farrow State Hospital (the state's geriatric psychiatric hospital) in the course of FY 1992–1993. These proposals were intended to encourage local ownership of the process of deinstitutionalization, rather than a top-down approach. These data from the consensus plans provided the base for decisions about program design and appropriateness for respondents to the Request for Proposals as well as baseline information for tracking the effectiveness of system interventions. A first wave of projects was funded in 1993, and a second wave followed with a modified RFP. As of May 1996, more than 250 consumers have been successfully transitioned from the state's long-stay institutions. A sophisticated program for consultation and evaluation of the initiatives was developed through a collaboration between DMH and the Medical University of South Carolina (see Chapter 19).

# Discussion

It should be noted that during much of the time that the activity described in this chapter has taken place, South Carolina has struggled under the same fiscal constraints as its sister states, and DMH has suffered significant losses to its base budget. Only through the assertive response of the state's Medicaid authority have we been able to absorb nearly $20 million in appropriations reductions in the past 2 fiscal years, while continuing to develop a truly community-based mental health system. We have been blessed by history in that our two largest long-term hospitals are located in the state capital, and in that DMH also operates an acute psychiatric hospital in Columbia, an inpatient alcohol and drug dependency facility, and a large nursing care facility. This has enabled DMH to drastically downsize hospital census without resorting to painful staff layoffs, by using attrition and local transfers to absorb employee reductions.

The mid-1990s have seen additional pressures on the system, with much attention being focused on preparing the integrated delivery system for a managed behavioral healthcare environment. Organizational consultants and DMH staff have been conducting analyses of DMH operations on the assumption that some sort of federal and/or state block granting of Medicaid will occur. The primary author of this chapter (Bevilacqua) stepped down as state director in August of 1995, and the second author

(Morris) was appointed interim director. As of May 1996, no permanent appointment had been made. Discussions continue about placing the department in the governor's cabinet.

In fairness, not all of our strategies have worked, and some of the most successful were initiated without the sort of sophisticated analysis that one would most desire. The support of advocates and key players external to the system has enabled us to avoid criticism when there have been mistakes and to provide credibility that state bureaucrats cannot command on their own. Flexibility and responsiveness have to be accepted as just as important as planning and analysis for real system change to occur and persist. No analysis of this type would be complete without some discussion of the core value that drives the activities we have described. The three organizational principles we posit are meaningless unless seen in the context of a strong commitment to community-based care because of what that care means to the people whom we serve. We believe that the actions we have described are the external manifestations of a consistent and clearly identifiable value orientation. It is too easy for change to occur mechanically or in reaction to outside forces, and it is a mistake to take for granted that value issues are easily understood, simply communicated, or readily accepted. Leadership and management activities, as well as financial and strategic planning, all must be driven by a clear sense of the underlying value. The challenge of having an organization of over 6,000 employees maintain a coherent, responsive commitment to a vision of improved patient care is an ongoing struggle. But results beget results, and systemwide momentum can be exhilarating for professionals who want to feel confident that their interventions are making a difference in patients' lives, and that the system wants them to succeed. In the final analysis, no system is better than the most fundamental contact that is its foundation: the face to face encounter between patient and provider. The quality of that interaction leads to the ultimate goal of any system of services for persons with mental illnesses: real improvement in quality of life, and truly local care.

# References

Bachrach L: Deinstitutionalization in the United States: promises and prospects, in Leona Bachrach Speaks: Selected Speeches and Lectures. San Francisco, CA, Jossey-Bass, 1987

Bevilacqua J: The changing federal-state human service system: perspectives from a State Commissioner of Mental Health and Mental Retardation. Consultation Magazine 2:1982

Bevilacqua J: The Galt Visiting Scholar in public mental health: a Virginia experience, in Working Together: State-University Collaboration in Mental Health. Edited by Talbott JA, Rabinowitz CB. Washington, DC, American Psychiatric Press, 1986, pp 111–120

Bevilacqua JJ: The NIMH public-academic liaison (PAL) research initiative: an update. Hosp Community Psychiatry 42:71–72, 1991

Bray JD, Bevilacqua JJ: A multidisciplinary public-academic liaison to improve public mental health services in South Carolina. Hosp Community Psychiatry 44:985–990, 1993

Bloom JD: State-university collaboration: the Oregon experience, in New Directions for Mental Health Services, Vol 44. Edited by Bloom JD. San Francisco, CA, Jossey-Bass, 1989, p 121

Boust SS: State-university collaboration in Nebraska: public psychiatry residency training in a rural area. Hosp Community Psychiatry 24:49–51, 1991

Davis KE: The challenge of state mental health systems and universities in Virginia: preparation of mental health professionals for work with the chronically mental ill. Interim Report. Richmond, Commonwealth of Virginia, Department of Mental Health, Mental Retardation and Substance Abuse, 1986

Drake RE, Wallach MA: Substance abuse among the chronically mentally ill. Hosp Community Psychiatry 40:1041–1046, 1989

Keefer BL, Kraus RF, Parker BL, et al: A state-university collaboration program: residents' perspective. Hosp Community Psychiatry 42:62–66, 1991

Morris J, Scales C: The group 3 experience: the public mental health hospital in a community-based system of care. Proceedings from a national conference, Columbia, SC, February 12–14, 1989. South Carolina Department of Mental Health, 1990

Musgrave RA, Musgrave PA: Public Finance in Theory and Practice. New York, McGraw-Hill, 1973

National Institute of Mental Health: Caring for people with severe mental disorders: a national plan of research to improve services (DHHS Publ No ADM-91-1762). Washington, DC, U.S. Government Printing Office, 1991

Neligh G, Shore JH, Scully S, et al: The program for public psychiatry: state-university collaboration in Colorado. Hosp Community Psychiatry 24:44–48, 1991

Peterson PD: State-university collaboration: next steps. Hosp Community Psychiatry 42:782–801, 1991

Scheffler R, Grogan C, Cuffel B, et al: A specialized mental health plan for persons with serious mental illness under managed competition. Hosp Community Psychiatry 44:937–942, 1992

Shurr M, Craft S, McEachern A (eds): The public mental hospital in a community-based system of care. Proceedings from a national conference, Columbia, SC, February 12–14, 1989. South Carolina Department of Mental Health, 1990

Talbott JA, Robinowitz CR (eds): Working Together: State-University Collaboration in Mental Health. Washington, DC, American Psychiatric Press, 1986

Talbott JA, Bray JD, Flaherty L, et al: State-university collaboration in psychiatry: the Pew Memorial Trust program. Community Ment Health J 27:425–439, 1991

Torrey EF, Wolfe SM: Care of the Seriously Mentally Ill: A Rating of State Programs. Washington, DC, Public Citizen Health Research Group, 1986

U.S. v State of South Carolina et al., Civil Action No. 3-861677-0, United States District Court for the District of South Carolina, August 14, 1990

Yank G, Barber JW, Vieweg WVR, et al: Virginia's experience with state-university collaboration. Hosp Community Psychiatry 24:39–44, 1991

Weintraub W, Nyman G, Harbin H: The Maryland plan: the rest of the story. Hosp Community Psychiatry 42:52–55, 1991

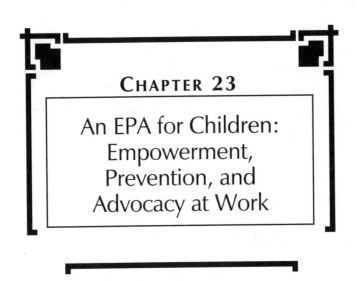

CHAPTER 23

## An EPA for Children: Empowerment, Prevention, and Advocacy at Work

**Cindy L. Hanson, Ph.D.**

Most innovative treatment models for children do not limit the definition of "health" as either physical or mental, but rather the well-being of youths is viewed at multiple levels, including physical, psychosocial, and spiritual, and within the multiple contexts of the family, community, and culture (Sciarillo 1993). Healing the lives of children involves health care efforts whose definitions of *health* are consistent with that of the World Health Organization, namely the promotion of physical, mental, and social health, in addition to the absence of disease (World Health Organization 1986) and also with the United Nations Convention on the Rights of the Child (1991), wherein mental, physical, and social conditions define the health and welfare of children. Similarly, on a national level, the distinctions between physical and mental health are slowly merging with the vision delineated in *Healthy People 2000: National Health Promotion and Disease Prevention Objectives* (U.S. Department of Health and Human Services 1990): to improve the healthy years of life of United States citizens. According to *Healthy People 2000,* "healthy life means a vital, creative, and productive citizenry contributing to thriving communities and a thriving Nation" (p 43). The status of children and their needs and rights to "healthy years of life" are discussed in this chapter to provide the framework for the critical importance of the new emerging models of health care that incorporate the family and community in their development, implementation, and ongoing evaluation and change, and that support the needs and rights of all children.

Traditionally (and still in many parts of the world), childhood chronic illness, disabilities, and diseases have been perceived as invoking or resulting from "deficits," weaknesses of the spirit, and/or unfavorable characteristics of children who live with disabilities or illnesses compared with other children. The pendulum has swung among many health care professionals who have examined the strengths and positive adaptation of youths who live with diseases and disabilities, particularly those who live within nurturing environments (Hanson 1992; Hanson et al. 1990). A shift is now needed from the world view of illness and disabilities as representing deficits, or, alternatively, adaptations, to a clear focus on the healing that must occur among us and within our communities. When the heart of the problem lies within the structures and values of society, then children, especially those who have significant health problems, become difficult to treat. As described later, the processes of empowerment, prevention, and advocacy denote the changes that are needed in the delivery of health care services to ensure the health and well-being of all children.

## Status of Health Care Services for Children in the United States

Reports summarizing the current status of health care services for children highlight the critical need for integrated systems of family- and community-based care that meet the mental, physi-

cal, and social needs of children (Burns 1991; Burns and Friedman 1990; Duchnowski and Friedman 1990; National Commission on Children 1991; Tuma 1989). The majority of children in
need are not receiving any services, and the services that are
provided are often inadequate, ineffective, inappropriate, or all
three (National Commission on Children 1991; U.S. Congress,
Office of Technology Assessment 1986). In 1983, the Child and
Adolescent Service System Program (CASSP) was initiated by the
National Institutes of Mental Health (NIMH) for the evaluation
of innovative and integrated delivery systems for underserved
children and adolescents labeled as severely or seriously emotionally disturbed (SED; Children's Mental Health Services Program 1992). As described by Lourie et al. (1990), efforts funded
by CASSP have resulted in progress across four central domains:
defining the systems of care that are needed for children with
mental health problems, creating interagency systems that monitor and facilitate the delivery of services, encouraging the development of a national movement of parents to promote
parent-professional partnerships to meet the needs of children,
and defining culturally sensitive systems of care. The excellent
work conducted for youths with SED (e.g., Stroul and Friedman
1986) and for youths with emotional and behavioral disorders
(e.g., Nelson and Pearson 1991) needs to be expanded to focus
on the broader spectrum of children and families to reduce the
prevalence of children at risk whether from environmental (e.g.,
homelessness), emotional (e.g., neglect, abuse), and/or physical
(e.g., debilitating diseases, violence) insults (National Commission on Children 1991).

## Questions of Needs, Risks, or Resources

With scarce resources, the question of who should be included in
innovative programs is controversial. No one would argue against
the idea that resources should be provided for those in highest
need. What characteristics define samples in highest need? Because our ideas are necessarily rooted in our frames of reference

and colored by our experiences, prioritizing levels of need is complex. Should more resources be allocated for those with the most medically burdensome diseases or for those with the fewest coping and social resources to meet the burdens of living with a chronic disease? Contrary to expectations that the youths with the most medically burdensome diseases would benefit the most from intensified home-based treatments, Jessop and Stein (1991) found such services were most beneficial for families with low coping and social resources, particularly families with less medically burdensome diseases. The findings also indicated that intensified treatment for families who do not need that level of help can be more aversive than standard care. Jessop and Stein suggested perhaps their intensified intervention did not adequately meet the needs of the families with youths who had the most burdensome diseases. Although compartmentalizing children and families into groups according to levels of risk on varying dimensions might be appealing to some, the issue is more complex and requires a comprehensive plan that is individualized and flexible.

Rather than ask "Who is at greatest risk?" Stark (1992) suggests that questions of need and risk emphasize the quick fix instead of addressing the more critical long-term resource questions. Resource questions illuminate the situations that cause inadequate resources and prevent children from reaching their potential. Stark proposes that the "quick fix" perspective reflects a patriarchal attitude that emphasizes the passivity of those waiting to be helped rather than enhancing the strengths and resources of those facing significant stressors. To avoid cumbersome semantic issues, the point is that as a society with individuals from diverse cultural and socioeconomic backgrounds, the health care system must use the resources and strengths of communities and families to promote positive well-being for all youths. The highest priority should be given to innovative health care services that are collaboratively planned and implemented by the family and community, developmentally appropriate, sensitive to cultural issues, individualized and flexible, interdisciplinary, cost-effective, and accessible to all children, especially those with circumstances that make care difficult to obtain. Empirical support for the effectiveness of these types of model programs is essential.

## The Changing Role of the Health Care Profession

Innovative models of health care are looking to change the roles of health care professionals and the resources available in the environment by respecting the ability of children and families to function effectively in supportive environments (e.g., Lash and Wertlieb 1993; Maternal and Child Health Coalition 1993). The most favorable family outcomes, feelings of self-efficacy, and positive family self-attributions among families who live with developmental disabilities have been linked to those helping styles and practices of health care professionals that are consistent with the principles of family support initiatives, namely those that emphasize the empowerment of people, underscore the importance of the consumer, and focus on the family regarding implementation of the program and the practices of case managers (Dunst et al. 1993). As another example, in the evaluation of sheltered care environments for adults with psychiatric disabilities (Carling 1990), the characteristics of communities were more important in predicting successful community participation by residents than were their individual characteristics (Segal and Aviram 1978; Tabor 1980).

Across a number of professional fields and lay communities, social and policy changes are redefining traditional roles in health care. Most child health care professionals in the public, private, and academic sectors have limited knowledge of national and international initiatives and are relatively unfamiliar with work outside of their specialty areas (Day and Roberts 1991; Roberts and Peterson 1984). It has become increasingly clear, however, that it is time to move on and meet the needs of children by directing, developing, and supporting child and family programs and initiatives (Roberts 1993).

The needs and rights of children cannot wait. The current health care models for children need to be revolutionized to incorporate families, schools, and communities in order to provide optimal development for children across physical, emotional, educational, and spiritual levels (Melton 1991). The inadequate integration of the behavioral, medical, and social sciences (e.g., social work, nursing, psychiatry, psychology, health policy), the poor interagency linkages, and the limited collaboration between health care professionals and community leaders and citizens has crippled many efforts to provide optimal environments for children. As only one example, considerable research indicates that the use of authoritarian child-rearing strategies has negative short- and long-term consequences for children and their families; however, this disciplinary style is frequently used by families and is sanctioned by many formal institutions (e.g., schools) and even by health care professionals (Straus 1992).

## Dissatisfaction and Distrust

The health care system in the United States functions best for healthy, insured, and financially secure people who occasionally have an acute illness. It is woefully deficient financially and structurally for those who need it the most: families with limited access or low income, and/or families who live with chronic illnesses and disabling conditions. Dissatisfaction with current models of health care in the United States is also reflected by the one out of four Americans who use unconventional, alternative, or traditional/indigenous medical practices (Eisenberg et al. 1993; Jing-feng 1987; Jonas 1993) for serious health problems. These medical practices may or may not be effective, and in some cases they are dangerous to children and adults, both because of the practice itself and because of the failure to seek out conventional methods whose efficacy has been demonstrated. Seven out of 10 individuals do not tell their medical doctors about the unconventional therapy (Eisenberg et al. 1993). At the same time that many of the helping professions in the United States are having identity problems and are engaging in turf battles and infighting, many people are leaving the battleground for something else.

Eisenberg et al. (1993) extrapolated that in 1990, Americans made 425 million unconventional medical visits, exceeding the 388 million visits made to all United States primary care physicians. Expenditures were similar to nonreimbursed medical expenses for all hospitalizations in the United States, and about half of what was spent for out-of-pocket physicians' services. On a positive note, some of the alternative medicine approaches are more family-centered and community-based, and view health as being multileveled. In other words, some of these approaches view health as involving strong interconnections between mind, body, and spirit. The innovative models of health care in Western medicine are not that "innovative" in many traditional medicines. As "peacemakers" and advocates for children, we need to develop practices that will demonstrate an understanding of the needs of children and families so that mutual trust can be rebuilt and effective collaborative programs can proliferate (Tyson and Said 1993).

## Balancing Cost-Effectiveness and Quality Care

From one perspective, the fulcrum that balances quality care and cost in the United States is cracking because of poor health outcomes, despite the high costs of clinical care. From another perspective, the foundation, or fulcrum on which quality care at reasonable cost is provided, is missing; that is, the services are driven primarily by the most salient needs at the given time. As Brooks and McGlynn (1991) remind us, "The principal goal of the U.S. health care system should be to maximize the health of the population; the goal is not to save money. . . . Put simply, health services research should distinguish between processes that produce health improvements and those that either produce no improvements or produce health decrements. Such information will assist policymakers in designing delivery and reimbursement systems capable of maximizing health" (p. 284).

The basic principles of empowerment, prevention, and advocacy are consistent with the many grass-roots efforts and federal initiatives that are building the fulcrum that can change the delivery of health care services for youths and families. Changes in the health care delivery system that involve using the strengths of children and their families (empowerment), that allow preventive action to facilitate optimal development of youths and families (prevention), and that provide the flexibility to meet the needs and rights of the youths and their families (advocacy) are needed for children's health care, particularly for those with chronic health conditions. These tenets will enable youths to obtain multilevel services that will foster their maximum development, according to the U.N. Convention on the Rights of the Child.

## Empowerment: Using the Strengths of Families and Communities

As a society with individuals from diverse cultural and socioeconomic backgrounds, the delivery of health care services must use the resources and strengths of the communities and families to promote positive well-being for all youths (i.e., empowerment). Empowerment has been used as a framework to facilitate positive health and well-being. Empowerment is similar to the concept of health promotion, the process of enabling people to increase control over and to improve their health (cf. Pederson et al. 1990). Pederson et al. (1990) list five strategies linked to health promotion: building healthy public policies, creating supportive environments, strengthening community action, developing personal skills, and reorienting health services toward health promotion and disease prevention. Empowerment denotes a sharing of responsibility through enabling others to perform optimally.

## Advocacy: A Necessary Ally of Empowerment

Empowerment does not replace the human responsibility to help others through advocacy. As such, the typical relationship between the health care provider and family changes from that of the health care provider helping to solve the problems of youths and their families to helping change the resources and environment in ways that facilitate people reaching their potential and following their own paths for good health (Meyers 1989), which is advocacy. Children must be provided with the opportunity to fulfill their rights to a long and healthy life. Although often conceptualized from an individual framework, the principles of empowerment and advocacy rely heavily on changes within social systems that facilitate changes at the individual level. Given that all ideas are culturally bound, empowerment and advocacy processes nevertheless seem to cut across cultural and economic environments (Stark 1992).

## Prevention: A Cornerstone for Change in Health Care Services

In addition to empowerment and advocacy, the third cornerstone of health care services change is prevention. Bond and Wagner (1988) highlight characteristics that differentiate effective and ineffective prevention programs. Many of the guidelines presented by Bond and Wagner for developing primary prevention programs are applicable to secondary and tertiary prevention efforts as well. The characteristics of the general orientation of effective prevention programs (Bond and Wagner 1988) include the multisystemic and multilevel perspective, the emphasis on promotion of competence, and sensitivity to developmental issues. The four distinguishing components of program development and refinement that are characteristic of effective prevention programs (Bond and Wagner 1988) include guidance by scientific theory, replicability, field experience, and longitudinal tracking. Coie et al. (1993) present a conceptual framework for the principles underpinning prevention programs and suggest directions for future research.

# A Shared Vision of Healing
# Within Our Communities

For those who share a dream of peace, a renewed spirit of change is beginning to emerge nationally and internationally. A heightened sense of unity is developing between peoples and within communities, and between nations and worlds. The dream of peace is a glimpse of a future that brings healing to its children. The nightmares and realities of war and violence, poverty, abuse, hunger, illness, disease, and premature death expose the failures of individuals and groups of people within the multiple and expanding layers of communities throughout our nation and the world. This chapter has highlighted some of the changes and shifts that are occurring that reflect a renewed commitment toward healing the lives of children globally.

# References

Bond LA, Wagner BM: What makes primary prevention programs work? in Families in Transition: Primary Prevention Programs That Work, Vol 11. Edited by Bond LA, Wagner BM. Newbury Park, CA, Sage, 1988, pp 343–354

Brooks RH, McGlynn EA: Maintaining quality of care, in Health Services Research: Key to Health Policy. Edited by Ginzberg E. Cambridge, MA, Harvard University Press, 1991, pp 284–314

Burns BJ: Mental health service use by adolescents in the 1970s and 1980s. J Am Child Adolesc Psychiatry 30:144–150, 1991

Burns BJ, Friedman RM: Examining the research base for child mental health services and policy. Journal of Mental Health Administration 17:87–98, 1990

Carling PJ: Major mental illness, housing, and supports: the promise of community integration. Am Psychol 45:969–975, 1990

Children's Mental Health Services Program: Grants for Comprehensive Community Mental Health Services for Children with Serious Emotional Disturbance. (Legislative Summary Series Number 12). Alexandria, VA, National Mental Health Association, 1992

Coie JD, Watt NF, West SG, et al: The science of prevention: a conceptual framework and some directions for a national research program. Am Psychol 48:1013–1022, 1993

Day C, Roberts MC: Activities of the child and adolescent service system program for improving mental health services for children and families. Journal of Clinical Child Psychology 20:340–350, 1991

Duchnowski AJ, Friedman RM: Children's mental health: challenges for the nineties. Journal of Mental Health Administration 17:3–12, 1990

Dunst CJ, Trivette CM, Starnes AL, et al: Building and Evaluating Family Support Initiatives: A National Study of Programs for Persons with Developmental Disabilities. Baltimore, MD, Brookes, 1993

Eisenberg DM, Kessler RC, Foster C, et al: Unconventional medicine in the United States: prevalence, costs, and patterns of use. New Engl J Med 328:246–252, 1993

Hanson CL: Developing systemic models of the adaptation of youths with diabetes, in Advances in Pediatric Psychology: Stress and Coping with Pediatric Conditions. Edited by La Greca AM, Siegel LJ, Wallander JL, et al. New York, Guilford, 1992, pp 212–241

Hanson CL, Rodrigue JR, Henggeler SW, et al: The perceived self-competence of adolescents with insulin-dependent diabetes mellitus: deficit or strength? J Pediatr Psychol 15:605–618, 1990

Jessop DJ, Stein REK: Who benefits from a pediatric home care program? Pediatrics 88:497–505, 1991

Jingfeng C: Toward a comprehensive evaluation of alternative medicine. Soc Sci Med 25:659–667, 1987

Jonas WB: Evaluating unconventional medical practices. The Journal of NIH Research 5:64–67, 1993

Lash M, Wertlieb D: A model for family centered service coordination for children who are disabled by traumatic injuries. The ACCH (Association for the Care of Children's Health) Advocate 1:19–41, 1993

Lourie IS, Stroul BA, Katz-Leavy J, et al: Advances in children's mental health. Am Psychol 45:407–408, 1990

Maternal and Child Health Coalition: Principles for maternal and child health care reform. The ACCH (Association for the Care of Children's Health) Advocate 1:11, 1993

Melton GB: Socialization in the global community: respect for the dignity of children. Am Psychol 46:66–71, 1991

Meyers J: The practice of psychology in the schools for the primary prevention of learning and adjustment problems in children: a perspective from the field of education, in Primary Prevention and Promotion in the Schools, Vol 12. Edited by Bond LA, Compas BE. Newbury Park, CA, Sage, 1989, pp 391–422

National Commission on Children: Beyond rhetoric: a new American agenda for children and families (publication no. HV741.N312). Washington, DC, U.S. Government Printing Office, 1991

Nelson CM, Pearson CA: Integrating services for children and youth with emotional and behavioral disorders (stock no. P364). Reston, VA, The Council for Exceptional Children, 1991

Pederson A, Roxburgh S, Wood L: Symposium reflections: conducting community action research. Office of Substance Abuse Prevention Monograph 4:265–285, 1990

Roberts MC: President's message: time to move on. Clinical Child Psychology Newsletter 8:1–3, 1993

Roberts MC, Peterson L (eds): Prevention of Problems in Childhood: Psychological Research and Applications. New York, Wiley, 1984

Sciarillo W: Editorial: advocacy.. professing one's conviction. The ACCH (Association for the Care of Children's Health) Advocate 1:4–5, 1993

Segal SP, Aviram U: The Mentally Ill in Community-Based Sheltered Care: A Study of Community Care and Social Integration. New York, Wiley, 1978

Stark W: Empowerment and social change: health promotion within the healthy cities project of WHO—steps toward a participative prevention program, in Improving Children's Lives: Global Perspectives on Prevention. Edited by Albee GW, Bond LA, Monsey TCV. Newbury Park, CA, Sage, 1992, pp 167–176

Straus MA: Corporal punishment: background and goals of the task force on the effects of corporal punishment on children. The Child, Youth, and Family Services Quarterly 15:1–2, 1992

Stroul BA, Friedman RM: A system of care for severely emotionally disturbed children and youth (monograph). Washington, DC, Georgetown University Child Development Center, CASSP Technical Assistance Center, 1986

Tabor MA: The social context of helping: a review of the literature on alternative care for the physically and mentally handicapped. Rockville, MD, National Institute of Mental Health, 1980

Tuma JM: Mental health services for children: the state of the art. Am Psychol 44:188–199, 1989

Tyson B, Said AA: Human rights: a forgotten victim of the cold war. Human Rights Quarterly 15:589–604, 1993

United Nations Convention on the Rights of the Child. New York, NY, United Nations Department of Public Information, 1991

U.S. Congress, Office of Technology Assessment: Children's mental health: problems and services—a background paper (OTA-BP-H-33). Washington, DC, U.S. Government Printing Office, 1986

U.S. Department of Health and Human Services: Healthy People 2000: National Health Promotion and Disease Prevention Objectives, Full Report, With Commentary. (DHHS Publication No. [PHS] 91-50512.) U.S. Government Printing Office, Washington, DC, 1990

World Health Organization: Ottawa Charter for Health Promotion. Copenhagen, Denmark, World Health Organization, 1986

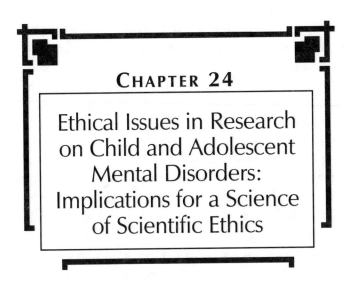

# CHAPTER 24

## Ethical Issues in Research on Child and Adolescent Mental Disorders: Implications for a Science of Scientific Ethics

**Kimberly Hoagwood, Ph.D., Peter S. Jensen, M.D., and Alan I. Leshner, Ph.D.**

In the face of the numerous reports documenting the very large numbers of children and adolescents who face serious problems in adaptation (American Medical Association 1990; Association for the Advancement of Health Education 1987; National Commission on the Role of the School and the Community in Improving Adolescent Health 1990; U.S. Congress, Office of Technology Assessment 1991), discussion of ethical issues in research with children and adolescents may appear at best peripheral, at worst, deflective. With current studies reporting prevalence rates of significant mental disorders among youth to be 20% and higher (Bird et al. 1988; Costello 1989; Offord et al. 1987), and with even basic questions about types

The opinions and assertions contained in this chapter are the private views of the authors and are not to be construed as official or as reflecting the views of the Department of Health and Human Services, the National Institute of Mental Health, or the National Institute on Drug Abuse.

and distribution of childhood disorders, service and treatment needs, and obstacles to treatment being actively studied but not yet answered (Barber et al. 1992; Bickman et al. 1995; Rosenblatt and Attkisson 1992), embarking on an analysis of ethical dilemmas may appear untowardly philosophical.

Yet, as will become clear later, analysis of ethical issues in research with children and adolescents cuts to the scientific bone, revealing both the raison d'etre for research and its essential dialectic. Ethical dilemmas arise when harm to participants, however minimal, is introduced as an element of a design or occurs unexpectedly, as, for example, an unforeseen consequence of a procedure. Because of the potential for science to improve the larger good, the essential tension becomes how to advance scientific study and maintain scientific integrity while simultaneously eliminating or minimizing individual discomfort, harm, or danger.

This essential dialectic is revealed starkly in research on children's mental disorders, especially studies conducted in naturalistic settings, with community-based samples, or involving innovative services, because it is here that the boundaries of science and practice, of knowledge and its applicability, are in closest proximity. The authors' purpose in this chapter is to describe key ethical dilemmas that may arise in research on children's mental health, especially studies of innovative treatments, in order to encourage investigators to give careful thought in advance of designing such intervention studies to the kinds of dilemmas that they may encounter. Legal regulations governing the protection of human subjects are introduced when applicable to clarify regulatory precedents. An overview of the principles from The Belmont Report (discussed in the next section) serves as a framework for organizing discussion about consent, confidentiality, voluntariness of participation, determination of risk, access to treatment, debriefing, recruitment, and randomization.

## The Belmont Report

The most complete discussion of ethical principles in research with human subjects is found in a report issued by the National

Commission for the Protection of Human Subjects of Biomedical and Behavioral Research (1979). In this report, the Commission described three major principles that dictate ethical practice in research with human beings. These principles form the backbone for ethical decision making in research with human subjects.

1. *Respect for persons.* This principle prescribes that all individuals should be treated as autonomous and should be protected from risk. Protection is especially important for persons with diminished autonomy, including children and adolescents. The extent of protection depends upon a calculation of both the potential risks involved in participating in research and the likelihood of benefit. Research issues related to informed consent, confidentiality, and voluntariness of participation are derived from this principle.

2. *Beneficence.* The Commission's report articulates the principle that not only must persons' decisions be respected and protected from harm, but that efforts to "secure their well-being" must be made (p. 4). Beneficence—producing good—is thus an obligation. Because producing ultimate good in research can entail some risks, the Code of Federal Regulations on the Protection of Human Subjects (1983) was written to establish the basic beneficence-related requirements for research. These requirements included establishment of Institutional Review Boards (IRBs), criteria for IRB approval, criteria for determining the hierarchy of risks, circumstances under which parental permission is needed or waivers can be obtained—issues especially important for research with adolescents—and special protections for children involved as subjects in research. These requirements stipulate that IRBs must determine for each research project the extent of risk and benefit for each research participant. The regulations make it clear that it is incumbent upon the researcher to minimize risk to the subject. Minimal risk is defined as that ordinarily encountered in daily life or during the performance of routine physical or psychological tests. Any research involving greater than minimal risk must

be justified by anticipated direct benefit to the subject. If there is no such direct benefit, the IRB must find that the research represents a minor increase over minimal risk. The research must also be likely to yield generalizable knowledge about the subject's condition.

From this principle of beneficence are derived several critical research issues, including determination of risk, linkages of research with access to treatment, and debriefing.

3. *Justice.*   This principle dictates that the benefits and burdens of research must be distributed fairly and equitably. This principle also suggests that research subjects should be chosen for reasons related directly to science and not for reasons of accessibility (Munir and Earls 1992). Correspondingly, persons with disabilities should not be asked to bear a disproportionate share of the burden. Potential participants in research are to be informed that their refusal to participate cannot affect their care. Research issues related to noncoercive recruitment procedures and to randomization of subjects are derived from this principle.

# Research on Child and Adolescent Mental Disorders

The interface between ethics, science, and the law is tenuous and is characterized by shifting standards and postmodern ambiguities (Blanck et al. 1992; Jameson 1991; Lyotard 1987). Yet the research investigator, especially if working with children, may be confronted with situations in which scientific objectives and ethical dictates may differ or in which the investigator may have entered uncharted ethical territory. This section describes specific research principles, the implementation of which may lead to ethical questions or issues. Legal regulations are cited when applicable.

## Respect for Persons

**Consent.**    Although Adair (1988) has argued that ethical dilemmas on consent arise most often from medical treatment studies, in fact, they seem to arise in many types of research, including service system, psychosocial treatments, and community-based studies. Informed consent is the major means of protecting the rights of research participants. Frequently cited guidelines for informed consent stipulate that involvement should be informed, voluntary, and rational (Freedman 1975).

Obtaining informed consent can become complex in research with adolescents because consent usually involves both the adolescent and the parent or guardian. In research involving minimal risk, it has sometimes been sufficient to obtain informed consent of one parent; however, in research with greater than minimal risk, obtaining permission of both parents (if available) may be advisable.

There are variations from state to state in the laws authorizing minors to consent to either treatment or participation in research. In all but three states (in which the age is 19), adolescents who are 18 or older are legally adults. However, in some states, adolescents younger than 18 are authorized to consent to care. There are circumstances under which minor children can give their own consent, based upon their status, the specific services sought, or the genre of study (in studies involving high-risk populations, for example) (English 1992). Some states allow minors who are living apart from their parents, such as minors who have run away from home or who are otherwise homeless, emancipated minors, mature minors, high school graduates, married minors, or minor parents to consent to care (English 1990; Gittler et al. 1990). Laws relating to consent for minors are in flux in many states and are subject to considerable variation within and across states. Consequently, it is advisable for the researcher to become well acquainted with the laws governing minor status and consent in the state in which the research is being conducted.

Research on HIV involving adolescents presents unique challenges to the investigator, which have been well articulated by

English (1990, 1992), Gittler et al. (1990), Melton and Gray (1988), North (1990), Rotheram-Borus and Koopman (1991), Sieber (1992), and Stanley and Sieber (1992), among others. In fact, most of the literature on ethical issues in research with youth has arisen from the experiences of investigators with this population of high-risk youth.

There are numerous HIV-specific laws, including statutes that govern consent for testing and treatment. Investigators studying HIV among adolescents should become familiar with the state statutes governing consent for diagnosis and treatment of communicable, contagious, or infectious diseases. For example, 11 states have statutes that explicitly authorize minors to consent to HIV testing; three of these states (e.g., Colorado, Iowa, and Michigan) also authorize minors to consent to treatment for HIV or AIDS infection (English 1992). Every state has a law enabling minors to consent to diagnosis and treatment of a sexually transmitted disease (STD) or venereal disease (VD), but not every state has classified HIV infection or AIDS as STD or VD (English 1990; North 1990). However, in the 13 states that do, minors could consent to testing and treatment of HIV (see English 1992 for a listing of states).

The Code of Federal Regulations on the Protection of Human Subjects (1983) allows for a waiver of parental permission if the research involves minimal risk (no more than the risks encountered in everyday life), if the research will not adversely affect the rights or welfare of the subjects, and if the research could not practicably be conducted without the waiver. For example, it may be impractical to contact parents if their children are living on the streets, if they are drug dealers, or if their parents may be dependent on their child's drug business (Sieber 1992; Stanley and Sieber 1992).

Evaluation of risk, especially in applied research areas, is complex and should include both risks associated with medical interventions and those associated with the social, emotional, or psychological impact of the intervention (Fisher and Rosendahl 1990), including the slippery concept of stigma. For example, simply being selected for participation in a study may suggest to some children that there is something "different" or possibly wrong with them. The psychological impact of diagnostic categories that may be applied to group selection in school-based research (such as a study of attentional deficits, for example) may carry stigmatizing aspects for the children involved.

When permission is waived, alternative mechanisms for protecting the adolescent need to be made. The specific mechanisms must relate to the particular risks involved in the research, taking into consideration the adolescent's maturity (Nolan 1992). For example, one method of reducing the risk (and increasing the benefit) of participation in a study of psychopharmacological treatment effectiveness could be to ensure that those adolescents who participate are automatically linked with services after the study (English 1992).

**Withdrawal.** The other aspect of informed consent that is derived from the principle of respect for persons involves participant withdrawal. Because investigator/subject relationships are inherently uneven, investigators need to be sensitive to power relationships, and child participants need to be informed clearly that they can withdraw at any time. Researchers working with adolescents need to be especially sensitive to these issues. Fisher and Rosendahl (1990) suggest that investigators be aware of behavioral indicators suggesting that the subject wants to terminate participation. Among adolescents, some of whom may be less inclined to express themselves verbally, awareness of their nonverbal cues signaling a disinclination to participate is particularly important.

**Confidentiality.** A third type of issue derived from the principle of respect and autonomy involves protection of the identity of research subjects and of information obtained from them during the course of research. One study found that children below the age of 12 could understand what they were asked to do, but that neither children nor adolescents believed that their performance would be kept confidential, despite assurances from the investigators (Abramovitch et al. 1991).

In research with adolescents, questions about protection of identity often arise about two issues: who has authority to disclose confidential information, and what constitutes the limits to confidentiality. Generally, the person or court with legal authority to make health care decisions can authorize the release of information (English 1992; Rennert 1991). Usually adolescents who are legally authorized to consent to HIV testing or treatment also have the right to control disclosure of related information (English 1990; Rennert 1991).

In all states, confidentiality is overridden by mandatory child abuse reporting laws and by the need to protect against the potential suicide of a client (English 1990). At this time, however, these laws do not mandate disclosure of adolescent HIV status (English 1990). Children and adolescents need to be provided with a clear explanation of the limits of confidentiality during the informed consent procedure in terms that they can understand.

Research on child abuse and issues of confidentiality can pose particularly thorny dilemmas for the investigator. Concerns about the use of information in research records, should they be subpoenaed, can lead investigators to limit their selection of instruments and questionnaires, to avoid asking possibly incriminating questions, and to neglect whole areas of research inquiry. In addition, the research community and clinical community often have differing perspectives on the values of child abuse research. From the research perspective, the clinical staff may seem unwilling to gather empirical data on their abused clients. The clinical staff, on the other hand, may believe that the researchers are not working to safeguard the interests of the child.

One protection that is available to research investigators in either federally or nonfederally funded projects is the Certificate of Confidentiality. The Department of Health and Human Services offers this certificate to protect researchers from being compelled to disclose identifying information about their research subjects. It protects research data from being subpoenaed, and it is a powerful protection. Application for the certificate is not automatic and must be sought (Hoagwood 1994; Melton 1990).

The certificate does not govern voluntary disclosure of identifying characteristics of research subjects. In other words, it does not prevent researchers from voluntarily disclosing child abuse or a subject's threat of violence to self or others. In fact, researchers usually include such information in their informed consent protocols. If the researcher intends to make such voluntary disclosures, the consent form must clearly indicate this. The certificate also does not authorize researchers to resist disclosure to a parent if the parent is the child's legal guardian and consents to the disclosure (e.g., in a custody dispute).

In the current climate of changing laws, standards, and practices, researchers investigating topics on child and adolescent mental health face their own dilemmas: they must ensure confidentiality knowing that the rationale guiding the procedures established to protect participants' disclosures is itself in flux (Bayer 1989; Blanck et al 1992). For example, Blanck et al. (1992) describe a study of HIV risk acts in which, at the beginning of the study, it was possible for the researchers to know the HIV serostatus of the participants; the participants could choose either to be informed or not to be informed of their status. Researchers were able to study the effect of knowledge of one's status upon subsequent behavior as a substudy of a larger project. However, a subsequent change in the policy by the funding agency prohibited researchers from withholding information from the participant on his or her status, regardless of the participant's preferences. This shift in policy, of course, precluded further investigation of the substudy. Investigators, particularly in applied research fields, will need to assume that standards and policies regulating informed consent and confidentiality may change and will need to think prospectively about ways to maximize protection for their child research subjects.

## Beneficence

**Risk/benefit.** Analysis of the risks and benefits of participation in research is made by the investigator and the appropriateness of the balance ascertained by the IRBs. The purpose of the research must include demonstration of the potential benefits of the study, as well as an explicit discussion of how the investigator will minimize risk. In assessing risks, investigators occasionally overlook some of the distinct advantages to participation in research. For example, in addition to the increased access to treatment that is available from participation in clinical trials, participation in research can also provide adolescents with information about the effectiveness of treatments, about the availability of community services, or about the perceptions or experiences of their peers or family.

**Treatment access.**    A second issue related to beneficence in research involves linkage and access to treatment. For adolescents with HIV, for example, the linkage between testing and treatment is critical (English 1992). If a clinical trial is proposed, but the control subjects cannot access treatment, the calculus between benefits and risks becomes skewed. Because testing for HIV can become an important avenue to early intervention, some have argued that access to treatment needs to be assured for any adolescent who tests positive, and that these assurances should be made in the informed consent process (English 1992).

**Debriefing and disclosure.**    A third issue that can pose ethical dilemmas for investigators entails informing participants about the research procedures after a study has been completed. Debriefing is meant to explain any deception that may have been involved in the conduct of the experiment and remove any deleterious psychological consequences, such as lessening the child's trust in adults (American Psychological Association 1992). Debriefing has become a broad term that includes a number of specific activities (and, in fact, the term *postinvestigation clarification* is preferred by some, e.g., Marans 1988). For example, some investigators recommend that children's reactions to planned procedures be carefully monitored, and that medical, psychological, or psychiatric consultants be made available if an adolescent becomes distressed during a procedure in the study (Fisher and

Rosendahl 1990). Debriefing can also include the provision of a list of medical, psychiatric, or community health resources to the adolescent participants.

Debriefing can provide a number of advantages to the researcher. For example, it offers the researcher an opportunity to determine the meaning of the study from the phenomenological perspective of the participants. It can be used as a means of sharing knowledge of the processes and problems involved in the study (Fisher and Rosendahl 1990). Debriefing enables the investigator to determine whether the experimental procedure was perceived as intended (Blanck et al. 1992). It can also be helpful in determining the effectiveness of clinical trials for drugs aimed at slowing diseases (e.g., whether HIV participants shared medications with each other). In addition, debriefing can provide researchers with ideas for follow-up studies, as well as help them identify problems with their current protocols (Blanck et al. 1992).

Many debriefing approaches are used, and some may be especially appropriate with adolescent populations. For example, Marans (1988) describes a debriefing and disclosure procedure that includes a limited debriefing with the subject immediately following the procedure; this debriefing reminds the participant of the purpose of the study and the importance of not discussing it with others. When the experiment is completed with all subjects, a complete disclosure procedure is provided in either an individualized or group format, wherein the investigator discusses the study and answers any questions about it. The group format may be especially effective with adolescents, who often respond well to group interactions. This two-pronged approach affords simultaneous protection of the internal validity of the study while enabling a full exploration of the adolescents' impressions of the study.

## Justice

**Recruitment of subjects.**   The last of the National Commission's principles, justice, implies that an equitable distribution of the advantages and disadvantages of participation in research across different groups should occur. Examples of activities in which this principle is exemplified include recruitment and randomization to experimental conditions. The direct effects of recruitment procedures, for example, can raise concerns for some youth because of potential stigmatizing effects (e.g., being identified as adopted, as the child of an alcoholic parent, as having a behavioral disorder or an illness). Investigators need to be sensitive to the potential of the recruitment procedures to precipitate distress that might not have occurred otherwise (Fisher and Rosendahl 1990); again this consideration is especially important in studies involving children or adolescents, who may be more distressed by unintended consequences of the study, such as potential stigmatizing effects, than would adult participants.

Recruitment issues also arise in connection with the appropriate use of volunteers. Studies of certain samples of children, such as institutionalized children with severe emotional disorders, raise questions about the voluntariness of their participation (Wells and Sametz 1985). Although from a methodological standpoint it is important to eliminate selection bias (Blanck et al. 1992; Suls and Rosnow 1981), there are also ethical problems in overzealous recruitment of volunteers. To increase generalizability of the findings of the study, the investigator may want to increase the diversity of the sample; however, recruitment needs to be accomplished without offering inducements that may be perceived either by the research community, or, more importantly, by the participants, as coercive. For example, participants can be more fully informed about the significance of the research and about the scientific rewards of contributing to an important activity. Blanck et al. (1992) argue persuasively that more attention to the scientific advantages of wider and noncoercive engagement of research participants will enhance the scientific integrity of research as well as distribute the advantages of participation more widely.

**Randomization.**   A second issue related to the principle of justice concerns random assignment of subjects. Random assignment is one means of ensuring equitable distribution of risks across groups. Some have argued that it exemplifies ethical practice in research (Henggeler 1994). Useful suggestions for handling the timing of random assignment in order to reduce attrition have been offered (Bickman 1992). Random assignment of participants to treatment and control groups, however, can also raise ethical questions. For example, how should an investigator handle participant preference for assignment to treatment or control groups? One solution is a design, proposed by Veatch (1987), called the semirandomized clinical trial, consisting of four experimental conditions of two randomized groups (consisting of participants who have agreed to be randomly assigned to the control and experimental group) and two nonrandomized groups (who have chosen not to be randomized but to be in either one or the other groups). The advantage of this design is that it respects participant autonomy.

Questions may also arise as to how to distribute the positive effects of an intervention while simultaneously maintaining scientific integrity. For example, if, in a longitudinal study, a treatment is found to be effective, how can this treatment be provided to the control group without jeopardizing experimental integrity? One suggestion is to use a midexperimental check: if the experimental group at midpoint is showing significant improvement over the control, then the decision can be made to provide treatment to control subjects (Fisher and Rosendahl 1990). Some investigators have found it necessary to accelerate presentation of the intervention to control groups when denial of a proven effective service cannot be clinically justified. Sometimes control subjects are referred to other services. Among children and adolescents, their rapid developmental changes in biological, social, and emotional areas suggest that particular attention be paid to the timing of the intervention: a shorter time period for evaluating the effectiveness of an experimental intervention and for providing it to the control group may be more necessary than among adult populations.

**Use of findings.** A final issue with respect to the ethical conduct of research concerns the extent to which the use of research findings should dictate the conduct of investigations. That is, should investigators consider potential applications of their research before generating results that may influence public practice or policy? This issue has been called the "scientist-citizen dilemma" (Veatch 1987), is particularly critical in applied research fields, and has generated different responses (Melton in press; Sarason 1984; Scarr 1990). Scientific knowledge, of course, can be used for good or ill; knowledge of the perseverance of belief systems (Anderson et al. 1980; Lepper et al. 1986), for example, could be used to manipulate public opinion or to change prejudicial beliefs. One approach to concerns about the possible misuse of scientific findings is to obtain community consultation. Melton et al. (1988) suggest that in studies involving socially sensitive issues, investigators may want to involve potential participants or surrogates in decisions about the study, formulating their concerns, for example, into researchable questions. In this way, a partnership between the investigators and the participants may be created.

## Summary

The increasing complexity of research methodologies and the growing need for research that can inform state and local policies create a situation wherein peripheralizing consideration of ethical issues in research is no longer tenable. Investigators in all fields of science, but most starkly in applied fields in which the uses of research findings are often immediate, need to give careful thought to potential ethical challenges that may arise. Although the report issued by the National Commission for the Protection of Human Subjects of Biomedical and Behavioral Research (1979) articulates principles to guide research involving human subjects, ambiguity about what constitutes harm for children confuses issues of ethical responsibility with legal issues of liability. Although several important studies have been conducted on children's compliance and voluntariness (Czajkowski and Koocher 1986, 1987; Gudas et al. 1991; Koocher and DeMaso 1990;

Weithorn and Scherer 1991), significant questions remain about the ability of children to assess the risks and benefits of research participation, about levels of research-related stress or satisfaction, and about perceptions of harm. The importance of these questions, their ripeness for empirical study, and their potential to advance scientific study by clarifying key aspects of children's perceptions about research participation suggest the need for a new genre of research: a science of scientific ethics in research on children.

The reciprocity between the domains of ethics and science suggests that the study of scientific ethics can shape investigations in important new ways. Such research can help to answer some of the complex ethical questions that are arising as our understanding of onset, course, and treatments for children with mental disorders expands. Investigations specifically focused upon research ethics may clarify the poles that constitute the essential dialectic of science.

# References

Abramovitch R, Freedman JL, Thoden K, et al: Children's capacity to consent to participation in psychological research: empirical findings. Child Dev 62:1100–1109, 1991

Adair JG: Research on research ethics. Am Psychol 43:825–826, 1988

American Medical Association: America's adolescents: how healthy are they? Chicago, IL, American Medical Association, 1990

American Psychological Association: Ethical principles of psychologists and code of conduct. Am Psychol 47:1597–1611, 1992

Anderson CA, Lepper MR, Ross L: Perseverance of social theories: the role of explanation in the persistence of discredited information. J Pers Soc Psychol 39:1037–1049, 1980

Association for the Advancement of Health Education: National Adolescent Health Survey. Reston, VA, Association for the Advancement of Health Education, 1987

Barber CC, Rosenblatt A, Harris LM, et al: Use of mental health services among severely emotionally disturbed children and adolescents in San Francisco. Journal of Child and Family Studies 1:183–207, 1992

Bayer R: Ethical and social policy issues raised by HIV screening: the epidemic evolves and so do the challenges. Aids 3:119–124, 1989

Bickman L: Designing outcome evaluations for children's mental health services: improving internal validity, in Evaluating Mental Health Services for Children. Edited by Bickman L, Rog DJ. San Francisco, CA, Jossey-Bass, 1992, pp 57–68

Bickman L, Guthrie PR, Foster EM, et al: Evaluating Managed Mental Health Services: The Fort Bragg Experiment. New York, Plenum, 1995

Bird HR, Canino G, Rubio-Stipec M, et al: Estimates of the prevalence of childhood maladjustment in a community survey in Puerto Rico. Arch Gen Psychiatry 45:1120–1126, 1988

Blanck PD, Bellack AS, Rosnow RL, et al: Scientific rewards and conflicts of ethical choices in human subjects research. Am Psychol 47:959–965, 1992

Code of Federal Regulations 45 CFR 46: Department of Health and Human Services. Protection of Human Subjects. Washington, DC, Government Printing Office, 1983

Costello EJ: Developments in child psychiatric epidemiology. J Am Acad Child Adolesc Psychiatry 28:836–841, 1989

Czajkowski DR, Koocher GP: Predicting medical compliance among adolescents with cystic fibrosis. Health Psychology 5:297–305, 1986

Czajkowski DR, Koocher GP: Medical compliance and coping with cystic fibrosis. J Child Psychol Psychiatry 28:311–319, 1987

English A: Treating adolescents: legal and ethical considerations. Med Clin North Am 74:1097–1112, 1990

English A: Expanding access to HIV services for adolescents: legal and ethical issues, in Adolescents and AIDS: A Generation in Jeopardy. Edited by Diclemente RJ. Newbury Park, CA, Sage, 1992, pp 262–283

Fisher CB, Rosendahl SA: Emerging ethical issues in an emerging field, in Annual Advances in Applied Developmental Psychology, Vol 4. Edited by Fisher CB, Tryon WW. Norwood, NJ, Ablex Publishing, 1990, pp 43–60

Freedman B: A moral theory of informed consent. Hastings Center Report 5:32–39, 1975

Gittler J, Quigley-Rick M, Saks MJ: Adolescent Health Care Decision Making: The Law and Public Policy. Washington, DC, Carnegie Council on Adolescent Development, 1990

Gudas LJ, Koocher GP, Wypij D: Perceptions of medical compliance in children and adolescents with cystic fibrosis. J Dev Behav Pediatr 12:236–242, 1991

Henggeler SW: Methodological issues in conducting treatment research in the juvenile justice system. J Clin Child Psychol 23:143–150, 1994

Hoagwood K: The Certificate of Confidentiality at the National Institute of Mental Health. Ethics and Behavior 4:123–131, 1994

Jameson F: Postmodernism or the Cultural Logic of Late Capitalism. Durham, NC, Duke University Press, 1991

Koocher GP, DeMaso DR: Children's competence to consent to medical procedures. Pediatrician 17:68–73, 1990

Lepper MR, Ross L, Lau RR: Persistence of inaccurate beliefs about the self: perseverance effects in the classroom. J Pers Soc Psychol 50:482–491, 1986

Lyotard JF: La Condition Postmoderne: Rapport sur le Savoir, Editions de Minuit. Minneapolis, University of Minnesota Press, 1987

Marans DG: Addressing research practitioner and subject needs: a debriefing-disclosure procedure. Am Psychol 10:826–827, 1988

Melton GB: Certificates of confidentiality under the Public Health Service Act: strong protection but not enough. Violence and Victims 5:67–71, 1990

Melton GB, Gray JW: Ethical dilemmas in AIDS research. Am Psychol 43:60–64, 1988

Melton GB, Levine RJ, Koocher GP, et al: Community consultation in socially sensitive research: lessons from clinical trials of treatments for AIDS. Am Psychol 43:573–581, 1988

Munir K, Earls F: Ethical principles governing research in child and adolescent psychiatry. J Am Acad Child Adolesc Psychiatry 31:408–414, 1992

National Commission for the Protection of Human Subjects of Biomedical and Behavioral Research: The Belmont Report: Ethical Principles and Guidelines for the Protection of Human Subjects of Research. Washington, DC, Government Printing Office, 1979

National Commission on the Role of the School and the Community in Improving Adolescent Health: Code Blue: Uniting for Healthier Youth. Chicago, IL, American Medical Association, 1990

Nolan K: Ethical issues: assent, consent, and behavioral research with adolescents. Am Acad Child Adolesc Psychiatry (Summer):7–10, 1992

North RL: Legal authority for HIV testing of adolescents. Journal of Adolescent Health Care 11:176–187, 1990

Offord DR, Boyle MH, Szatmari P, et al: Ontario Child Health Study: six-month prevalence of disorder and rates of service utilization. Arch Gen Psychiatry 44:832–836, 1987

Rennert S: Aids/HIV and Confidentiality: Model Policies and Procedures. Washington, DC, American Bar Association, 1991

Rotheram-Borus MJ, Koopman C: HIV and adolescents. Journal of Primary Prevention 12:65–82, 1991

Rosenblatt A, Attkisson CC: Integrating systems of care in California for youth with severe emotional disturbance, in A Descriptive Overview of the California AB377 Evaluation Project. Journal of Child and Family Studies 1:93–113, 1992

Sarason SB: If it can be studied or developed, should it? Am Psychol 39:477–485, 1984

Scarr S: Race and gender as psychological variables: social and ethical issues. Am Psychol 43:56–59, 1990

Sieber JE: Community intervention research on minors, in Social Research on Children and Adolescents: Ethical Issues. Edited by Stanley B, Sieber J. Newbury Park, CA, Sage, 1992, pp 162–187

Stanley B, Sieber JE: Introduction: The Ethics of Social Research on Children and Adolescents. Newbury Park, CA, Sage, 1992, pp 1–6

Suls JM, Rosnow RL: The delicate balance between ethics and artifacts in behavioral research, in New Directions for Methodology of Social and Behavioral Science: Ethics of Human Subject Research. Edited by Kimmel AJ. San Francisco, CA, Jossey-Bass, 1981, pp 55–67

U.S. Congress, Office of Technology Assessment: Adolescent Health, Summary and Policy Options, Vol I (OTA-H-468). Washington, DC, U.S. Government Printing Office, 1991

Veatch RM: Medical Ethics. Boston, MA, Jones and Bartlett, 1987

Weithorn LA, Scherer DG: Children's involvement in research participation decisions: psychological considerations, in Children as Research Subjects: Science, Ethics, and the Law. Edited by Grodin MA, Glantz LH. Cary, NC, Oxford University Press, 1994

Wells K, Sametz L: Involvement of institutionalized children in social science research: some issues and proposed guidelines. Journal of Clinical Child Psychology 14:245–251, 1985

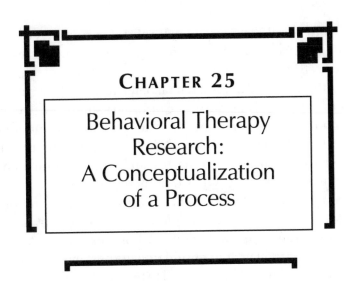

CHAPTER 25

# Behavioral Therapy Research: A Conceptualization of a Process

**Lisa Simon Onken, Ph.D., Jack D. Blaine, M.D., and Robert J. Battjes, D.S.W.**

R esearch on psychotherapy and other forms of behavioral therapy is abundant. Thousands of clinical trials have been performed comparing the efficacy of one type of therapy to another, or to medication in various populations with various disorders. Hundreds of forms of psychosocial and behavioral therapy have been pitted against other forms to see which therapy is best, to determine whether a therapy is better than treatment as usual, or to determine interactions with patient characteristics. Some have argued that comparative behavioral therapy research should not be conducted at all—that instead, we should be looking at the mechanism of action of behavioral therapy, or the efficacious components of therapy. Still others argue that we should not be performing controlled clinical trials of behavioral therapies—that, ultimately, the lack of control is so significant that to even attempt a controlled experiment in this area is folly, and that we should be evaluating the effective-

477

ness of behavioral therapies in naturalistic settings. As these arguments intensify, the debate continues over whether psychotherapy is efficacious at all.

The ultimate goal of research on behavioral and psychosocial therapies for mental and addictive disorders should be to delineate which therapies work best for which individuals under what conditions. As Paul (1967) stated, "In all its complexity, the question towards which all outcome research should ultimately be directed is the following: What treatment, by whom, is most effective for this individual with that specific problem, and under which set of circumstances. . . . With careful application of appropriate methodology and strategy, hope exists that 25 more years of research will no longer find psychotherapy characterized as "an undefined technique applied to unspecified problems with unpredictable outcome" (p. 117).

Twenty-seven years of research have passed, and Paul's hope has not been fully realized. For many mental and addictive disorders, we are not much further along than we were 27 years ago. Why has the acquisition of knowledge progressed so slowly? The answer is in part because of the inherently difficult nature of research in this area. Operationally defining a therapy in a therapy manual is, in itself, a major undertaking that does not even begin to ensure that the therapy will be administered properly. There must be intensive monitoring and assessment of the therapy and, of course, the assessment must be valid and reliable. After the therapy has been well defined, studying its efficacy presents a whole new array of issues. The dilemmas inherent in undertaking clinical trials in behavioral therapy are well documented, and it is not our intention to summarize them here. Suffice it to say that the difficulties are extensive and complex, and many have no perfect, practical, or realistic solutions.

However, few would assert that no progress at all has been made. In fact, many psychotherapies and behavior therapies have been operationally defined in therapy manuals, clinical trials have been performed, and for certain disorders, such as panic disorder, it could well be argued that a behavioral "therapy of choice" exists. This is, no doubt, at least in part due to the adaptation of a technological model of psychotherapy research (Carroll and Rounsaville 1990; Docherty 1984) exemplified by the studies begun in the 1970s, such as the NIMH Treatment of Depression Collaborative Research Project (Elkin et al. 1985; Elkin et al. 1988a, 1988b) and the University of Pennsylvania study on psychotherapy for opiate addicts (Woody et al. 1983).

We contend, however, that progress in the field could be further accelerated by a goal-oriented, systematic approach to the development and testing of behavioral therapies—therapies ultimately to be used by clinicians in the field. Although Rush (1984) proposed a conceptualization of the phases of psychosocial treatment research, there is no universally accepted conceptualization of behavioral and psychosocial therapy research as a process, consisting of a series of stages, all of which must be supported to maximize the breadth and depth of information obtained about a particular therapy. Such a conceptualization would allow the scientific community to easily assess the stage of development of a therapy, the state of the research on that therapy, and what needs to be accomplished before other types of research can occur.

Such an approach could be considered analogous to the process used by the pharmaceutical industry to develop medications. It would allow for the establishment of a mechanism for the support of therapy development, including a process for the peer review and approval of therapies prior to their widespread dissemination to the clinical community.

A systematic, well-delineated conceptualization of the stages of behavioral therapy research would facilitate the grant application process; investigators involved in behavioral therapy research could easily identify what needs to be studied next and avoid the temptation of jumping ahead with research that is premature (e.g., efficacy testing before competence and adherence measures for a therapy have been fully developed). If investigators, members of grant review committees, and scientific administrators have clear and congruent ideas about the process of behavioral therapy research, research progress should be greatly advanced.

# Conceptualization of the Stages of Behavioral Therapy Research

In this chapter, a conceptualization of the stages of behavioral therapy research is presented. As mentioned previously, Rush (1984) presented an initial conceptualization of the phases of psychosocial treatment research. The conceptualization presented here was developed as part of the National Institute on Drug Abuse Behavioral Therapies Development Program, launched in 1993, which we three authors headed. Many of the ideas presented in this chapter resulted from an interactive exchange with experts in the psychotherapy, behavior therapy, and drug dependence treatment research fields, including the following participants at a meeting held October 6, 1993: Drs. Richard Bootzin, John Docherty, Marc Galanter, Alan Kraut, Howard Liddle, G. Alan Marlatt, A. Thomas McLellan, Karla Moras, Bruce Rounsaville, A. John Rush, Jose Schapoznik, Charles R. Schuster, Andrea Solarz, Maxine Stitzer, Elizabeth Wells, Fred Wright, and Debra Zarin. The ideas described here should be considered as evolving, rather than as being carved in stone. In fact, further meetings with experts in the field are planned to help refine the concepts presented here. The ideas described in this chapter are intended to stimulate thought about the process of behavioral therapy research, its various essential components, and the most logical and pragmatic ways in which this process and its components can be viewed.

## Stage I

Behavioral therapy research has been conceptualized as consisting of three phases. Stage I, the earliest phase of behavioral therapy research—therapy development—involves identifying promising behavioral and psychosocial clinical and research findings relevant to treatment, generating and formulating new therapies, operationally defining the therapies in manuals, developing valid and reliable competence and adherence measures, refining the therapies based upon feedback from patients and clinicians, and pilot testing the therapies. It is essentially a multistage, iterative process consisting of all the preliminary work necessary before a well-designed and controlled clinical trial on the therapy can take place.

Until recently there has been little support for the time-consuming and costly process of Stage I. This lack of support for therapy development placed researchers in a Catch-22 situation. That is, paradoxically, researchers could get support for the controlled efficacy testing of a fully developed therapy, but could not get support to develop their therapy. Support for Stage I was initiated by the National Institute on Drug Abuse with the release of the program announcement, "Development of Theoretically Based Psychosocial Therapies for Drug Dependence," and by the National Institute of Mental Health with the program announcement, "Exploratory/Developmental Grants (R21) for Psychosocial Treatment Research." Despite the fact that support is now available for Stage I research at the National Institute on Drug Abuse and the National Institutes of Mental Health, writing a grant application for Stage I research is a challenging task. The applicant must convince a review committee that a therapy that has not yet been developed or shown any efficacy (from a scientific point of view) is worth being funded for development. Therefore, an explicit, logical, consistent, and coherent statement describing the rationale for the proposed therapy must be written. If there is no basis for the therapy in the behavioral science literature, there is little chance that it will receive a competitive priority score.

Investigators must also address how they intend to measure what is actually occurring in the therapy they are proposing to develop, adding to the difficulty of writing a Stage I research grant application. The credibility of any treatment research depends on the ability to determine the extent to which that treatment was actually administered, and administered correctly. In the development of any therapy, therefore, emphasis should be placed upon the development of psychometrically sound instruments measuring the integrity and fidelity of the therapy.

Pilot efficacy testing of newly developed and modified therapies should be considered an integral part of any therapy development process. Although most researchers agree that a pilot test need not have the statistical power and should not have the cost of a full-scale clinical trial, there is little agreement as to what constitutes a sound pilot study. This is an issue that needs attention in the fields of psychotherapy and behavior therapy research, and, we believe, will receive this attention if a staged model of behavioral and psychosocial therapy research is adopted by the scientific community. In spite of the lack of agreement in the field regarding pilot studies, it is clear that a pilot study must indicate that the new therapy can produce clinically meaningful results. If this is not the case, there is little point in proceeding to Stage II.

## Stage II

Stage II research establishes the efficacy of therapies and the efficacious components of therapies. Most of the behavioral treatment research that the federal government has supported in the past has been Stage II research. It consists of small-scale clinical trials of promising therapies identified in Stage I, as well as studies that attempt to determine the mechanism of action of therapies. Stage II also involves the replication, at other sites, of efficacy studies with positive results. When planning a Stage II clinical trial of a behavioral or psychosocial therapy, it is important to consider possible interactions of therapist or patient characteristics with therapy type and to design the study to assess the relative contribution of relevant therapist and patient characteristics, and the contribution of type of therapy to outcome. Wherever possible and practical, designing a study to determine not only if a therapy works, but why it works, is a worthwhile goal.

As a rule, in Stage II research, comparison interventions should be operationally defined, standardized, and manualized. However, there is a lack of consensus in the field regarding appropriate control and comparison groups. There is no perfect placebo control. Early in Stage II, it may be appropriate to compare a therapy with an attention-control group, a nonspecific intervention, or even a nonmanualized treatment as usual, to determine with relatively little cost if the new therapy is at least as good as the standard treatment currently in use. If the newly developed therapy does not compare favorably with the attention-control group or nonspecific intervention, even when administered by the individual who developed it, there may be little justification to proceed. Proceeding with a more costly study in which both the experimental and control therapies are manualized requires careful consideration. Component analysis studies might be appropriate, depending upon the research questions being asked. The point here is that investigators should have clearly delineated research questions and should carefully choose their control and comparison groups to answer those specific questions. The field at large needs to directly address the issue and come to some consensus regarding what control and comparison groups are desirable, appropriate, and acceptable at which points in Stage II.

At the end of Stage II, a manualized therapy for a well-defined population should exist that has been shown, through at least one controlled clinical trial and a replication, to be efficacious.

## Stage III

At this point, a Stage III study is needed to determine a therapy's transferability and usefulness in community-based drug abuse treatment programs. An example of a Stage III study might involve an investigator, using a therapy that has been rigorously tested in a replicated controlled clinical trial, packaging that therapy, including development of training manuals and other training materials, to be used in a community setting. The investigator might then pilot the therapy in the community clinic, refine the therapy package, and ultimately test the usefulness of the packaged therapy in the community setting. Dissemination to clinicians would occur after a panel of experts examines the Stage II and Stage III research and concludes that there is substantial evidence for the efficacy of a particular behavioral therapy for particular patient populations. Training of clinicians and/or technical assistance to treatment programs may most appropriately occur outside the National Institutes of Health through organizations such as the Substance Abuse and Mental Health Services Administration (SAMHSA).

It is our belief that for research on behavioral therapies to succeed, it is critical that all stages of behavioral therapy research receive sufficient attention. The conceptualization of the phases of behavioral therapy research, as presented here, should accelerate the progress made in the field by allowing researchers, review committee members, and funding organizations to target for investigation, in a systematic way, essential areas of research on behavioral therapies for various mental and drug abuse disorders.

# References

Carroll KM, Rounsaville BJ: Can a technology model of psychotherapy research be applied to cocaine abuse treatment?, in Psychotherapy and Counseling in the Treatment of Drug Abuse. Edited by Onken LS, Blaine JB. NIDA Research Monograph #104, Department of Health and Human Services Publication Number (ADM) 90-1722, 1990, pp 91–104

Docherty JP: Implications of the technological model of psychotherapy, in Psychotherapy Research: Where Are We and Where Should We Go? Edited by Williams JBW, Spitzer RL. New York, Guilford, 1984, pp 139–149

Elkin I, Parloff MB, Hadley SW, et al: NIMH treatment of depression collaborative research program: background and research plan. Arch Gen Psychiatry 42:305–316, 1985

Elkin I, Pilkonis PA, Docherty JP, et al: Conceptual and methodological issues in comparative studies of psychotherapy and pharmacotherapy, I: active ingredients and mechanisms of change. Am J Psychiatry 145:909–917, 1988a

Elkin I, Pilkonis PA, Docherty JP, et al: Conceptual and methodological issues in comparative studies of psychotherapy and pharmacotherapy, II: nature and timing of treatment effects. Am J Psychiatry 145:1070–1076, 1988b

Paul GL: Outcome research in psychotherapy. J Consult Psychol 31:109–118, 1967

Rush AJ: A phase II study of cognitive therapy of depression, in Psychotherapy Research: Where Are We and Where Should We Go? Edited by Williams JBW, Spitzer RL. New York, Guilford, 1984, pp 216–234

Woody GE, Luborsky L, McLellan AT, et al: Psychotherapy for opiate addicts: does it help? Arch Gen Psychiatry 40:639–645, 1983

# Index

*Page numbers printed in **boldface** type refer to tables or figures.*